Biomechanical Principles on Force Generation and Control of Skeletal Muscle and their Applications in Robotic Exoskeleton

Advances in Systems Science and Engineering

Series Editor:
Li Da Xu

PUBLISHED

Enterprise Integration and Information Architecture:

A Systems Perspective on Industrial Information Integration
by Li Da Xu
ISBN: 978-1-4398-5024-4

Systems Science: Methodological Approaches
by Yi Lin, Xiaojun Duan, Chengli Zhao, and Li Da Xu
ISBN: 978-1-4398-9551-1

Biomechanical Principles on Force Generation and Control of Skeletal
Muscle and their Applications in Robotic Exoskeleton
by Yuehong Yin
ISBN: 978-0-367-34398-9

Biomechanical Principles on Force Generation and Control of Skeletal Muscle and their Applications in Robotic Exoskeleton

Yuehong Yin

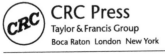

CRC Press
Taylor & Francis Group
Boca Raton London New York

CRC Press is an imprint of the
Taylor & Francis Group, an **informa** business

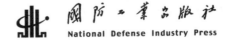

国 防 工 业 出 版 社
National Defense Industry Press

CRC Press
Taylor & Francis Group
6000 Broken Sound Parkway NW, Suite 300
Boca Raton, FL 33487-2742

First issued in paperback 2022

© 2020 by Taylor & Francis Group, LLC, under exclusive license granted by National Defense Industry Press for English language throughout the world except Mainland China.
CRC Press is an imprint of Taylor & Francis Group, an Informa business

No claim to original U.S. Government works

ISBN: 978-1-03-240119-5 (pbk)
ISBN: 978-0-367-34398-9 (hbk)
ISBN: 978-0-429-33062-9 (ebk)

DOI: 10.1201/9780429330629

Visit the Taylor & Francis Web site at
http://www.taylorandfrancis.com

and the CRC Press Web site at
http://www.crcpress.com

Contents

Foreword

Force sensing and control technology is essentially a kind of bionic behavior and belongs to behavioral intelligence. It has long been considered a research hotspot in science and engineering field and has been widely applied in the fields of robotics, artificial intelligence, and intelligent ultra-precision manufacturing. However, since its birth, force sensing and control technology has faced many challenges and bottlenecks in force perception, force generation, and force control. As the power source of the human body, research on force generation mechanism, sensing, and control have always been one of the most attractive and challenging research topics.[*]

In the past two decades, Professor Yuehong Yin has conducted in-depth research on the mechanism and regulation of skeletal muscle contraction. He has a good understanding of this subject and made some innovative achievements in biomechanical modeling of skeletal muscle, human–machine interaction interface and exoskeleton robot technology, bionic skeletal muscle design method, etc. A relatively complete academic system has been developed. This book is a systematic summary of these research results. Based on the anatomical morphology of skeletal muscle and the excitation–contraction coupling process, Chapters 1 and 2 summarize the control and driving mechanism of muscle contraction and the mechanism of force generation and a method for microscopic to macroscopic biomechanical modeling is proposed. It includes models of skeletal muscle mechanics based on the collective operation mechanism of molecular motors and semi-phenomenological models of sarcomere. Chapter 3 discusses the application of surface-electromyography (sEMG) signal in the prediction of skeletal muscle contraction state and a differential extraction method and a novel energy kernel extraction method to realize real-time and accurate recognition of human motion intentions are proposed. Chapters 4 and 5 summarize the key technologies of the lower-extremity exoskeleton rehabilitation robot. Through the two-way human–computer interaction interface including the motion control channel and the information feedback channel, the coordinated control of the human exoskeleton robot is realized. Research on the systematic application of clinical rehabilitation is also done based on the exoskeleton robot. Chapter 6 focuses on the bionic skeletal muscle technique and uses the shape memory alloy (SMA) as the key technology of bionic muscle material to design the artificial skeletal muscle with drive–sensing–structure integration, including SMA self-sensing model and hysteresis model. Most of the research results are published in international mainstream academic journals, and their innovation and contribution to the field of biomechanical mechanisms have been fully recognized. A series of related models and algorithms have been implemented and have achieved good application results, reflecting the close combination of theory and practice.

This book reflects the independent innovation achievements of Chinese scholars in basic research on exoskeleton robots and related biomechanics. I hope that the publication of this book will positively promote the development of the related fields.

April. 4. 2019.

---

[*] Zhongqin Lin is the president of Shanghai Jiao Tong University and academician of the Chinese Academy of Engineering.

Author

Yuehong Yin received his B.E., M.S., and Ph.D. degrees from Nanjing University of Aeronautics and Astronautics, Nanjing, China in 1990, 1995, and 1997, respectively, all in mechanical engineering. From December 1997 to December 1999, he was a Postdoctoral Fellow with Zhejiang University, Hangzhou, China, where he became an Associate Professor in July 1999. Since December 1999, he has been with the Robotics Institute, Shanghai Jiao Tong University, Shanghai, China, where he became a Professor and Tenure Professor in December 2005 and January 2016, respectively. His research interests include robotics, force control, exoskeleton robotics, molecular motor, artificial limb, robotic assembly, reconfigurable assembly system, and augmented reality. Dr. Yin is a fellow of the International Academy of Production Engineering (CIRP).

1 Force Generation Mechanism of Skeletal Muscle Contraction

In a narrow sense, the aim of studies on the mechanism of force generation of skeletal muscle is to give theoretical explanations to the dynamic characteristics and phenomena of muscular contraction and to promote the relevant experimental researches in an iterative way of verification and correction. In a broad sense, it aims to provide theoretical guidance to practical applications in the fields such as biomechanics and biomedicine, including diagnosis and evaluation of muscle diseases, human–machine integrated coordinated control of exoskeleton robots, dynamic modeling of human motion, bionic design of artificial muscle and humanoid robot, etc. Thus, there are both great theoretical significance and wide application foreground concerning the study of force generation mechanism of skeletal muscle.

In this field, the earliest breakthroughs were made by Hill [1] and Huxley [2], both of them Nobelists. Their work laid the foundation for the study on mechanism of muscular contraction. Recently, with the development of micro/nano technology and single-molecule manipulation technique, deeper understandings were achieved about the microscopic mechanism of skeletal muscle contraction. Physiology, physical chemistry, molecular biology, statistical thermodynamics, cybernetics, nonlinear mathematics, etc., are all involved in the study of force generation mechanism of skeletal muscle, which is typical interdisciplinary research. In consequence, both the degrees of complexity and difficulty are very high, resulting in theoretical and technical challenges. In this chapter, the morphological structure of skeletal muscle under various scales is introduced first. On that basis, the biomechanical principle of muscular contraction, i.e., the excitation–contraction coupling (ECC) process, is systematically illustrated. Finally, receptors in skeleton muscle and proprioceptive feedback of human motion are discussed, aiming to provide readers with elementary-to-profound understanding of the mechanism and process of skeletal muscle contraction.

1.1 ANATOMY OF SKELETAL MUSCLE

For a biological system, structure and function are inseparable; i.e., most of the functions are basically determined by its structure. Thus, the activities of skeletal muscle contraction are based on its particular structure. An overall comprehension of its structure from macroscopic to microscopic is necessary in the first place, in order to have deeper understanding on the mechanism of contraction and force generation. In this book, the spatial scale is divided as follows: macroscopic scale (greater than $10^2\,\mu m$), mesoscopic scale (10^{-1}–$10^2\,\mu m$), and microscopic scale (less than $10^{-1}\,\mu m$).

1.1.1 MACROSTRUCTURE

The macrostructure of skeletal muscle is illustrated in Figure 1.1a. According to the above scale division, the macrostructure scales from muscle to single fascicle. A muscle is wrapped up by epimysium consisting of blood vessels and nervous tissues. The epimysium goes into the muscle and divides it into fascicle tissues. Each fascicle, wrapped by epimysium, consists of tens or hundreds of muscle fibers, i.e., the myocyte. Thus, the maximum diameter of fascicle is approximately several hundred μm. There are different morphologies of skeleton muscle, such as paralleled muscle, musculi fusiformis, single-pennate muscle and multi-pennate muscle, etc., depending on various fiber arrangements. Payne angle and physiological cross-sectional area are the two parameters that are often used to describe muscle's structural characteristics. Payne angle is the angle between fiber and

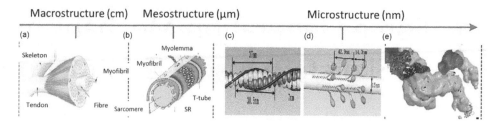

FIGURE 1.1   Skeletal muscle under different space scales (from left to right): (a) macrostructure; (b) meso-structure; (c) microstructure—thin filament; (d) microstructure—thick filament; (e) microstructure—head group of molecular motor.

tendon, while the physiological cross-sectional area is the maximum cross-sectional area of muscle. Thus, the bigger the area is, the more muscle fibers in the muscle.

1.1.2   MESOSTRUCTURE

The mesostructure of skeletal muscle is illustrated in Figure 1.1b. It ranges from fiber to sarcomere. Skeletal muscle mainly consists of parallel fibers, which are connected by endomysium and wrapped by sarcolemma with a diameter of about 1–2 μm. Inside the sarcolemma, there are tens or hundreds of myofibrils. Tissues, such as motion proprioceptor, neuromuscular junction, and the opening of transverse tubule (T-tubule), are adhered to the sarcolemma. Each myofibril, wrapped by sarcoplasmic reticulum (SR), consists of many sarcomeres in series, each of which is surrounded by two rings of T-tubules.

1.1.3   MICROSTRUCTURE

The microstructure of skeletal muscle refers to the structure of sarcomere, including the thin filament (Figure 1.1c), thick filament (Figure 1.1d) and myosin motor (also called as molecular motor) (Figure 1.1e). The horizontal and vertical spatial relationships are illustrated in Figure 1.2a,b. M-line has been recognized as the center of sarcomere. Thick filaments start from the M-line and extend to both ends of sarcomere. Thin filaments start from the Z-line at the two extremes of sarcomere and extend to the M-line. Thus, the thin and thick filaments overlap with each other. The thin filament, also called as actin filament, mainly consists of single actins in the form of α-double helix. Tropomyosin (Tm) and troponin (Tn) twine around the thin filaments periodically. The thick filament is formed by the tails of molecular motor twining with each other. The molecular motor binds with thin filaments periodically, consuming the energy released by the hydrolysis of adenosine triphosphate (ATP) in cytoplasm to do work, thus pulling the thin filaments and making the Z-line get closer to the M-line. In this way, sarcomere contraction is realized. As both M-line and

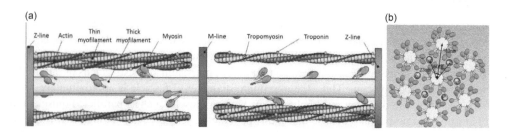

FIGURE 1.2   (a) Horizontal structure of sarcomere; (b) vertical structure of sarcomere.

Z-line are three-dimensional structures, they are also called as M-band and Z-band, respectively, in horizontal view. Moreover, the spatial arrangement of thin and thick filaments appears to be a hexagonal structure; i.e., the molecular motor on each thick filament can bind with six adjacent thin filaments, and each thin filament can be bound by three thick filaments.

1.2 FORCE GENERATION MECHANISM OF SKELETAL MUSCLE CONTRACTION: THE EXCITATION–CONTRACTION COUPLING

Molecular motor is the power source of muscular contraction. Thus, stimuli released by a motoneuron must be able to drive the molecular motor to do work, and this process is called the excitation–contraction coupling (ECC) [3]. The process is briefly illustrated in Figure 1.3. First, the motor intent activates the corresponding motoneurons. The control signal is sent to the neuromuscular junction on sarcolemma in the form of action potential (AP) and further generates new AP on sarcolemma. Next, AP arrives at T-tubule, releasing the high-concentration Ca^{2+} in SR into cytoplasm and then into the deeper part of sarcomere. Finally, Ca^{2+} binds to Tn on the thin filaments, thus making it possible for the motor head to bind with thin filaments and consume ATP to do work and start the contraction. Besides, information of length, velocity, and force of contraction are fed back by the proprioceptor to the central nervous system, brain, and even the motoneuron itself to form a local closed loop.

1.2.1 MOTONEURON AND NEUROMUSCULAR JUNCTION

1.2.1.1 Action Potential
It is recognized that motoneuron is the end of control signal for skeletal muscle contraction. The control signal, encoded by the AP, is sent to the neuromuscular junction through the axon of neuron. AP is the basic unit of nerve signal. The earliest systematic and quantitative research on AP was

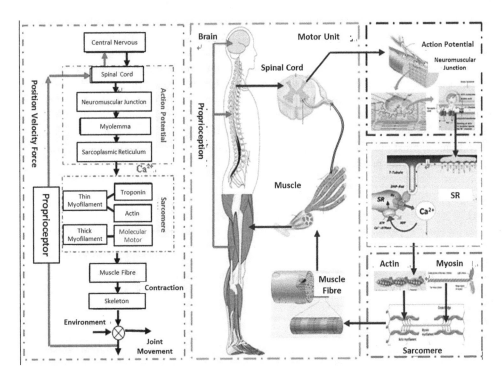

FIGURE 1.3 The excitation–contraction coupling process of skeletal muscle [3].

conducted by Hodgkin and Huxley [4] using squid's giant axon. There are numerous ion channels on the membrane of neuron, including Na^+ channel, K^+ channel, Cl^- channel, and Ca^{2+} channel. The ion concentration is unequal inside and outside the membrane and is generally kept constant by the cell. For instance, the K^+ concentration inside the membrane ($[K^+]_i$) is higher than that outside the membrane ($[K^+]_o$). Oppositely, $[Na^+]_o$ and $[Ca^{2+}]_o$ are higher than $[Na^+]_i$ and $[Ca^{2+}]_i$, respectively, and $[Cl^-]_o$ and $[Cl^-]_i$ can be treated as equal. The ion concentration (charge concentration) difference across the membrane contributes to the formation of membrane potential. AP is actually a special kind of membrane potential.

The change of membrane potential is dominated by the open and close of ion channels. When a specific channel is open, driven by transmembrane and chemical potential, the ions inside (outside) the membrane spread quickly to the opposite side of the membrane, leading to the change of charge concentration across the membrane and accordingly the change of membrane potential. There are two types of ion channels, namely the receptor type and voltage-sensitive type. The former opens when binding with specific acceptor, and the latter opens when the membrane potential rises. The voltage-sensitive Na^+ channel and K^+ channel play a key role in the generation and spread of AP. There are two significant potentials for the neuron membrane: the resting potential (about $-80\,mV$) and the threshold potential (about $-70\,mV$). The excitation in the soma of motoneuron raises the membrane potential near the axon (depolarization), thus opening the high-density voltage-sensitive Na^+ channels here. The inward flow of Na^+ brings about the further rise of the membrane potential. When the membrane potential is higher than the threshold potential, the opening of the numerous Na^+ channels leads to a huge leap in the membrane potential (tens of mV). However, there is a delay in the opening of K^+ channels compared to that of Na^+ channels. Thus, after the jump of the membrane potential, K^+ ions start to flow out due to the opening of K^+ channels, so this current is called delayed rectifier K^+ current. This makes the membrane potential decrease to the resting potential (repolarization) or even lower than the resting potential temporarily (hyperpolarization). The waveform of a typical AP is illustrated in Figure 1.4a. When one AP bursts, the adjacent Na^+ and K^+ channels will open in series, transferring the AP to the distal end of axon. It should be noted that inactivation mechanism exists for the voltage-sensitive Na^+ and K^+ channels; i.e., when AP is generated somewhere on the membrane, there is a refractory period for the ion channels lasting for several milliseconds (ms), which is also called absolute deactivation period. Then, the threshold potential would decrease exponentially with time, and the unidirectional conduction of AP is also guaranteed by the inactivation mechanism. However, if there are continuous intensive excitations somewhere on the membrane (membrane potential is constantly high), back propagation of AP would occur. There is another significant kind of ion channel on the membrane, the active type ion channel or the ion pump. The ion pump would consume the energy of ATP and transport ions across the membrane against the concentration gradient to maintain the transmembrane ion concentration difference at the resting potential.

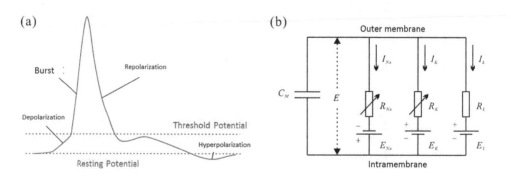

FIGURE 1.4   (a) Typical waveform of AP; (b) electrical model of membrane potential.

One important feature of AP is the *all-or-none* principle; i.e., AP either bursts or does not burst, so there is no intermediate state. It is similar to the digital quantity (they are also either one or zero), and the amplitude of an AP is approximately constant in a short period for some specific membrane or axon. It means that the control signal is characterized by the firing frequency. There are various models that describe the membrane potential during the research history of AP, and they can be divided into two categories, the *electrical model* and the *mathematical model.*

i. Electrical Model: Currently, the electrical model has been widely applied in the mathematical description of the membrane potential, as illustrated in Figure 1.4b. The core idea is to take the neuron or its axon as electric capacity (C_M) and the ion channel as electric resistance or conductance. In Figure 1.4b, E is the membrane potential and R_{Na}, R_K, and R_L are the resistances of Na$^+$ channel, K$^+$ channel, and leakage current, respectively. Na$^+$ and K$^+$ channels can be expressed as variable resistances, owing to the fact that their opening probability changes with the membrane potential, but the leakage current is relatively constant. It should be noted that the resistances in the model hold statistical significance instead of single-channel resistance. E_{Na}, E_K, and E_L are equilibrium potentials of Na$^+$, K$^+$, and leakage currents, respectively. The so-called equilibrium potential is the membrane potential when the transmembrane chemical potential and electric potential reach dynamic equilibrium during the transmembrane transfer of some specific ions. The total transmembrane current I can be expressed as

$$I = C_M \frac{dE}{dt} + \frac{E - E_K}{R_K} + \frac{E - E_{Na}}{R_{Na}} + \frac{E - E_L}{R_L}. \tag{1.1}$$

According to Eq. (1.1), electrical model actually treats the changes of membrane potential as the charge–discharge process of cell capacitance by ion current. The complexity over normal engineering electrical models stems mostly from the diffusion process of ions and the complicated gating behavior (resistance) of ion channels, which add notable nonlinear features to the model. In the research of neuron activities and computing mechanism, electrical model, including the derived *Cable Theory* [5] that describes AP transfer, is by far the most acceptable method for modeling and simulation. Currently, finite element analysis [6] of neuron activities and even large software are all based on this model.

ii. Mathematical Model: Mathematical model describes the membrane potential dynamics mainly based on nonlinear mathematical theories, usually Dynamic Systems [7]. Fitzhugh was the first to propose to describe the firing feature of AP in time domain using the van der Pol functions [8]; thus, this kind of model was named the Bonhoeffer-van der Pol (BVP) model. The BVP model can be expressed by two coupled differential equations:

$$\begin{cases} \dot{x} = c\left(y + x - x^3/3 + z\right) \\ \dot{y} = -(x - a + by)/c \end{cases}, \tag{1.2}$$

in which a, b, and c are all constant parameters; z, x, and y stand for exciting current, membrane potential, and transmembrane current, respectively. After choosing certain parameters, the phase portrait of the system in x–y plane would be a closed periodic orbit (the limit cycle); thus time-domain response of x would be used to express the periodic wave of AP. Due to the fact that the form is simple and the mathematical structure of the functions contain the nonlinear features of AP, the model has been popularized to do the finite element modeling of large-scale membrane. For instance, Rogers and McCulloch [9] conducted the finite element modeling of the spread of AP in myocardium based on the work of Fitzhugh and Nagumo. Aiming at overcoming the defect that the proportional

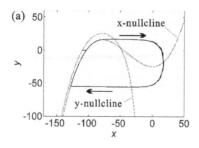 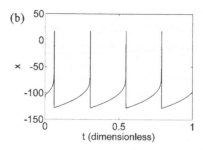

FIGURE 1.5   (a) The phase portrait of the dynamical system; (b) the time-domain feature of variable x.

relation between exciting current and AP cannot be faithfully reflected by the BVP model, Hindmarsh and Rose further modified Eq. (1.2) as

$$\begin{cases} \dot{x} = -a[f(x) - y - z] \\ \dot{y} = b[f(x) - q\exp(rx) + s - y] \end{cases}, \tag{1.3}$$

in which $f(x) = cx^3 + dx^2 + ex + h$; z, x, and y still stand for exciting current, membrane potential, and transmembrane current, respectively. All the other parameters are constant. The phase portrait of Hindmarsh–Rose model and time-domain response of membrane x are illustrated in Figure 1.5a,b, respectively, in which the x-nullcline and y-nullcline are represented by the dotted line. It should be noted that the corresponding amplitude and time are all transformed to a dimensionless form. The proportional relation between the oscillating frequencies of z and x can be well expressed. On this basis, three first-order–coupled differential functions were used to model the burst firing of neuron by Hindmarsh, the results of which also fit well with the experimental data [10].

The electrical model and the mathematical model are actually the typical representatives of mechanism models and phenomenological models, respectively; i.e., the former emphasizes the biophysical mechanism of the membrane potential, and the latter focuses on the abstract mathematical form instead of the biological principles. Due to the radical difference of their core modeling notions, the advantage and disadvantage of each method are also obvious. Given all the parameters, the electrical model is able to simulate and predict the neuron's discharge activity precisely. However, the resulting computational complexity of the finite element models is unacceptable, making it impossible to simulate complex or long-term neuron activities. On the other hand, there are fewer parameters in the mathematical model, whose nonlinear features were embed in its mathematical structure instead of its parameters. Thus, the computational efficiency is higher. However, because it is highly simplified, general behaviors of the membrane (e.g., the response of membrane potential under the threshold), including the fusion and spreading of AP, cannot be described accurately. Moreover, it is also difficult for the two models to be compatible with each other. Currently, how to develop an efficient and accurate membrane potential model is still a big problem. One possible solution is to consider the spreading of the membrane potential or AP as the nonlinear wave.

In summary, the influencing factors of the membrane potential are very complex, including the density distribution of various ion channels and the geometric structure of the different parts of neuron. Thus, the membrane potential is not only influenced by the oscillating characteristic of potential in time, but also influenced by the distribution feature of the membrane potential in space. The two aspects are closely related to each other through the spreading of AP, reflecting typical wave characteristics. As AP is closely related to the electromyography (EMG) signal which will be introduced in the next chapter, the generation mechanism, research methods, and current status for AP will be discussed in this section, aiming at providing readers with comprehensive understanding so that the subsequent contents can be better understood.

1.2.1.2 The Acceleration of Ion Diffusion Due to Electromagnetic Effects of Ion Currents in Ion Channels

Ion channel has been extensively studied as nanochannel and is well-recognized that there are many unique effects when microfluid goes through nanochannels [11,12]. In nanoscale, traditional hydrodynamics is inapplicable due to intermolecular forces between the channel and fluid particles [13]. Thus, more studies in recent years have been concentrated on the effect of ionic reaction to viscosity and the velocity of fluid in the channel [14]. Driven by numerous relevant experiments and molecular dynamic simulation [15], significant progresses have been made on nanochannels. However, there are still many problems and puzzles. After a long-term development, ion channel has been recognized as the best nanochannel as well as an excellent material for studying the features of nanochannel. Despite the force between molecule bond and electrovalent bond involved in the fluid–fluid interaction and fluid–channel interaction, insufficient attention has been paid to the overall physical field effect in ion channel. Thus, it is necessary to study the features of electromagnetic field produced by the ion current.

Na^+ channel and K^+ channel are significant in the spreading of AP based on the introduction in the former sections. Molecular conformation and composition of these channels, including the mechanism of opening, inactivation, and closing, have been revealed substantially [16]. Benefitting from these fundamental studies, the effect of ion channel activities to ion current is much clearer. However, due to the fact that the analysis about electrochemistry is insufficient in current studies, the understanding of dynamic effect of the ion current is still limited. Thus, it becomes vital to analyze the physical features of ion current and its influence on ionic motion. It has been well-recognized that varying current produces electromagnetic field in its surrounding space and influences the motion of charged particles. Therefore, there must be corresponding electromagnetic effects whose features are determined by the ion current. On the contrary, the electromagnetic field will also influence the ions in and around the channel.

1.2.1.2.1 Electromagnetic Field Induced by Ion Current

The model and calculation of electromagnetic field are based on the membrane current data obtained by Hodgkin and Huxley in their experiments on squid giant axons and their mathematical analyses [4], which are reliable and representative. The simulation of membrane currents during the formation of one single AP is shown in Figure 1.6a, in which the time step is 0.01 ms. The change of membrane potential in this process is shown in Figure 1.6b, and the curve demonstrates a typical shape of AP. Both results in Figure 1.6 are consistent with that of the original paper.

i. Modeling of the Microscopic Electromagnetic Field:

While establishing the physical model of the electromagnetic field around the ion channel, the physical conditions and space scales should be carefully identified. The membrane current data mentioned above were obtained with voltage clamp, so the cross-sectional area passed by membrane currents in our model should be the head area of the voltage clamp. As the currents run through the membrane, the path length of the currents can be regarded as equal to the thickness of the membrane. The head of a voltage clamp is a cone-shaped tube with an inner diameter of 1–3 μm [17]; therefore, without losing generality, we define the area as a circle of radius 1 μm. As for the thickness of the membrane, it is recognized as 5–8 nm by physiology, so we choose the upper limit (8 nm) for the squid giant axon membrane. Within this area, there may exist tens to hundreds of

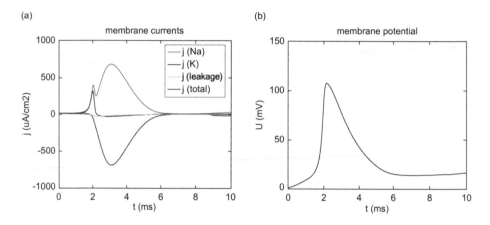

FIGURE 1.6 (a) Membrane current response of single AP; (b) membrane potential change caused by membrane current.

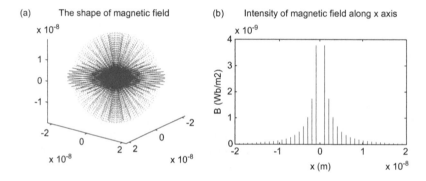

FIGURE 1.7 (a) The shape of magnetic field; (b) intensity of magnetic field along x axis.

channel proteins, so the currents are integrated, and the electromagnetic effects need to be calculated with the data of total current. The diameter of ion channel is about 1.5 nm, and the channels are unevenly distributed on the membrane, with mutual distance ranging from several to tens of nanometers. Here, we choose the center of the circle area as the origin, and the calculation is conducted within the 20 nm-radius sphere; moreover, the duration of calculation is that of a single AP.

Figure 1.7 shows the shape and coordinate of the microscopic current model. The field can be described by Maxwell's equations, which will not have wave-like solutions for the reason that what we consider here is the field during one single AP; thus, the decay of field intensity due to the refractive index of cytoplasm can also be neglected. Moreover, in the space near an ion channel, no unidirectionally polarized dielectric exists, so the solutions will provide considerably accurate distribution of the fields. At microspace scale, the vector potential of the field can be stated as

$$A = \frac{2\vec{j}(t)S}{4\pi\varepsilon c^2} \cdot \ln\frac{d - 2z + \sqrt{d^2 - 4dz + 4R^2}}{-d - 2z + \sqrt{d^2 + 4dz + 4R^2}}, \qquad (1.4)$$

where $j(t)$ is the current density and S is the cross-sectional area, while ε, c, and d correspond to the dielectric constant of water, the speed of light, and the thickness of the membrane, respectively. In Eq. (1.4), $R^2 = x^2 + y^2 + z^2$, and the coefficient "2" ahead of the equation is introduced for complementing the leakage current and the radius error. In order to simplify the expression, we write

$$\sqrt{d^2 - 4dz + 4R^2} = \sqrt{-}$$

$$\sqrt{d^2 + 4dz + 4R^2} = \sqrt{+}$$

Thus, Eq. (1.4) can be rewritten as

$$A = \frac{2\vec{j}(t)S}{4\pi\varepsilon c^2} \cdot \ln \frac{d - 2z + \sqrt{-}}{-d - 2z + \sqrt{+}}.$$

Thus, we get the expressions of magnetic field in x, y, and z directions:

$$B_x = \frac{8y\vec{j}(t)S}{4\pi\varepsilon c^2} \cdot \left[\frac{1}{\sqrt{-}\left(-d - 2z + \sqrt{-}\right)} - \frac{1}{\sqrt{+}\left(-d - 2z + \sqrt{+}\right)} \right]$$

$$B_y = -\frac{8x\vec{j}(t)S}{4\pi\varepsilon c^2} \cdot \left[\frac{1}{\sqrt{-}\left(-d - 2z + \sqrt{-}\right)} - \frac{1}{\sqrt{+}\left(-d - 2z + \sqrt{+}\right)} \right]. \qquad (1.5)$$

$$B_z = 0$$

The electric field can be calculated via scalar potential ϕ and vector potential A, and since we find that the vector potential term is infinitesimal during calculation, the electric field is expressed as

$$E = -\nabla\phi.$$

Thus, we get the electric field in x, y, and z directions:

$$E_x = \frac{16xS \int \vec{j}(t)\,dt}{4\pi\varepsilon} \cdot \left[\frac{-1}{\left(\sqrt{-}\right)^2 \left(d - 2z + \sqrt{-}\right)} \right.$$

$$\left. + \frac{d - 2z + 2\sqrt{-}}{\left(\sqrt{-}\right)^3 \left(d - 2z + \sqrt{-}\right)} + \frac{d + 2z}{\left(\sqrt{+}\right)^3} \right]$$

$$E_y = \frac{16yS \int \vec{j}(t)\,dt}{4\pi\varepsilon} \cdot \left[\frac{-1}{\left(\sqrt{-}\right)^2 \left(d - 2z + \sqrt{-}\right)} \right. \qquad (1.6)$$

$$\left. + \frac{d - 2z + 2\sqrt{-}}{\left(\sqrt{-}\right)^3 \left(d - 2z + \sqrt{-}\right)} + \frac{d + 2z}{\left(\sqrt{+}\right)^3} \right]$$

$$E_z = \frac{8S \int \vec{j}(t)\,dt}{4\pi\varepsilon} \cdot \left[-\frac{1}{\sqrt{+}} + \frac{(d + 2z)^2}{\left(\sqrt{+}\right)^3} - \frac{d - 2z}{\left(\sqrt{-}\right)^3} \right]$$

Here, we have got the complete expressions for the electromagnetic field; next we need to take simulations based on the data shown in Figure 1.6a so as to facilitate the observations of the field shapes.

ii. Simulation of the Electromagnetic Field:

The purpose of the simulation is to investigate the shapes of the fields and to represent the integrated effects of ion currents within the calculation area; thus, the data we use is the total current (the black line in Figure 1.6a). We need to linearly interpolate the data for the reason that our current data is discrete, and to facilitate the observation, we first calculate the fields at the time 2.2 ms, because the total current increases rapidly and its magnitude is relatively large at this moment.

The simulation result of the magnetic field is shown in Figure 1.7a, from which we can see that the shape of the field is like a sphere. The lengths of the line segments in the figure characterize the field intensity, and their directions correspond to the field directions. The field is stronger at the membrane plane ($z = 0$), and it decays rapidly while leaving the membrane. Actually we need to investigate the field intensity quantitatively, and the intensity distribution along x axis is shown in Figure 1.7b, from which we can see that the field decays exponentially while leaving the current center. At 10 nm from the center, it is 1.442×10^{-22} μWb nm^{-2}, and it decreases to 3.809×10^{-23} μWb nm^{-2} at 20 nm; therefore, we can tell that the magnetic field is very weak, and it can hardly affect the ions in the ion channel; however, due to the properties of electromagnetic field, the electric field should be much stronger; thus, we next discuss the electric field.

The shape of the electric field at this moment is represented in Figure 1.8a, which appears very special. The field radiates from the current center, and just like the magnetic field, it is also intense near the membrane plane; however, at both sides of the plane, there are cone-shaped radiation fields, and there are weaker fields in the neighborhood of the current center. Obviously, the electric field is quite directional. We still need to investigate the intensity distribution of the electric field along x axis (due to the symmetry), as shown in Figure 1.8a. We can see that the field also decays exponentially but more slowly than the magnetic field. More significantly, the electric field is quite strong, and it reaches 3.395×10^6 mV nm^{-1} at the current center, and it is 4.975×10^5 mV nm^{-1} at 10 nm from the center, while at 20 nm, it decreases to 1.387×10^5 mV nm^{-1}. This means the potential drop is very large with the increase of distance from the current center, and we can predict that such fields will certainly affect ion motion and even influence the activities of ion channel.

Based on the analyses above, we conclude that the electric field is dominant; thus in the continuing analysis, we neglect the effect of the magnetic field. Here, we have observed the electric field at one specific moment, but theoretically speaking, the field should grow

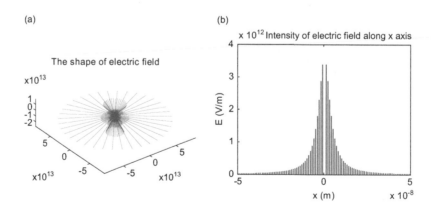

FIGURE 1.8   (a) The shape of electric field; (b) intensity of electric field along x axis.

stronger with the increase of the total current and decay when the current decreases. After the simulation of the complete time range, we find that the electric field indeed acts like this. As previously mentioned, the electric field will affect ion motions for the reason that charged particles near the current center will be driven by electric force; more specifically, Na^+ will be pushed out from the channel center due to the radiating electric field. Such behavior makes us aware that the field will considerably accelerate the diffusion of Na^+ concentration beneath the membrane and thus speed up the propagation of APs.

1.2.1.2.2   Analysis of Acceleration Effect

In order to investigate the acceleration effect of the electric field on the diffusion of Na^+, we need to analyze the drift property of ions under electric force. Actually even without the electric field, Na^+ can also diffuse in the cytoplasm due to chemical concentration gradient and Brownian motion. If we call the diffusion under chemical potential as "passive diffusion" and that under electric force as "active diffusion", our purpose is then to compare the diffusion speed between the passive diffusion and the combined diffusion (passive plus active) and finally tell to what extent the electric field accelerates Na^+ diffusion.

i. Physical Model for Passive Diffusion:
   To start, we choose a specific direction for analysis, e.g., the x direction; then the diffusion flux of special particles (the ions we considered) among the background particles is

$$J_D = -D\frac{\partial n}{\partial x},\tag{1.7}$$

where n denotes the molar concentration of ions and D is the diffusion coefficient. The dynamical equation of concentration changes can be expressed as

$$\frac{\partial n}{\partial t} = D\frac{\partial^2 n}{\partial x^2}.\tag{1.8}$$

ii. Physical Model for Active Diffusion:
   If there is an extra field force (in our case, the electric force) exerting on the particles except their intrinsic thermal motions, they will go through a net drift, and the flux of the active diffusion can be stated as

$$J_E = \mu q n \cdot E_x,\tag{1.9}$$

where μ, q, and E_x denote the drift rate, the charge carried by a single particle, and the electric field in x direction, respectively. Thus, the combined diffusion flux is

$$J_x = J_D + J_E = -D\frac{\partial n}{\partial x} + \mu q n \cdot E_x,\tag{1.10}$$

and the dynamical equation of combined diffusion becomes

$$\frac{\partial n}{\partial t} = D\frac{\partial^2 n}{\partial x^2} - \mu q E_x \frac{\partial n}{\partial x} - \mu q n \frac{\partial E_x}{\partial x}.\tag{1.11}$$

iii. Numerical Simulation of the Diffusion Process:
   The objects of simulation are the dynamics expressed in Eqs. (1.8) and (1.10), and they need to be numerically solved due to the complexity of the differential equations. Before calculation, the parameters involved should firstly be identified. The environmental

TABLE 1.1

Parameters Involved in the Simulation

Parameter	k (J/K)	q (C)	τ (s)	μ
Value	1.38×10^{-23}	1.6×10^{-19}	1.81×10^{-13}	4.75×10^{12}

temperature of squid cells is ~6.3°C, so the absolute temperature $T = 279.8$ K; besides, the mass of Na^+ is ~3.82×10^{-26} kg. Other values of parameters are listed in Table 1.1.

In the table, the parameter τ characterizes the average collision time interval between Na^+ and water molecule, and it is approximated by that between water molecules. On the other hand, the initial conditions and boundary conditions should be given. We reasonably assume that the Na^+ concentration at the center of the channel is equal to that outside the membrane and based on the experimental data [18]; the concentrations inside and outside the membrane are 50 mmol/L and 500 mmol/L, respectively. We further assume that the initial concentration distribution is parabola-shaped, with extension distance of 5 nm, as shown in Figure 1.9. As for the boundary conditions, at $x = 0$, the concentration n is constant, $n = 500$ mmol/L, while at the far end $x = \infty$, n is always set to zero. Finally, considering the convergence of the calculation, the spatial interval and the temporal interval are set as $\Delta x = 1$ nm, $\Delta t = 0.01$ ns, and the simulation proceeds for 10 ns after the time $t = 2.2$ ms.

The electric field we are using now is that 500 nm under the membrane, and the concentration distribution after 10 ns is shown in Figure 1.10a. The dotted line and the solid line represent the concentration distribution without or with active diffusion; besides, note that here the original Na^+ concentration at rest state level (50 mmol/L) inside the membrane is not included, so Figure 1.10a only shows the difference of the diffusion speed. Actually, if we observe the diffusion process with animation, we will find that the wave front of the solid line always leads that of the dotted line, indicating faster diffusion with the effect of electric field. Furthermore, we need to know the speed difference quantitatively; therefore we choose the data points of 20 mmol/L above the rest state level on these two curves and compare their displacement values. For the dotted line, such concentration is ~39 nm away from the current center, while it is ~125 nm for the solid line, so we can see that the diffusion speed under the effect of the electric field is three times of that under pure chemical effects, and the average spreading speed during this time interval is ~12.5 m/s.

According to the previous calculation results, we know that the field intensity should decrease with the increasing distance from the membrane. Figure 1.10b shows the

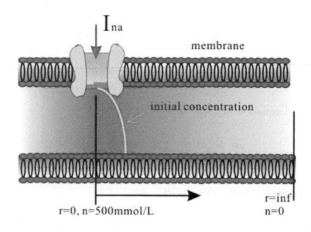

FIGURE 1.9   Initial condition and boundary condition.

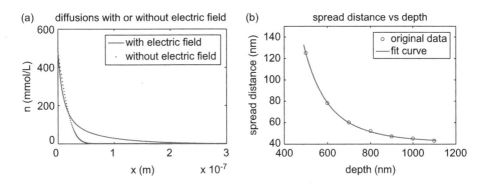

FIGURE 1.10 (a) Concentration distribution with the membrane depth of 500 nm; (b) the furthest distance distribution of the some concentration under different membrane depths.

distribution of the farthest positions of the same concentration (20 mmol/L above the rest state level), from which we can see that the distance decreases exponentially when leaving the membrane and gradually approaches the distance of pure chemical diffusion. Actually Figure 1.10b also demonstrates the diffusion speeds of Na^+ concentration of different depths under the membrane; i.e., the diffusion is slower at positions farther away from the membrane, and it is faster at positions closer to the membrane due to the stronger effect of electric field. This result is quite reasonable because the channel proteins are embedded in the membrane, so in order to transfer the membrane excitations more efficiently, the ions near the membrane should spread faster; thus the depolarization sensitivity of the membrane can be greatly enhanced.

Based on the above analyses, we conclude that the electromagnetic effects can remarkably accelerate the diffusion of ions and such effects are essential for the spread of Na^+ concentration in biological systems. The spreading speed of membrane excitations (like APs) may dramatically fall without the help of electric field, and the Na^+ concentration beneath the membrane will rapidly drop due to the high efficiency of Na/K pumps, so it is difficult to activate channels farther away, leading to the low success ratio of signal conduction on the membrane. On the other hand, our analyses are microscopic (the head area of the voltage clamp); therefore, the results we obtained can be regarded as local electromagnetic effects, and if the whole cell membrane is involved, it is not hard to imagine that these many local fields will interfere with each other. Such integrated effects actually represent the distribution of electromagnetic signals on the membrane, and they can affect the expressions of membrane potential information when treating with EMG.

1.2.1.3 Postsynaptic Response on Sarcolemma

To activate the muscle fiber, the AP propagating on motoneuron axon must be transformed first through the neuromuscular microstructures, as shown in Figure 1.11. When the AP arrives at the axon terminals (presynaptic membrane), the voltage-sensitive Ca^{2+} channels will be activated and open. Thus, massive numbers of Ca^{2+} are able to get into the cell and bind to the calcium-binding proteins (x), turning them into the activated conjugated proteins (x*). The proteins then bind with the vesicle located on the presynaptic membrane to make the vesicle exocytosis start. In the vesicle of motoneuron, there is high-concentration acetylcholine (Ach), which is an important messenger for information transfer between neuron and muscle fiber. There are ion channel receptors for Ach on the wrinkle top of postsynaptic membrane (sarcolemma). The receptors will open quickly when binding with the Ach released by exocytosis, thus allowing for the inward flow of Na^+ and depolarizing the postsynaptic membrane, on which there are lots of voltage-sensitive Na^+ channels and K^+ channels. When the membrane potential rises, they will open in series to generate new AP

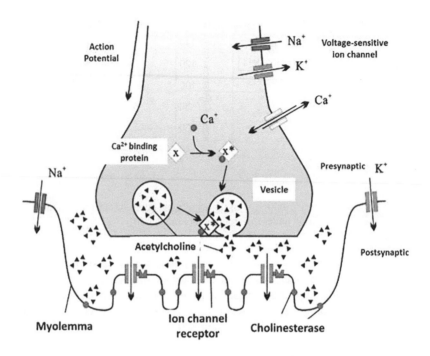

FIGURE 1.11   Information transfer at the neuromuscular junction.

spreading on sarcolemma. The distance between postsynaptic and presynaptic membranes (synaptic cleft) is approximately 50 nm. Most of the Ach released into the synaptic cleft will be resolved by the cholinesterase in the wrinkle of presynaptic membrane and will be resynthesized as Ach for next exocytosis. The above process belongs to the typical chemical synaptic transmission, during which the direction of transfer is irreversible with a response time of approximately 0.5–1 ms.

Neuromuscular junction is responsible for transferring AP from motoneuron to muscle fiber. Thus, it is the freight station for neural signal that controls skeleton muscle. Some scholars describe the information-transfer process as "copying action potential from neuron to sarcolemma". However, in a strict sense, it is not a simple copying process. Note that during the stimuli-transfer process, the information changes from "digital quantity" (AP) to "analog quantity" (Ach transmitter concentration) and back to "digital quantity" (AP). The frequency of AP on the presynaptic membrane only determines directly the transmitter concentration in synaptic cleft and then influences the input current strength on postsynaptic membrane. However, the input current itself cannot determine the AP frequency on sarcolemma. As mentioned before, the waveform and frequency of the AP also depend on the distribution of voltage-sensitive ion channels, membrane morphology, and stimulation history. Thus, the AP's frequency and waveform on the postsynaptic membrane are usually different from those on the presynaptic membrane. In a strict sense, the frequency of the AP on sarcolemma and the firing rate of neuron are positively correlated. In fact, the transformation between firing rate and transmitter concentration is very common in human's daily physiological activities (the information exchange between neurons, for example). Thus, it remains a question whether to choose "analog quantity" or "digital quantity" for studying neural cybernetic principles.

1.2.2   T-Tubule and SR

1.2.2.1   Contraction Drive: RyR Channel and DHPR

T-tubule transfers excitation from sarcolemma to the deeper part of muscle fiber through the connecting point of T-tubule and SR. The T-tubule with the SR (longitudinal tubule) on its two sides is

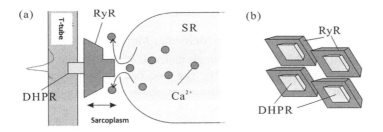

FIGURE 1.12 (a) Ca^{2+} release mechanism of thribble; (b) space structure of tetrame.

called the thribble structure. The T-tubule connects with SR terminal cisterna through the coupling structure of dihydropyridine (DHPR) and ryanodine receptor (RyR) (tetramer) [19]. Tetramer is actually an electrically and mechanically coupled L-type Ca^{2+} channel. When the AP on T-tubule reaches the terminal cisterna, DHPR will take conformational change when the potential rise is detected. Then it drives RyR to move from SR to open the channel so that the high-concentration Ca^{2+} in SR could be released to cytoplasm. It can be seen that the tetramer channel acts like a molecular stopper. The motion of the stopper is controlled by the potential of T-tubule. The structure of tetramer is illustrated in Figure 1.12b. Each group of RyR is arranged like a parallelogram, corresponding to the four DHPRs, respectively. Through the electrically and mechanically coupled L-type Ca^{2+} channel, the AP spreading on sarcolemma is able to control $[Ca^{2+}]$ in sarcoplasm to activate muscle contraction.

1.2.2.2 Ca^{2+} Dynamics in Sarcoplasm

Tetramer dominates the quick release of Ca^{2+} in sarcoplasm. However, there exists a complex and complete regulation mechanism for Ca^{2+} kinetics in sarcoplasm, and it maintains the muscle fiber in good condition and the resting $[Ca^{2+}]$. Several major buffers are illustrated in Figure 1.13. Besides the tetramer channel, Ca^{2+} pump is another important organelle on SR. It consumes the energy of ATP to recycle the released Ca^{2+} in sarcoplasm back to SR quickly to maintain the gradient across SR membrane so that enough Ca^{2+} in SR could be normally released when the AP in T-tubule arrives. The regulation factors of the operational efficiency of Ca^{2+} pump is relatively complex, as it is affected by both the membrane potential of SR and $[Ca^{2+}]$ in sarcoplasm. Moreover, Tn, ATP, parvalbumin, etc. are also important buffers for Ca^{2+}. They constantly bind and dissociate with Ca^{2+} in sarcoplasm, forming the compounds such as [CaTn], [CaATP], and [CaParv]. Thus, the $[Ca^{2+}]$ is maintained by a dynamic equilibrium all the time. Baylor and Hollingworth [20] modeled the dynamics of the system in detail using Markov process.

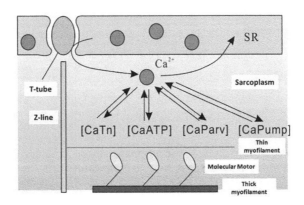

FIGURE 1.13   Dynamic equilibrium of Ca^{2+} in sarcoplasm.

1.2.3 MYOSIN MOTOR

1.2.3.1 Operation Mechanism of Single Molecular Motor: Lymn–Taylor Cycle

It has been recognized that the operation of single molecular motor is a mechanochemical coupling cycle, also known as Lymn–Taylor cycle [21]. The so-called mechanochemical coupling implies that motor's chemical state during ATP hydrolysis is closely coupled to its mechanical state. The complete cycle is illustrated briefly in Figure 1.14. "A" denotes actin, and "M" stands for myosin. In state ① (A,M), actin and the molecular motor are still in "rigor state" after a work cycle of the motor; then, ATP binds to the head of molecular motor, which changes the conformation of the motor so that the molecular motor dissociates with actin to form state ② (M.ATP). This process is called "recovery stroke". Then the ATP hydrolyzes into ADP.Pi, and molecular motor turns into state ③ (M.ADP.Pi). When the Ca^{2+} in sarcoplasm binds the Tn on the thin filament to make the binding site on the Tm open, the molecular motor is able to bind to actin and to reach state ④ (A.M.ADP.Pi). The process is called the "pre-power stroke". The inorganic phosphorus Pi is released from the head of motor so that the motor head binds strongly with the actin to form state ⑤ (A.M.ADP). The neck region of molecular motor begins to bend; the relative sliding of thick and thin filaments starts, and the motor reaches the "power stroke". Then, the motor head further releases ADP to bend more to generate displacement and returns to state ①; then, the whole cycle is completed. The evolution of the above cycle is statistically significant; i.e., the process should be described by probability (such as the Markov process). Thus, in a more microscopic time scale, there are occasionally reversed evolutions of the motor's states; e.g., the motor is possible to return to weak binding state from strong binding state.

1.2.3.2 Collective Working Mechanism of Molecular Motors

The contraction of one sarcomere is accomplished by the collective operation of many molecular motors, and this requires the study on collective working mechanism. There are radical differences between the collective behavior and individual behavior of molecular motors, because in a system of multiple molecular motors, the operation of each molecular motor is not independent but correlated. Thus, the collective working mechanism involves typical probabilistic description. Currently, there are two interpretations. The first one is based on the work by Huxley [2]. The core idea is to obtain

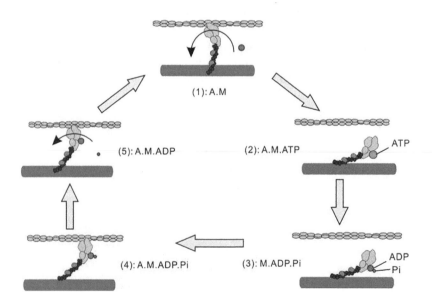

FIGURE 1.14 Lymn–Taylor cycle of single molecular motor.

the average force of single molecular motor through probability density function of molecular motor's binding location and then calculate the contraction force of a sarcomere by summing up all the motors in that sarcomere. The second one is based on statistical thermodynamics. It treats the molecular motor as Brownian ratchet and obtains the probability flow of motor state transition by correlation function, Fokker–Planck [22] function, and the dynamical function of the system.

The working mechanism of individual motors and the collective molecular motor will be discussed in detail in Chapter 2. In the working cycle, energy released by ATP hydrolysis transforms into heat and potential energy for conformational change in motor's head. The potential energy then transforms into the elastic energy of motor's head, which is the main driving force of the motor. Finally, the elastic energy transforms into the kinetic energy of the relative sliding of the thick and thin filaments.

1.2.4 RECEPTOR

In skeletal muscle, besides the fibers responsible for muscular contraction, there are also perceptive organs, or receptors, that sense the muscle's working state. Receptors are able to transmit the information of length, velocity, and force of muscle as proprioceptive feedback to central nervous system (CNS) without visual support. Thus, it is the physiological basis of reflex and muscle memory. There are two major types of receptors: muscle spindle and tendon organ.

1.2.4.1 Muscle Spindle

The main functions of muscle spindle are detecting and feeding back muscle length and contraction velocity. It can be divided into nuclear bag type and nuclear chain type, and the structures are illustrated in Figure 1.15a and b, respectively. It can be seen that these two types are very similar, and only differ in the response characteristics. Muscle spindle is in parallel with muscle fiber and is located in muscle belly. There are also contractile fiber tissues in muscle spindle. They are located on both ends of the muscle spindle and are called as "intra-spindle muscle". Correspondingly, the muscle fibers are called "extra-spindle muscle". The contractions of intra-spindle muscle and extra-spindle muscle are dominated by γ and α motoneurons, respectively.

Generally, the firing rate of γ motoneuron is proportional to that of α motoneuron; i.e., the stronger muscle fiber contracts, the stronger intra-spindle muscle contracts so that the stiffness of muscle spindle increases and the spindle's sensitivity for mechanical deformation can be enhanced. The ending (primary ending) of type-Ia afferent nerves twines around the middle part of muscle

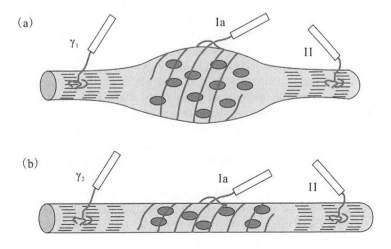

FIGURE 1.15 (a) Nuclear bag muscle spindle; (b) nuclear chain muscle spindle.

spindle, and the ending (secondary ending) of type-II afferent nerves twines around the ending part of muscle spindle. These two types of afferent nerves are responsible for transforming mechanical deformation of muscle spindle into AP so that it can be transmitted to central nervous system. The former could detect dynamic (velocity) and static (length variation) tensile reflections, but the latter could only detect the static one. The firing rates of the two endings are proportional to the velocity or length of stretching. Note that the nuclear bag muscle spindle contracts relatively slower with less strength and thus is often found in slow-twitch fiber. On the contrary, the nuclear chain type is often found in fast-twitch fiber.

1.2.4.2 Tendon Organ

Tendon organ, also called as Golgi tendon organ, is the receptor that feeds back muscle contraction force. It is located on the joint part between skeletal muscle and muscle tendon. Different from muscle spindle, they are not dominated by motoneuron, and the ending afferent nerve is Ib type. Besides, tendon organ is sensitive to the changing rate of contraction force instead of absolute magnitude. The firing strength of the afferent ending is proportional to the increasing rate of contraction force. In stretch reflex, the excitation of muscle spindle is positive feedback; i.e., it enforces the firing of motoneuron, thus strengthening the contraction to resist stretching. The excitation of tendon organ is negative feedback through interneuron, in order to restrain the firing of α motoneuron and to avoid muscle strain.

1.2.5 A Dynamical System: Markov Model for Active Postsynaptic Responses of Muscle Spindle Afferent Nerve

The operation of skeletal muscle is a typically bioelectrochemical closed-loop control process, which is regulated by the AP fired by motoneurons. The contraction length/speed and tension of the muscle are fed back by the afferent nerves of muscle spindles and tendon organs within it, and these signals are simultaneously transmitted to the CNS and the motoneuron itself [23,24]. As an important receptor, the muscle spindle is equivalent to the displacement/speed transducer of skeletal muscle, as the real-time firing rate of its afferent nerves (Ia afferents) varies with the length and contraction speed of the muscle. We have proposed the bioelectrochemical frequency-regulating control mechanism for skeletal muscle based on the characteristics of the APs on muscle fibers [25]; i.e., the working process of muscle is regulated by the frequency of AP in real time. The afferent signals influence the firing behavior of motoneurons; thus, the feedback of a muscle spindle to the motoneuron forms a local closed loop, which is pivotal to the stability of muscle operation. The researches on the working mechanism of skeletal muscle have lasted for many decades, while the regulation and control mechanisms of muscle are seldom touched; therefore, our understanding of the control principium is far from satisfactory. On the other hand, in order to explore the closed-loop control properties, the key point is to take extensive researches on the feedback effects of the afferents, and this involves the synaptic transmission between Ia afferents and motoneurons.

Motoneurons are myelinated neurons with their dendrites and somas located in the spinal cord [26]. The signals of muscle spindles are excitatory afferents, whose terminals extend into the spinal cord and are connected with the dendritic shafts or spines of motoneurons, and the dendritic tree of one motoneuron can receive thousands of inputs [27]. The investigations on excitatory synapses show that a single input can depolarize the postsynaptic membrane by 0.2–0.4 mV [28]. Synaptic signals regulate the firing behavior of the axon of a motoneuron via a mechanism called synaptic integration, and the control information is contained in the frequency of AP [25], while because of the *all-or-none* feature of AP, the quantity regulated by the afferents via synaptic interactions should also be the firing rate of the postsynaptic neuron. Despite of the extensive experimental observations on the process of synaptic integration [29], relevant researches are still at the qualitative stage, and the cybernetic model based on frequency information has not been extracted and proposed. Moreover, the frequency-regulating feedback mechanism of the afferents is closely related to the postsynaptic responses, and researches on excitatory/inhibitory synapses have been massively carried out [30,31]. Dendrites used to be regarded as purely passive; i.e., postsynaptic currents can only diffuse passively within them. Based on such assumptions, Rall et al. [32] proposed the passive cable theory of membrane, and Hines et al. [33] further developed the NEURON code aimed at calculating the membrane potential responses of the whole neuron. However, recent studies have proved that dendrite structures possess active features, and voltage-sensitive ion channels exist on the dendritic tree [6]. Particularly, the dendritic Ca^{2+} currents of motoneurons play a key role in their synaptic integration [34]. The passive cable model can hardly simulate the active properties of dendrites, not to say investigating the influence of the non-uniform distribution of channel density on signal processing. For the fact that many difficulties remain in the measurements of the electrical/chemical responses in a single segment of dendrites, theoretical analyses are indispensable for the exploration of the interactions of dendritic information [35], while efficient models being able to easily simulate the active responses of dendrites have not been proposed till today. In effect, the essence of the propagation of membrane potential is the diffusion of cytoplasmic ion; thereby finite element method (FEM) is favorable for the analysis of the non-uniformity of the membrane. Finite element analysis has already been applied in the research of AP propagation on cardiac muscle [9], while for synaptic integration, the main trouble is the high calculation cost of the cable model during the implementation of finite element analysis. It is noteworthy that the dimensionless dynamical system model reflecting the changing characteristics of membrane potential has been proposed [8], and such models can spontaneously simulate the active features of membrane. Besides, based on the chemical kinetics of ion channels, Destexhe et al. [36,37] proposed that postsynaptic responses can be expressed by Markov models. These two models are able to reduce the calculation cost to a large extent; consequently, by means of combining existent research results, this chapter aims at establishing a highly efficient computational model that can be used to describe the active postsynaptic responses of Ia afferents and laying the foundation for further research of synaptic integration and the frequency-regulating feedback mechanism of motoneurons.

1.2.5.1 The Synapse of Ia Afferent Nerve

The synapse of Ia afferent nerve belongs to chemical type, whose structure is shown in Figure 1.16. After APs fired by the afferent nerve arrive at presynaptic membrane, the voltage-sensitive

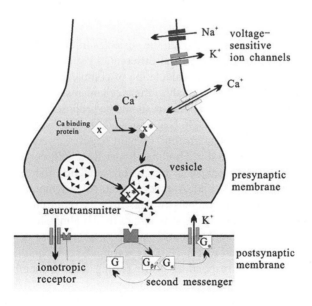

FIGURE 1.16 The structure of chemical synapses.

Ca^{2+} channels will open when sensing the rise of membrane potential, and presynaptic Ca^{2+} concentration ($[Ca^{2+}]$) will increase. The vesicles containing neurotransmitters reside at the presynaptic active zone, and when Ca^{2+} binds with relevant protein complexes (x), their activated state (x*) will be formed. These proteins further combine with the vesicles, causing them to exocytose, and neurotransmitter can be released [38]. For the synapses of Ia afferents, the main type of neurotransmitter is glutamate [28], and postsynaptic membrane is densely occupied by ionotropic receptors and metabotropic receptors (also called second-messenger–type receptors) that can receive glutamate transmitter. Ionotropic receptor directly opens the ion channel coupled to it after binding with transmitter and lets Na^+, K^+, and Ca^{2+} pass through the membrane; thus, it dominates the rapid transmission of synaptic signal. Metabotropic receptor mainly contributes to the slow and long-term regulation of postsynaptic responses, while for the feedback activities of motoneurons during normal operation of muscle, the instantaneous dynamic response is more significant, so this chapter only deals with ionotropic receptors. On the other hand, ionotropic receptors can be classified into two categories according to the types of transmitter that they receive [28]: one category is called N-methyl-D-aspartate (NMDA) receptor; i.e., this kind of receptors bind with NMDA-type transmitter to open; and the other class is non-NMDA receptor. These two types of receptors coexist in the synapses of motoneurons; therefore, the excitatory postsynaptic current during rapid signaling is the superposition of their respective currents. It should be noted that the exocytosis of vesicles requires the increase of presynaptic $[Ca^{2+}]$, which is caused by presynaptic depolarization. We see that for chemical synapses, there always exists a cycle in which presynaptic potential induces postsynaptic current, which is transferred into presynaptic potential again; thus, it is necessary to build a dynamic model for membrane potential first.

1.2.5.2　The Dynamical System Model for Membrane Potential

Since the generation mechanism of AP was discovered, several kinds of mathematical models describing the dynamical features of membrane potential have been proposed. The earliest systematic and quantitative researches on AP were conducted by Hodgkin and Huxley [4], who concluded the coupling relationships among membrane potential and channel conductance and time based on the chemical characteristics of ion channels, and the resultant model was named as the H–H model. This model succeeded in the dynamic description of membrane potential; however, the H–H model includes four state variables, and the computation involves four coupled differential equations. The passive cable model is similar to the H–H model for the reason that it belongs to electrical models as well. Although the variables in the cable model are fewer, solving temporal and spatial coupled parabolic partial differential equations is needed [32]; as a result, electrical models are not suitable for the calculation of complex activities of neurons. As previously mentioned, in order to elaborately analyze the mechanisms of synaptic integration, a model aimed at complicated finite element computation should be proposed. FitzHugh et al. [8] proposed a dynamical system model (the FitzHugh–Nagumo model) composed of two differential equations, which can both represent the main time-domain features of AP and considerably reduce the complexity of computation. Besides, Hindmarsh and Rose [10] corrected the defect that the FitzHugh–Nagumo model is not capable of reasonably reflecting the relation between AP frequency and control current (f–I relation). Another advantage of dynamical system models is that computation can be carried out dimensionlessly, degrading the requirements on temporal and spatial iteration steps. This chapter adopts the structure of the Hindmarsh–Rose model to implement the real-time calculation of membrane potential, and the model can be described by two coupled differential equations, as illustrated by Eq. (1.3). By setting the two equalities in Eq. (1.3) to zero, the fixed point of the system corresponding to the resting state of membrane can be obtained. Although the calculation of Eq. (1.3) can be dimensionless, and the fixed point can be freely chosen from the perspective of mathematics, here we let y and z be zero and x be negative when the system is at equilibrium (with no stimulation current and net membrane current and resting potential being negative), so that the system is consistent with the actual physiological features of membrane. Thus, at equilibrium, the system can be written as

$$\begin{cases} f(x_{ep}) = 0 \\ -q\exp(rx_{ep}) + s = 0 \end{cases}, \tag{1.12}$$

where x_{ep} is the x-coordinate of the fixed point, so we have

$$x_{ep} = \frac{1}{r}\ln\left(\frac{s}{q}\right). \tag{1.13}$$

In order to assure the resting potential being negative, there must be $s < q$. The parameters of the two equalities in Eq. (1.4) can be decided independently, and finally we chose the dimensionless resting potential as ~ -110; i.e., the fixed point is $(-110, 0)$, and the parameters of the system in this case are listed in Table 1.2. If we iterate the system with the fourth-order Runge–Kutta method, the phase portrait of the system ($z = 10$) can be drawn as shown in Figure 1.17a, in which the dashed lines characterize the x- and y-nullclines. The state of the system will go through a periodic orbit when it deviates from the fixed point, and this corresponds to the reciprocating change of the membrane potential when AP train occurs (Figure 1.17b). Furthermore, it can be noted from Eq. (1.3) that the parameters a and b determine the changing rates of x and y, respectively. Due to the rapid change of x and the slower change of y, the system is very sensitive to b. We see from the second equality of Eq. (1.1) that the parameter b actually decides the changing rate of membrane currents; thereby b can be considered as corresponding to the densities of Na/K/Ca channels on the membrane; i.e., under the same injection current, the firing rate of AP should be positively correlated to the value of b. Figure 1.3a shows the frequencies of AP when b is 30, 60, and 90, respectively, with the same injection current ($z = 10$). It must be noted that if b is simply fixed, we are actually adjusting the densities of all the types of channels simultaneously, while during the practical application of the model, sometimes only one of these densities need to be changed. For a certain membrane domain, the number of K^+ channels relative to that of Na^+/Ca^+ channels determines the amplitude, duration, and frequency of AP [39]; therefore the parameter characterizing the density of K^+ channels needs to be separated. As for the total membrane current, Na^+ channels and Ca^+ channels mainly contribute to the rising phase of the current, while its falling phase attributes to the effect of K^+ channels [4], so when $\dot{y} \geq 0$,

$$f(x) - q \cdot \exp(rx) + s \geq y.$$

We see that the value of y is under its nullcline when the current is increasing. The value of b in this case corresponds to the densities of Na^+/Ca^+ channels, and we denote it as b_1. When $\dot{y} < 0$,

$$f(x) - q \cdot \exp(rx) + s < y.$$

TABLE 1.2

Parameters in the Dynamical System Model of the Membrane

Parameter	Value	Parameter	Value
a	4×10^3	h	-14.297
b	30	q	1.464×10^3
c	1.7×10^{-4}	r	1×10^{-1}
d	2×10^{-2}	s	2.4×10^{-2}
e	1×10^{-2}		

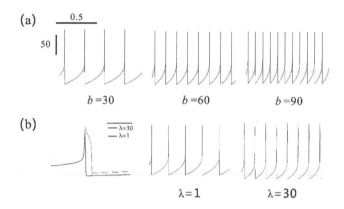

FIGURE 1.17   (a) The phase portrait of the dynamical system; (b) the time-domain feature of variable x.

This implies when the current is decreasing, y is above its own nullcline, and now b corresponds to the density of K$^+$ channels, which is denoted by b_2. Hence, the non-uniform distribution of channel densities can be simulated via adjusting the values of b_1 and b_2 in different domains of the membrane. Furthermore, if defining $\lambda = b_1/b_2$, the ratio between the number of Na channels and the number of K channels is represented by λ. We take $b_1 = 30$ and $z = 12$; then Figure 1.17b shows the comparisons of the time-domain properties of a single AP and the frequencies of AP trains when $\lambda = 1$ and $\lambda = 30$, respectively. It can be checked that with the increase of λ, the amplitude, duration, as well as the frequency of AP will all grow in response, and this feature coincides with the electrophysiological principles of the membrane.

Identifying the physical meaning of b is significant to the research on the frequency-regulating feedback mechanism of neurons, for the reason that the channel densities at different locations of a neuron may differ a lot, forming the unique function of information modulation [39]. In the remaining part of this chapter, if not particularly specified, the parameter b corresponds to the situation where $\lambda = 1$. One extra thing worth noting is that the dynamical system model represented by Eq. (1.3) characterizes the response of a closed membrane domain to the injection current, while for an open domain, the diffusion effect of the charges inside the membrane should be considered.

On the other hand, according to Figure 1.17b, when AP is induced, the peak value of x is ~18, corresponding to the real spike of AP (40 mV), while at equilibrium, the value of x (−110) corresponds to the resting potential (−65 mV); therefore the transformation between the dimensionless voltage V_{dim} and the real voltage V_{mV} in the unit of mV can be obtained as

$$k \cdot V_{dim} + \Delta = V_{mV}, \tag{1.14}$$

where the ratio constant $k = 0.82$ and $\Delta = 25.24$. In the same way, if we match the dimensionless time with physical time, the model can be applied to the firing behavior analysis of neurons in different frequency domains.

1.2.5.3   The Kinetic Model for Postsynaptic Receptors

As shown in Figure 1.16, the open state of the ionotropic receptors on the postsynaptic membrane requires their binding with corresponding transmitter, and the receptors will experience closed and/ or desensitization states. The transition rates between these states may depend on the surrounding transmitter concentration. Markov models can be used to describe chemical kinetic systems whose transition rates do not vary with time, and relevant studies [40] have shown that Markov models can provide reasonable descriptions for ligand-gated ion channels like postsynaptic receptors. Besides, the open fraction of the receptors is directly related to the transmitter concentration in the synaptic gap, while the release quantity of transmitter is determined by presynaptic [Ca^{2+}],

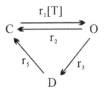

FIGURE 1.18   The Markov model for non-NMDA receptors.

so if we build the model according to the physiological open process of the receptors, the relations between presynaptic [Ca²⁺] and ion currents, the dynamic recycling process of Ca^{2+} by ionic pumps, the activation process of Ca^{2+} binding protein complex, as well as the releasing and recycling kinetics of transmitter [36] should all be taken into account. In this way, too many state variables and differential equations are involved; thus, it is very difficult to get a kinetic model of receptors for complex computation and whole cell simulation from the perspective of detailed physiology. There has been detailed modeling for postsynaptic responses via Markov models with six state variables to describe the open fraction of receptors [41]; however, Destexhe et al. [36] found that a three-state Markov model is enough to grasp the main features of the open kinetics via comparisons between computational results and experimental data, and the dependence of transition rates on transmitter concentrations can be simplified into a piecewise pulse function; therefore this chapter describes the open kinetics of receptors with three-state models.

1.2.5.3.1   Non-NMDA Receptors

The three-state Markov model for non-NMDA receptors is shown in Figure 1.18, where C, O, and D characterize the open, closed, and desensitization states, respectively, and the transition rates are denoted by r_i ($i = 1, 2, 3, 5$), in which r_1 is the function of transmitter concentration $[T]$. We assume that $[T]$ is a pulse function with the pulse width of 1 ms. When an AP train occurs at the presynaptic membrane, if the membrane potential exceeds 0 mV at the rising phase of AP, $[T] = 1$ mM, and it returns to zero after 1 ms [18]. Thus, r_1 is a piecewise function with each segment constant, and the advantage is that the analytical solutions of the time-varying open fraction of receptors can be obtained.

The presynaptic AP train can be generated by the dynamical system model illustrated in Eq. (1.3). Let the dimensionless time 0.004 correspond to 1 ms; then we can calibrate that the dimensionless injection current needed for producing an AP train of 20 Hz is $z = 12$, and the real stimulus is ~0.1 nA according to experimental data [41]. So the relation between the dimensionless time t_{dim} and the physical time t_{real} in the unit of s is

$$k_t \cdot t_{dim} = t_{real}, \tag{1.15}$$

where $k_t = 0.25$. The relation between the dimensionless current I_{dim} and the real current I_{real} in the unit of nA can be listed as

$$k_I \cdot I_{dim} = I_{real}, \tag{1.16}$$

where $k_I = 8.33 \times 10^{-3}$. When $[T] = 1$ mM, the solution of the Markov model in Figure 1.18 can be written as

$$\begin{cases} O(t-t_0) = O_\infty + K_{1h} \exp\left[-(t-t_0)/\tau_1\right] + K_{2h} \exp\left[-(t-t_0)/\tau_2\right] \\ D(t-t_0) = D_\infty + K_{3h} \exp\left[-(t-t_0)/\tau_1\right] + K_{4h} \exp\left[-(t-t_0)/\tau_2\right] \end{cases}, \tag{1.17}$$

where O denotes the open fraction and D is the desensitization fraction. The time when $[T]$ changes is denoted by t_0, and the parameters involved are as follows:

$$O_\infty = \frac{-\delta r_1}{\alpha\delta - \beta\gamma}$$

$$K_{1h} = \frac{\left(O_0 - O_\infty\right)\left(\alpha + \tau_2^{-1}\right) + \beta\left(D_0 - D_\infty\right)}{\tau_2^{-1} - \tau_1^{-1}}$$

$$K_{2h} = \left(O_0 - O_\infty\right) - K_{1h}$$

$$z_\infty = \frac{\gamma r_1}{\alpha\delta - \beta\gamma}$$

$$K_{3h} = K_{1h}\frac{-\alpha - \tau_1^{-1}}{\beta}$$

$$K_{4h} = K_{2h}\frac{-\alpha - \tau_2^{-1}}{\beta}$$

$$\tau_{1,2}^{-1} = -\frac{\alpha+\delta}{2} \pm \frac{1}{2}\sqrt{(a-\delta)^2 + 4\beta\gamma}$$

where O_0 and D_0 are the initial values of the open fraction and desensitization fraction and we have $\alpha = -r_1 - r_2 - r_3$, $\beta = -r_1$, $\gamma = r_3$, and $\delta = -r_5$. When $[T] = 0$, the solution is

$$\begin{cases} O(t-t_0) = K_{1l}\exp\left[-(t-t_0)/\tau_3\right] \\ D(t-t_0) = K_{2l}\exp\left[-(t-t_0)/\tau_3\right] + K_{3l}\exp\left[-(t-t_0)/\tau_4\right] \end{cases}, \tag{1.18}$$

$$K_{1l} = O_0$$

$$K_{2l} = \frac{\gamma K_{1l}}{-\delta - \tau_3^{-1}}$$

$$K_{3l} = D_0 - K_{2l} .$$

$$\tau_3^{-1} = \beta - \alpha$$

$$\tau_4^{-1} = -\delta$$

By adjusting the transition rates between states in the model, it can be applied to the descriptions of the open kinetics of different non-NMDA receptors.

1.2.5.3.2 NMDA Receptors

The activation properties of NMDA receptors are distinct from that of non-NMDA ones, because their open and desensitization rates are both slower. The corresponding Markov model is shown in Figure 1.19, from which we see that for NMDA receptors, the open state can only turn into the closed state instead of the desensitization state, which, on the contrary, can be transferred into both the open and closed states. The transition rates are still r_i ($i = 2, 4, 5, 6$), in which r_6 depends on $[T]$, which is

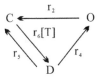

FIGURE 1.19 The Markov model of NMDA receptors.

the same pulse function defined above. When $[T] = 1\,\text{mM}$, the form of the solution of the Markov model in Figure 1.19 is the same as that presented in Eq. (1.17), except that O_∞ and D_∞ become

$$O_\infty = \frac{\beta r_6}{\alpha\delta - \beta\gamma},$$

$$z_\infty = \frac{-\alpha r_6}{\alpha\delta - \beta\gamma},$$

where $\alpha = -r_2$, $\beta = r_4$, $\gamma = -r_6$, and $\delta = -r_4 - r_5 - r_6$. When $[T] = 0$, the solution becomes

$$\begin{cases} O(t - t_0) = K_{1l}\exp\left[-(t - t_0)/\tau_3\right] + K_{2l}\exp\left[-(t - t_0)/\tau_4\right] \\ D(t - t_0) = K_{3l}\exp\left[-(t - t_0)/\tau_3\right] \end{cases}, \tag{1.19}$$

$$K_{1l} = \frac{\beta K_{3l}}{-\delta - \tau_3^{-1}}$$

$$K_{2l} = O_0 - K_{1l}$$

$$K_{3l} = D_0 \qquad .$$

$$\tau_3^{-1} = \gamma - \delta$$

$$\tau_4^{-1} = -\alpha$$

1.2.5.4 The Model for Postsynaptic Responses

The open kinetics of non-NMDA and NMDA receptors directly influence the postsynaptic responses, i.e., the excitatory postsynaptic current (EPSC) and the excitatory postsynaptic potential (EPSP). For the postsynaptic neuron, EPSC is equivalent to the injection current z in Eq. (1.3), and EPSP corresponds to x. With a certain total conductance of postsynaptic receptors, the instantaneous value of EPSC is decided by the present EPSP based on the Ohm's law. However, according to Eq. (1.3), EPSP is also dynamically influenced by EPSC, so these two quantities need to be iterated in a coupled way during computation. On the other hand, based on the superposition principle of currents, EPSC is composed of the currents of non-NMDA and NMDA receptors, and remarkable differences exist in their magnitudes and modulation factors.

1.2.5.4.1 EPSC

i. **The current of non-NMDA receptors**: At physiological conditions, the behavior of non-NMDA receptors can only be modulated by transmitter concentration; thereby the EPSC can be calculated as

$$I_n = \bar{g}_n \cdot O_n \cdot (E - E_{rev}), \tag{1.20}$$

where I_n is the non-NMDA current, and $\bar{g}_n$ is the maximum conductance of receptors. From the physiological data [6], the single-channel conductance of non-NMDA receptors is far

TABLE 1.3

The Transition Rates in the Markov Models of Non-NMDA and NMDA Receptors

Receptor type	r_1 (s⁻¹ (mmol/L)⁻¹)	r_2 (s⁻¹)	r_3 (s⁻¹)	r_4 (s⁻¹)	r_5 (s⁻¹)	r_6 (s⁻¹ (mmol/L)⁻¹)
Non-NMDA	1,000	10	50	/	2	/
NMDA	/	6.9	/	160	4.7	190

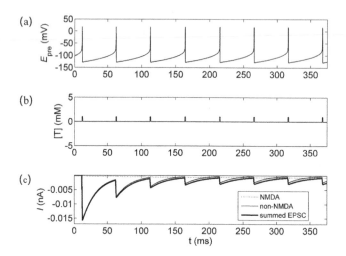

FIGURE 1.20 (a) Presynaptic AP train; (b) transmitter concentration [T]; (c) the summed EPSC, NMDA, and non-NMDA currents.

less than 20 pS, while the maximum postsynaptic conductance is about $\bar{g}_n = 0.4\,\text{nS}$. The open fraction is represented by O_n, E is the postsynaptic potential, and the reversal potential (equilibrium potential) is denoted by E_{rev}. For glutamate ionotropic receptors, $E_{rev} = 0$.

Non-NMDA current is dominant in EPSC [42], especially at the initial increasing stage of the current. However, non-NMDA receptors desensitize rapidly; thus their currents decay very fast under the repetitive stimulations of the AP train. In order to match the non-NMDA current generated by the model with experimental results, the transition rates of the model shown in Figure 1.18 are chosen as listed in Table 1.3. Assume that the frequency of the presynaptic AP train is 20 Hz; then its waveform can be calculated with Eq. (1.3) (Figure 1.20a), and the pulse train of [T] generated by the model is shown in Figure 1.20b. The response of non-NMDA current can be further obtained with Eq. (1.17) and (1.18) (Figure 1.20c, thin solid line). It should be noted that the excitatory current (inward current) is defined negative. Figure 1.20c shows that the amplitudes of the current as well as the open fraction are higher under the stimulations of the first 2–3 pulses, while they decay rapidly and approach the steady state. This result is consistent with the relevant voltage-clamp experiments on postsynaptic membrane [36].

ii. **The current of NMDA receptors**: The modulation process of NMDA receptors is much more complicated than that of non-NMDA receptors, for the reason that their open process is affected by three factors: the transmitter concentration, postsynaptic potential, and extracellular [Mg^{2+}]. When the membrane is at the vicinity of the resting potential, the pores of the ion channels of NMDA receptors are occupied by Mg^{2+} [6]; consequently, even if the receptors are bound with neurotransmitter, the channels remain closed. These channels can be opened only if the depolarization of the postsynaptic membrane occurs and

Mg^{2+} leaves the pores under the effect of electromotive force across the membrane. Thus, when calculating NMDA current, a function related to membrane potential and extracellular $[Mg^{2+}]$ needs to be introduced [43]:

$$G = \frac{1}{1 + ([Mg]_o/3.57)\exp(-0.062E)}, \tag{1.21}$$

where $[Mg]_o$ denotes the extracellular $[Mg^{2+}]$, which can be regarded as constant at physiological state: $[Mg]_o = 1$ mM. E is the membrane potential in mV, so the NMDA current I_N can be written as

$$-I_N = \bar{g}_N \cdot G \cdot O_N \cdot (E - E_{rev}), \tag{1.22}$$

where the meaning of E stays the same and the reversal potential $E_{rev} = 0$. The maximum conductance of NMDA receptors is denoted by $\bar{g}_N$, and the single-channel conductance is ~50 pS [28]. Compared with non-NMDA receptors, the conductivity of NMDA receptors is larger, because they allow Ca^{2+} to pass beside Na^+ and K^+. However, experiments show that the contribution of NMDA current to EPSC is very small [24], and it only takes effect during the late components of EPSC for rapid signaling. Therefore, the number of NMDA receptors on the postsynaptic membrane is much smaller than that of non-NMDA ones. By setting their density ratio per unit area to be 1:100, we have $\bar{g}_N = 0.5$ nS. In the CNS, the main function of NMDA receptors is to generate long-term potentiation (LTP) effect [44], while for Ia afferents of muscle spindles, our purpose is to investigate the fast dynamic responses; i.e., the LTP effect will not be considered in this chapter.

The transition rates involved in the model of NMDA receptors are also listed in Table 1.3. The presynaptic stimulus is the same as previously described, and the NMDA current can be computed with Eqs. (1.17) and (1.19), as shown in Figure 1.20c (dashed line). The total EPSC is formed by the summation of the non-NMDA and NMDA currents (Figure 1.20c, bold solid line), from which we see that EPSC faithfully reserves the frequency information of presynaptic AP. By comparing the total current with the NMDA current, it is easy to find that at the rising stage of the current, NMDA current imposes little effect, while at the falling phase, it contributes to the tail current of EPSC. Moreover, after repetitive stimulations, NMDA current gradually becomes remarkable and stable, consistent with experimental phenomena [42].

1.2.5.4.2 EPSP

EPSP refers to the depolarization responses of dendrites or the soma under the effect of EPSC. As mentioned above, due to the active properties of dendrites, EPSP can differ a lot from that in passive conditions where EPSP rapidly attenuates with the increasing distance from the synapse, while for active dendrites, the amplitude of EPSP can be kept constant or even be amplified [6] during its propagation. The dynamical system model can conveniently simulate the active features of the membrane, so if we take EPSC as the injection current z, the model represented by Eq. (1.3) can still be applied to the calculation of EPSP. For the fact that a single excitatory synapse can only depolarize the postsynaptic membrane by less than 1 mV, compared with the axon, the Na/K channel densities of the postsynaptic membrane are 40 folds lower [39]; as a result, the parameter b needs to be readjusted so as to reflect the actual physiological characteristics of the membrane, and we take $b = 30/40 = 0.75$. On the other hand, Figure 1.20c shows that after repetitive stimulations by the presynaptic AP train, EPSC becomes stable, and this is equivalent to a constant average injection current I_i. As discussed previously, Eq. (1.3) represents the response of a closed membrane domain to the injection current; therefore at the steady state, the variation of the charge inside postsynaptic membrane can be denoted as

$$\bar{Q} = I_i t + Q_0, \tag{1.23}$$

where Q_0 is the initial charge. The instantaneous membrane potential is proportional to the difference of the positive charge densities across the membrane [25], so the mean postsynaptic potential $\bar{U}$ can be expressed as

$$\bar{U} = k_c(\bar{Q}/V - \rho_0) = \left(k_c/V\right)I_i t + C_0,   \tag{1.24}$$

where k_c is a constant ratio, V is the effective volume of the closed membrane domain, and the extracellular charge density is denoted by ρ_0, which can be assumed constant. C_0 is also a constant, and $C_0 = (k_c/V)Q_0 - k_c\rho_0$. Equation (1.24) shows that when EPSC reaches the steady state, EPSP will linearly grow with time due to charge accumulation. However, under actual physiological conditions, the charge injected into the postsynaptic membrane will diffuse to farther regions, and when the steady state is achieved, there should be no net current in the finite volume of postsynaptic region; i.e., the equilibrium between the injected current and diffusing current is reached. Thus, when computing EPSP, the steady-state mean current I_i needs to be removed so as to match with the real situation. The variation of EPSP can be obtained by substituting the resultant EPSC into Eq. (1.3), as shown in Figure 1.21. Figure 1.21a and b separately shows the comparisons between the computed EPSP and experimental results [45] under the presynaptic stimulus of 5 and 40 Hz. It should be noted that the experimental EPSP in Figure 1.21 was measured at the soma and the amplitude attained several millivolts, which implied that EPSP was amplified during its propagation from dendrites to the soma [45]. In order to better verify the model, we magnify the theoretical EPSP by the same extent, and it is clear that the dynamic features presented by the simulation results are consistent with that of actual cases. Furthermore, experimental researches have revealed that the decay rate of EPSP under high-frequency stimulus is larger than that stimulated by lower frequency [45], and by comparing the results of 5 and 40 Hz, we see that our model faithfully represented such dynamical features as well.

On the other hand, relevant researches show that the steady-state amplitudes of EPSP (like the last two EPSP spikes in Figure 1.21a) depend on the frequency of presynaptic stimulus, i.e., the higher the frequency, the lower the steady state amplitude, which decays exponentially as the general trend, and this effect is called the redistribution of synaptic efficacy [45]. For the model in this chapter, if we investigate the EPSP under different stimulus frequencies and denote the steady-state EPSP as $\mathrm{EPSP_{st}}$, the relation between the frequency f and the $\mathrm{EPSP_{st}}$ can be obtained as shown in Figure 1.22a, in which the data can indeed be expressed by an exponential function and the trend

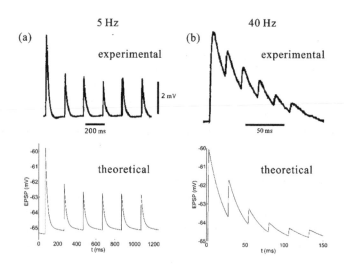

FIGURE 1.21   The comparisons between theoretical and experimental EPSP. (a) 5 Hz; (b) 40 Hz.

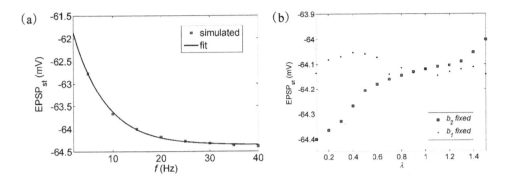

FIGURE 1.22 (a) The relation between $EPSP_{st}$ and f; (b) the relation between $EPSP_{st}$ and λ when b_1 and b_2 are respectively fixed at 0.75.

is the same as that of experimental results. Thus, the effectiveness of the model has been further verified, and the fit function for the curve in Figure 1.22a is

$$EPSP_{st} = c_1 \exp(-c_2 f) + c_3, \qquad (1.25)$$

where $c_1 = 3.376$, $c_2 = 0.152$, $c_3 = -64.36$. Figure 1.22b shows the variation trend of $EPSP_{st}$ with λ when b_1 and b_2 are respectively fixed at 0.75, under the presynaptic stimulus of 20 Hz. We see that $EPSP_{st}$ almost does not vary with λ when b_1 is fixed, while when b_2 is fixed, $EPSP_{st}$ approximately grows linearly with the increasing λ. As previously discussed, for the reason that b_1 mainly characterizes the density of Na^+ channel and b_2 represents the density of K^+ channel, under the stimulation of constant frequency, the amplitude of $EPSP_{st}$ is dominated by the value of b_1, while b_2 is mainly responsible for the kinetics of the decreasing phase of EPSP. In other words, different changing modes of λ will lead to distinct influences on $EPSP_{st}$, and this is consistent with the principles of depolarization response of the membrane.

Different from the traditional passive cable theory, this model does not simply treat the membrane as a coupled structure of capacitors and resistors; instead, based on the intrinsic properties of the dynamical system, the model calculates the dynamic responses of the potential of a membrane region under the effect of the stimulating current. Particularly, we identified the physical meaning of relevant parameters (b, λ), making it possible to independently adjust the physiological characteristics (the densities of Na/K/Ca channels) of a certain membrane domain with these parameters, which enabled the model to simulate the active electrophysiological features of nonuniform membrane. Although this paper only involved the simulation of the potential in a closed region, actually if we express the injection current (z) as a diffusion item, the spread of the current and the interactions of the potential among different membrane domains can be computed. Thereby, the modeling method we proposed can be easily applied in the finite element analysis of motoneurons, and the disadvantage of the electrical model which cannot reflect the detailed features of the membrane can be overcome. For postsynaptic responses, we employed the simplified Markov model, which covered the main features of EPSC, and at the same time avoided introducing too many differential equations and state variables, so that the computation cost can be greatly saved. When calculating EPSP, we combined the Markov model with the dynamical system model to make the model capable of simulating the active propagation property of the postsynaptic membrane. Thus, from the generation of presynaptic AP train to the response of EPSP, we need only to solve twice the first-order system of differential equations (Eq. (1.3)), and EPSC can be obtained directly from the analytical expressions (Eqs. (1.17)–(1.19)). The model can be applied to the real-time computation of synaptic responses; i.e., we can get the postsynaptic response under the presynaptic stimulus of dynamically varying frequency. Moreover, despite that the calculations in this chapter are transferred into dimensional form so as to compare with the experimental data, the final purpose is to extract essential mathematical rules of synaptic integration and information processing during actual complicated computations; therefore the model can be completely dimensionless so that the calculation efficiency and the simulation scale can be further enhanced.

REFERENCES

1. Hill A. The heat of shortening and the dynamic constants of muscle. *Proc. R. Soc. London Series B*, 1938, 126: 136–195.
2. Huxley A F. Muscular contraction. *J. Physiol.*, 1974, 243: 1–43.
3. MacIntosh B R, Gardiner P F, McComas A J. *Skeletal Muscle-Form and Function*, Yu Z, Li Q, Xu P, et al., eds. Xi'an: The Fourth Military Medical University Press, 2010.
4. Hodgkin A L, Huxley A F. A quantitative description of membrane current and its application to conduction and excitation in nerve. *J. Physiol.* (London), 1952, 117: 500–544.
5. Dayan P, Abbott L F. *Theoretical Neuroscience*. Cambridge, MA: MIT Press, 2001.
6. Hausser M, Spruston N, Stuart G J. Diversity and dynamics of dendritic signaling. *Science*, 2000, 290: 739–744.
7. Robinson R C. *An Introduction to Dynamical Systems: Continuous and Discrete*. Beijing: China Machine Press, 2005.
8. Fitzhugh R. Impulses and physiological states in theoretical models of nerve membrane. *Biophys. J.*, 1961, 1: 445–466.
9. Rogers J M, McCulloch A D. A collocation-galerkin finite element model of cardiac action potential propagation. *IEEE Trans. Biomed. Eng.*, 1994, 41: 743–757.
10. Hindmarsh J L, Rose R M. A model of the nerve impulse using two first-order differential equations. *Nature*, 1982, 296: 162–164.
11. Pu Q, Yun J, Temkin H, Liu S. Ion-enrichment and ion-depletion effect of nanochannel structures. *Nano Lett.*, 2004, 4: 1099–1103.
12. Qiao R, Aluru N R. Charge inversion and flow reversal in a nanochannel electro-osmotic flow. *Phys. Rev. Lett.*, 2004, 92: (198301) 1–4.
13. Sbragaglia M, Benzi R, Biferale L, Succi S, Toschi F. Surface roughness-hydrophobicity coupling in microchannel and nano channel flows. *Phys. Rev. Lett.*, 2006, 97: (204503) 1–4.
14. Qiao R, Aluru N R. Ion concentrations and velocity profiles in nanochannel electroosmotic flows. *J. Chem. Phys.*, 2003, 118: 4692–4701.
15. Fan X J, Phan-Thien N, Yong N T, Diao X. Molecular dynamics simulation of a liquid in a complex nano channel flow. *Phys. Fluids*, 2002, 14: 1146–1153.
16. Guy H R, Seetharamulu P. Molecule model of the action potential sodium channel. *Proc. Natl. Acad. Sci. USA.*, 1986, 83: 508–512.
17. Hamill O P, Marty A, Neher E, Sakmann B, Sigworth F J. Improved patch clamp techniques for high-resolution current recording from cells and cell-free membrane patches. *Pflugers Arch.*, 1981, 391: 85–100.
18. Levitan I B, Kaczmarek L K. *The Neuron Cell and Molecular Biology*. 2nd ed. New York: Oxford University Press, 1997.
19. Stern M D, Pizarro G, Rios E. Local control model of excitation-contraction coupling in skeletal muscle. *J. Gen. Physiol.*, 1997, 110(4): 415–440.
20. Baylor S M, Hollingworth S. Calcium indicators and calcium signalling in skeletal muscle fibres during excitation-contraction coupling. *Prog. Biophys. Mol. Biol.*, 2011, 105(3): 162–179.
21. Lymn R W, Taylor E W. Transient state phosphate production in the hydrolysis of nucleoside triphosphates by myosin. *Biochemistry*, 1970, 9(15): 2975–2983.
22. Yin Y, Guo Z. Collective mechanism of molecular motors and a dynamic mechanical model for sarcomere. *Sci. China: Technol. Sci.*, 2011, 54(8): 2130–2137.
23. Pecho-Vrieseling E, Sigrist M, Yoshida Y, et al. Specificity of sensory-motor connections encoded by sema3e-plexinD1 recognition. *Nature*, 2009, 459(7248): 842–846.
24. Yin Y, Guo Z, Chen X, Fan Y. Operation mechanism of molecular motor based biomechanical research progresses on skeletal muscle. *Chinese Sci. Bull.*, 2012, 30: 2794–2805 (in Chinese).
25. Yin Y, Chen X. Bioelectrochemical principle of variable frequency control on skeletal muscle contraction - Operation mechanism of molecular motor based biomechanical mechanism of skeletal muscle (II), *Sci. China: Technol. Sci.*, 2012, 42(8): 901–910 (in Chinese).

26. Kernell D. Principles of force gradation in skeletal muscles. *Neural Plast.*, 2003, 10: 69–76.
27. Magee J C. Dendritic integration of excitatory synaptic input. *Nature Rev. Neurosci.*, 2000, 1: 181–190.
28. Kandel E R, Siegelbaum S A. *Principles of Neural Science*. 4th ed. New York: McGraw-Hill/Appleton and Lange, 2000: 207–228.
29. Grillner S. The motor infrastructure: From ion channels to neuronal networks. *Nature Rev. Neurosci.*, 2003, 4: 573–586.
30. Capaday C, Stein R B. The effects of postsynaptic inhibition on the monosynaptic reflex of the cat at different levels of motoneuron pool activity. *Exp. Brain Res.*, 1989, 77: 577–584.
31. Wong A Y C, Graham B P, Billups B, et al. Distinguishing between presynaptic and postsynaptic mechanisms of short-term depression during action potential trains. *J. Neurosci.*, 2003, 23(12): 4868–4877.
32. Goldstein S, Rall W. Changes of action potential shape and velocity for changing core conductor geometry. *Biophys. J.*, 1974, 14: 731–757.
33. Hines M L, Carnevale N T. The neuron simulation environment. *Neural Comput.*, 1997, 9: 1179–1202.
34. Heckman C J, Lee R H, Brownstone R M. Hyperexcitable dendrites in motoneurons and their neuromodulatory control during motor behavior. *Trend. Neurosci.*, 2003, 26: 688–695.
35. Segev I, London M. Untangling dendrites with quantitative models. *Science*, 2000, 290: 744–750.
36. Destexhe A, Mainen Z F, Sejnowski T J. An efficient method for computing synaptic conductances based on a kinetic model of receptor binding. *Neural Comput.*, 1994, 6: 14–18.
37. Destexhe A, Mainen Z F. Synthesis of models for excitable membranes, synaptic transmission and neuromodulation using a common kinetic formalism. *J. Comput. Neurosci.*, 1994, 1: 195–230.
38. Lin R C, Scheller R H. Mechanisms of synaptic vesicle exocytosis. *Ann. Rev. Cell Biol.*, 2000, 16: 19–49.
39. Kole M H P, Stuart G J. Signal processing in the axon initial segment. *Neuron*, 2012, 73: 235–247.
40. Colquhoun D, Hawkes A G. On the stochastic properties of single ion channels. *Proc. R. Soc. London Series B*, 1981, 211: 205–235.
41. Standley C, Ramsey R L, Usherwood P N R. Gating kinetics of the quisqualate-sensitive glutamate receptor of locust muscle studied using agonist concentration jumps and computer simulations. *Biophys. J.*, 1993, 65: 1379–1386.
42. Pennartz C M A, Boeijinga P H, Lopes da Silva F H. Contribution of NMDA receptors to postsynaptic potentials and paired-pulse facilitation in identified neurons of the rat nucleus accumbens in vitro. *Exp. Brain Res.*, 1991, 86: 190–198.
43. Jahr C E, Stevens C F. Voltage dependence of NMDA-activated macroscopic conductances predicted by single-channel kinetics. *J. Neurosci.*, 1990, 10(9): 3178–3182.
44. O'Connor J J, Rowan M J, Anwyl R. Tetanically induced LTP involves a similar increase in the AMPA and NMDA receptor components of the excitatory postsynaptic current: Investigations of the involvement of mGlu receptors. *J. Neurosci.*, 1995, 15(3): 2013–2020.
45. Markram H, Tsodyks M. Redistribution of synaptic efficacy between neocortical pyramidal neurons. *Nature*, 1996, 382: 807–810.

2 Biomechanical Modeling of Muscular Contraction

Biomechanical models of skeletal muscle are closely related to the research of muscle's contractile mechanism, and their core significance lies in explaining the dynamic contractile characteristics and phenomena of skeletal muscle, including describing the input–output relations among stimulus intensity, load, contractile force, velocity, and muscle length, as well as predicting muscle force and the corresponding contractile status. Therefore, biomechanical models are applied widely in the biomechanical modeling of human kinetics and hold important merits in biomedical engineering (diagnosis, rehabilitation, etc.) related to musculoskeletal system.

The studies on biomechanical models of skeletal muscle have been developed for many years. The earliest widely accepted model originated from Hill's pioneering work [1] in 1938, and the resulting model was named as Hill-type model by the following researchers. Hill-type model was derived from the contraction heat experiments. It clarifies that the contraction energy is composed of contraction heat and mechanical work and provides the Hill's equation describing the force–velocity relationship based on the linear influence of load on muscle's total power. Further, Hill proposed a three-element model indicating that muscle can be characterized by a contractile element, a series element, and a parallel elastic element. Hill's work laid a solid foundation for the biomechanical research on skeletal muscle. Later, many scholars have made improvements and modifications. For instance, Zajac et al. [2] added the factor of the angle between the directions of muscle fibers and tendon to Hill's model. Due to the simplicity, these models are still being used in biomechanical and medical fields. However, Hill-type model only describes the quasi-static features of muscle because it is deduced from the macroscopic experimental phenomena. Moreover, Hill's model only contains elastic elements and neglects the damping of muscle; thus, it is unable to make precise estimation or prediction of dynamic muscle force. Limited by the unclear understanding of the microscopic structure of muscle at Hill's time, Hill-type model is inevitably oversimplified, leading to a moderate overall precision.

By 1954, H. E. Huxley et al. [3] observed the structure of sarcomere and thick/thin filaments for the first time, and proposed the sliding-filament theory of muscular contraction based on the bright and dark band feature of muscle fibers. At the meantime, the key morphology of myosin was also unveiled. In 1957, A. F. Huxley proposed the famous cross-bridge model on *Nature* and made clear for the first time that the sliding between thin and thick filaments is due to the attaching and working of myosin motors, so the actomyosin structure is referred to as "cross-bridge". From then on, the models based on cross-bridge assumption have been called as Huxley-type model. Further, Huxley identified the viscoelastic element in muscle via step stretch and release experiments on tetanized muscle fibers and declared the existence of damping. From the perspective of free energy, he proposed that at least two states take part in the working of molecular motors and estimated that a cross-bridge can produce a distance of 8–10 nm during one stroke. The assumption of cross-bridge also explains well the force–length relationship of skeletal muscle [4]. Huxley-type model provides a deeper understanding for muscular contraction via explaining the microscopic working mechanism of molecular motors. It attributes most of the sarcomere stiffness to cross-bridge, and the thick filament is regarded as purely rigid during stretch, while other stiffness comes from the connective tissue like titin. Based on the cross-bridge model, more sophisticated models have sprung up. The lever-arm model proposed by Spudich [5] identifies that molecular motor pulls the thin filament by rotating its neck region (conformational change) and specifies the utilization phases of the energy released by ATP hydrolysis. Piazzesi et al. [6] provided a more detailed explanation towards

Huxley's step stretch and release experiments using a five-state model. Compared with Hill-type model, Huxley-type model has introduced the viscous and damping effect of muscle, thus being able to describe the dynamic force response of the sarcomere under various speeds, so it is no more a quasi-static model. However, Huxley-type model is based on the microscopic working mechanism of molecular motor, while actually there are remarkable differences between the working features of molecular motor and those of sarcomere or whole muscle; e.g., Hill's equation is hyperbolic, but the force–velocity of a single motor is linear. In addition, Huxley-type model does not account for the passive characteristics of muscle. For these issues, statistical model has provided the possible solutions, while the question of how to transit statistical model and Huxley-type model correctly to the macroscopic scale is still not answered satisfactorily.

The biomechanical models developed in recent years are mostly derived from Hill-type model or Huxley-type model. In order to describe the mechanical features of muscle globally, finite element method (FEM) has been used widely in the modeling of skeletal muscle [7]. Finite element models usually treat muscle as a special type of active material, and the three-dimensional meshing is relatively random. For each element, the tensor description form in material mechanics is used, and the difference is that the nonlinear activation, elastic, and damping characteristics are all introduced into the model. Finite element model is able to describe the mechanical responses of a whole muscle, including the local mechanical states at different times and positions, while such kind of models are complex and not based on the fundamental contractile mechanism of skeletal muscle. Therefore, finite element model is only an empirical engineering model hard to be compatible with the microscopic contractile dynamics of muscle; i.e., it also fails to achieve the truly unified description of microscopic and macroscopic scales.

Referring to the contractile mechanism and the emphases of current models, a truly dynamic and uniform biomechanical model should be able to elucidate the following problems or links, as shown in Figure 2.1:

- The activation kinetics (Act) of sarcomere, i.e., the dynamic transfer relation from the stimulus intensity (firing rate, f) of action potential (AP) to the activation degree ($[Ca^{2+}]$, β) of sarcomere;
- The working kinetics of the active element (AE, molecular motor) and the dynamic dependence of the non-Newton damping of the passive element (PE) on the velocity v (red);
- The dynamic dependence of AE's kinetics and PE's nonlinear stiffness on the sarcomere length L (blue);
- The dynamic properties of the system formed by the serial and parallel combination of massive sarcomeres.

As a matter of fact, when considering the most basic sense and goal of a biomechanical model of skeletal muscle, on one hand it should be consistent with (or at least can reproduce) the fundamental contractile mechanism, and on the other hand it should hold sufficient engineering value to provide effective theoretical guidance for the diagnosis, rehabilitation, and bionics of muscle. Currently, the development of traditional biomechanical models has reached a bottleneck, and the real-time application research of the model is nearly absent, while a biomechanical model capable of unifying reasonably the above links has not been reported yet.

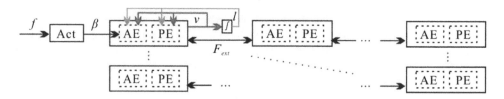

FIGURE 2.1   The key links a biomechanical model of skeletal muscle should account for.

This chapter is composed of three parts. The first part introduces the modeling research of the driving and control of muscular contraction and discusses in detail the bioelectrochemical variable-frequency control mechanism of sarcomere contraction proposed by the authors. The second part is dedicated to the force-producing model of muscle, from the classical models to the working cycle of a single myosin motor. This part includes (1) the coupling mechanism of multi-force interaction mechanism of a single motor approaching the actin filament via studying van der Waals (vdW) force, Casimir force, electrostatic force, and Brownian force; (2) the dynamical model of sarcomere established via the analysis of collective mechanical features of myosin motors using statistical mechanics; (3) the macroscopic model based on the serial and parallel structures of sarcomeres established via combining the activation and contraction processes of muscle. Finally, detailed discussions are dedicated to the engineering phenomenological models and the novel semiphenom-enological model proposed by the authors.

2.1   MODELING OF DRIVING AND CONTROL PROCESSES

The driving mechanism of skeletal muscle explains how motor neurons excite muscle fibers and ignite the working cycles of the myosin motors in a sarcomere and regulate the contraction of muscle fibers. This is a typical bioelectrochemical process. When the AP of motor neuron arrives at the neuromuscular junction, it will be "copied" onto the sarcolemma. This indicates that the APs produced by the sarcolemma and motor neurons reflect the motion intention of human and contain the control information of muscular contraction. As is mentioned earlier, the prerequisite for myosin motors to start their power stroke is the combination of Ca^{2+} and the troponin (Tn) on the thin filament. Under the normal operation condition, [ATP] in the cytoplasm is nearly saturated, so $[Ca^{2+}]$ would determine whether the myosin motors are working or not; i.e., the activities of Ca^{2+} contain the driving information of myosin motors.

Figure 2.2a shows the detailed excitation–contraction coupling (ECC) process [8]. The Ca^{2+} in the cytoplasm is recycled by the Ca-ATPase on sarcoplasmic reticulum (SR) [9], making the $[Ca^{2+}]$ always in a homeostasis in a sarcomere. During the normal working of muscle fibers, the channels and Ca-ATPase on SR dominate the cytoplasmic $[Ca^{2+}]$. Since the track number of working molecular motors characterizes the activation degree as well as the power of muscle fibers, which is featured by the cytoplasmic $[Ca^{2+}]$, the key problem would be the quantitative modeling of the ECC mechanism for the research of the driving process of muscle. Yin et al. [10] found the physical coupling of the calcium channels on SR; i.e., the depolarization and repolarization of the membrane can make the channels open or close massively and rapidly, justifying that the control source of $[Ca^{2+}]$ is AP. Stern et al. [11] conducted physical modeling toward the ECC in sarcomere based on the physiological structure of the sarcolemma. Cannell et al. [12] made simulations about the Ca^{2+}

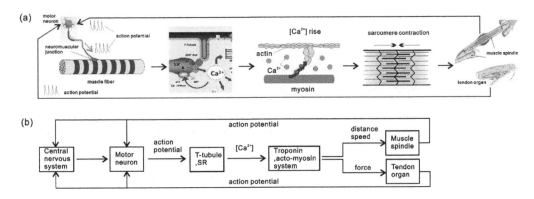

FIGURE 2.2   (a) The biological process of muscular contraction; (b) the cybernetic process of muscular contraction.

movements in the sarcomeres of frog, while the model neglects the detailed physiological features of sarcolemma. Stuyvers et al. [13] investigated the static relationship between the firing rate of AP and [Ca^{2+}].

At present, the studies on the driving properties of sarcomere are mostly focused on the static features of cytoplasmic [Ca^{2+}] or the static relationship between firing rate and [Ca^{2+}], while the problems of how [Ca^{2+}] spreads and changes dynamically and how AP dynamically regulates [Ca^{2+}] are seldom involved. Furthermore, experiments have shown that the firing rate of AP on sarcolemma is positively correlated to the isometric force of muscle [14], indicating that a similar relation exists between the firing rate and sarcomere [Ca^{2+}]. In other words, the cytoplasmic [Ca^{2+}] is regulated and controlled by the firing rate of AP. Moreover, the precision of the open-loop system is not high when neglecting the feedback effect of the proprioceptors, making it hard to represent the true motion intention of human. Thus, it is necessary to further investigate the closed-loop control mechanism of skeletal muscle.

From the perspective of cybernetics, muscular contraction is a typical closed-loop control process. Nervous signal generated by the central nervous system (CNS) passes down through corticospinal tracts in the form of AP and then ignites new APs in motor neurons to control muscular contraction, as shown in Figure 2.2b. Consequently, AP can be considered as the information carrier of human's motion intention, and the control information of molecular motors is contained in the APs released by motor neuron. As the hardware foundation for detecting the contraction states of muscle, proprioceptors provide CNS with motor information and realize the coordinated control via perceiving the contraction speed, force, and length of the muscle. The proprioception is fed back to the CNS or motor neuron in the form of AP as well. The proprioceptors of muscle mainly include muscle spindle and tendon organ, acting as the position/speed and force sensors, respectively.

It can be seen that biological neural network is the information feedback pathway of motor information as well as the central control unit [15], wherein the basic unit is motor neuron. Therefore, it becomes very important to investigate how a motor neuron accepts the synaptic feedback input, processes the information, and regulates the output. Relevant studies have shown that the distribution density and geometric form of ion channels influence largely the amplitude, conduction speed, and frequency of AP, and these quantities are usually coupled together. In addition, due to the "all-or-none" property of AP's firing, the frequency of AP is pivotal to the control information of molecular motors. Thus, one needs to identify what factors/physical quantities would impact frequency and to explore the feedback and integration mechanism of AP's frequency information, because it is closely related to the problem of how the APs fed back by the muscle spindle/tendon organ are modulated by motor neuron to stabilize the system and how the dynamic control of muscular contraction is finally realized. On the other hand, our current understanding about how biological neural network implements adaptive self-learning according to the proprioception feedback is far from sufficient, resulting in the big difficulty in constructing an adaptive motion controller by mimicking biological neural networks. However, this would be one of the focuses of future research on the control mechanism of skeletal muscle.

2.1.1 BIOELECTROCHEMICAL CONTROL MODEL WITH VARIABLE-FREQUENCY REGULATION FOR SARCOMERE CONTRACTION

As mentioned above, the understanding of macroscopic and microscopic mechanisms of muscle contraction has become clearer, and physical explanation has also been provided toward how the control-signal–like APs transform into drive signal [16]. While there have been plenty of studies revealing the relationship between [Ca^{2+}] and tension or stimulation rate of AP and tension, the correlation between wave characteristics of AP and [Ca^{2+}] variation remains unclear; i.e., the understanding of the control principium of how the control signal modulates the drive signal is still not complete. Due to the above problem, there are difficulties in the description of harmonic work of massive muscle fibers, as well as how motion intention is realized. Therefore, elucidating this regulation mechanism is closely related to the unification of the microscopic and macroscopic skeletal muscle dynamics. Most studies on the relation between AP frequency and sarcomere tension were based on experiments, including studies on mammalian cardiac muscle fibers [13]. These works did not extract refined theoretical model or focus on control theory; as a result, there was no strong correlation between the above studies and motion control of muscle. To solve these problems, one needs to build a complete bioelectrochemical model describing AP, the release of Ca^{2+}, and the diffusion of $[Ca^{2+}]$, based on the physiological structures of skeletal muscle fibers, and to further discuss the mode and features of the control signal regulating the drive signal so as to indirectly provide the description of how APs control muscle tension.

2.1.1.1 Modeling of Action Potentials on Sarcolemma

The resting potential of sarcolemma is $\sim-85\,mV$, and the threshold for Na^+ channel to open is $14\,mV$ higher than that. The peak value of AP is $\sim39\,mV$ [16], and its conduction speed along muscle fibers is $\sim4\,m/s$, while the radial speed from the surface of a muscle fiber to its center is about several centimeters per second [17]. Consequently, the excitations of sarcomeres in different myofibrils are not synchronized, and in order to obtain the drive properties of a single sarcomere, we take the myofibril closest to sarcolemma as the modeling object. The purpose of the model is to get the mathematical description of the AP shape on sarcolemma and facilitate the investigation of its influence on $[Ca^{2+}]$, as the duration of single AP directly affects the open interval of Ca^{2+} channels on SR. Na^+ currents coming into the membrane and K^+ currents going out of it form the physical basis of sarcolemma electric activities, which are governed by the opening and closing of Na^+ channels and K^+ channels, while the instantaneous potential of sarcolemma is decided by the charge density (concentrations of different types of ions) inside and outside of it. It should be noted that voltage sensitive Na^+ channels distribute on sarcolemma while most voltage-sensitive K^+ channels are located at T-tubules. According to such distribution features of channels, we can flatten the sarcolemma and the cylindrical muscle fiber, and select the cytoplasm between neighboring T-tubules (also between sarcolemma and SR) as the modeling region, as shown in Figure 2.3. With general sense, we take the central point of this region as the ion concentration reference point inside the membrane (ion concentrations outside are approximately constant); i.e., the membrane potentials on sarcolemma can be characterized by the potentials at the central points between successive T-tubules. Once APs arrive at these points, the membrane potential will immediately jump to the peak value, while its rate of decrease is decided by the speed of K^+ diffusing out of the membrane, and this is related to the K^+ channel density on T-tubules, i.e., the higher the density, the faster the diffusion. During the analysis, we use the area ratio of total K^+ channel opening to the wall of

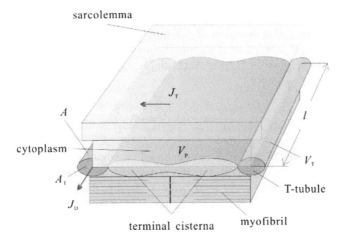

FIGURE 2.3 $[K^+]$ calculation model of the cytoplasm near sarcolemma.

T-tubule per unit area to represent the K^+ channel density and denote it as η_K. The K^+ channels on T-tubules will rapidly open when they feel potential rise. During the flowing out of K^+, they will firstly fill into T-tubules and then diffuse to extracellular regions through the T-tubule openings on sarcolemma; i.e., the rate of decrease of $[K^+]$ in cytoplasm is determined by the diffusion speed of K^+ at the openings. We set $[K^+]$ as n_K and the K^+ current from cytoplasm to T-tubule as J_T; thus from diffusion dynamics, we know that J_T can be described by the concentration gradient at the T-tubule wall:

$$J_T = -D_K \frac{\partial n_K}{\partial r}, \tag{2.1}$$

where D_K is the diffusion coefficient of K^+ and $D_K = \mu k_B T$, where μ is the drift speed of the considered particle and $\mu = \tau/m_k$, in which τ denotes the average time interval between successive particle collisions during Brownian motion. Under mammalian body temperature, the mean free path of a particle can be approximately regarded as of the order of Å; with the theorem of energy equipartition, we can get $\tau = {\sim}1.8 \times 10^{-13}$s. The mass of K^+ is denoted by m_k, and $m_k = {\sim}6.477 \times 10^{-26}$kg, while $k_B = 1.38 \times 10^{-23}$ J/K, being the Boltzmann constant. We take $T = 310.15$ K as the human body temperature. Finally, we get $D_K = {\sim}1.196 \times 10^{-8}$. The r in Eq. (2.1) represents the radial direction of a T-tubule, inside of which the change of $[K^+]$ with time can be written as

$$\frac{\partial n_K}{\partial t} = -J_T \frac{\eta_K A}{V_T}, \tag{2.2}$$

where A is the total area of the wall of a T-tubule, whose volume is V_T. With Eq. (2.2), $[K^+]$ becomes

$$n_K = \frac{\eta_K A}{V_T} |J_T| t + \text{Const.} \tag{2.3}$$

It can be seen from Eq. (2.3) that n_K is proportional to η_K at the same radial position of a T-tubule and the same time. On the other hand, the loss rate of K^+ in the cytoplasm is decided by the diffusion speed at T-tubule openings; it is still related to the $[K^+]$ gradient at the opening. Consequently, the higher the $[K^+]$ in a T-tubule, the larger the gradient at the opening; i.e., the $[K^+]$ gradient is also proportional to η_K. The diffusion flux of K^+ at the opening is

$$J_D = -D_K \frac{\partial n_K}{\partial x}\bigg|_{x=l_T}, \tag{2.4}$$

where x denotes the tangential direction of a T-tubule, whose perimeter is represented by l_T. It has been mentioned that T-tubules wrap around the myofibril, whose diameter is ${\sim}1$–$2\,\mu$m. When taking it as $1.5\,\mu$m, we get $l_T = {\sim}4.712\,\mu$m. Accordingly, the variation of $[K^+]$ in cytoplasm can be written as

$$\frac{\partial n_K}{\partial t} = -J_D \frac{A_T}{V_p} = -J_D \frac{1}{L}, \tag{2.5}$$

where A_T is the cross-sectional area of T-tubule, based on whose physiological geometric parameters the value of A_T is calculated [12]. For the reason that the area can be approximated by a rectangle of 125 nm by 25 nm, $A_T = {\sim}3.1 \times 10^{-3}\,\mu$m^2. V_p denotes the cytoplasm volume of the region shown in Figure 2.2. The distance between neighboring T-tubules is about half of the length of a sarcomere [2], so we take it as $1\,\mu$m, and due to the less than 3 nm layer between sarcolemma and SR, we can set it as 2.5 nm; thus, $V_p = {\sim}11.78 \times 10^{-3}\,\mu$m^3. $L = V_p/A_T$, which is an effective length, and it is easy to get $L = 3.78\,\mu$m. Based on the properties of diffusion dynamics and the proportional relation between concentration gradient and η_K mentioned above, we can assume that the gradient in Eq. (2.4) decreases with time exponentially, i.e.,

$$\left.\frac{\partial n_K}{\partial x}\right|_{x=l_T} = -\eta_K a_1 \exp(-b_1 t), \tag{2.6}$$

where both a_1 and b_1 are undetermined parameters, a_1 is constant, and $a_1 > 0$; meanwhile the coefficient of decrease $b_1 > 0$. Substituting Eq. (2.6) into Eq. (2.5) and integrating it, we get the expression of [K+] in cytoplasm as

$$n_K = \frac{D_K \eta_K a_1}{L b_1} \exp(-b_1 t) + \text{Const.} \tag{2.7}$$

The [K+] inside and outside the sarcolemma are 160 mmol/L and 4 mmol/L, respectively [18]; therefore when t approaches infinity in Eq. (2.7), n_K should be 4 mmol/L, from which we get Const. = 4 mmol/L. When $t = 0$, $D_K \eta_K a_1/(L b_1) = 156$, and because D_K, a_1, and L are all constants, the coefficient of decrease b_1 gains with η_K. Besides, when $t = 0$ and $\eta_K = 1$, the [K+] gradient should be at maximum, and if we denote it as S_0, we obtain $a_1 = |S_0| = 156/\lambda$, in which λ is the decay length (passing through this length, [K+] decreases to the value outside from that inside). On the other hand, because the value of membrane potential is decided by the potential difference between inside and outside the membrane, it can actually be regarded as proportional to the effective positive ion concentration difference

$$E_m = \eta_E \left(\Delta\left[Na^+\right] + \Delta\left[K^+\right] + E_r \right), \tag{2.8}$$

where E_m is membrane potential with the unit of mV and η_E is a proportion constant. With the calibration of the relation between the resting potential and [Na+], [K+] inside and outside the membrane, we get $\eta_E = \sim 1$. $\Delta[Na^+]$ and $\Delta[K^+]$ are [Na+] change and [K+] change inside the membrane, with the unit of mmol/L. For sarcolemma, the resting [Na+] inside is ~10 mmol/L [18], and it increases to 135 mmol/L when APs happen, so $\Delta[Na^+] = 125$ mmol/L while $\Delta[K^+] = n_K - 160$ mmol/L. E_r is the resting potential of the sarcolemma (−85 mV). During the simulation of the AP, we take $\lambda = 1$ μm; thus, the AP shapes when η_K changes from 0.1 to 0.5 can be obtained, as shown in Figure 2.4, from which we can see that the larger the channel density, the faster the AP decreases, and with η_K approaching

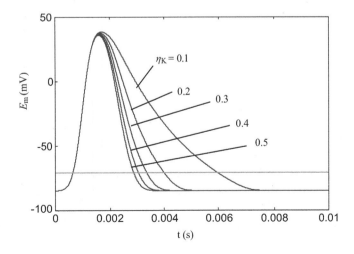

FIGURE 2.4 AP shapes under different K+-channel densities.

1, the AP shape converges. As mentioned previously, we know that the K⁺ channel density is very high on T-tubules, so η_K can be regarded as 0.5. If we assume that the open condition for Ca²⁺ channels on SR is that the membrane potential is higher than the threshold for APs to happen (−71 mV, the horizontal red line in Figure 2.4), it is apparent that the duration of Ca²⁺ channel opening is directly related to that of AP, due to the very slow deactivation of Ca²⁺ channels. For our situation where $\eta_K = 0.5$, this time interval is ~1.8 ms, and the shape of the AP can be fitted as

$$E_{AP} = \frac{t}{a_2}\exp(-t/b_2) + c_2, \tag{2.9}$$

where $a_2 = 1.569 \times 10^{-6}$, $b_2 = 5.016 \times 10^{-4}$, and $c_2 = -85$. Equation (2.9) describes the dynamical feature of a single AP at a certain point on sarcolemma.

2.1.1.2   [Ca²⁺] Variation Inside Sarcomeres Caused by AP

If we consider a single sarcomere, it is very small compared with the longitudinal and radial conduction speeds of APs; thus, the conduction time of them on T-tubules can be neglected, and it can be considered that almost all the Ca²⁺ channels on SR will open only if the membrane potential is higher than their open threshold. The [Ca²⁺] in sarcomeres at resting state is ~10⁻⁴ mmol/L, and it can be 100 times higher up to 10⁻² mmol/L, when stimulated [19]. The [Ca²⁺] on the surface of an excited sarcomere can be regarded as 10⁻² mmol/L for the reason that sarcomeres are tightly wrapped by SR. Moreover, sarcomere contraction is closely related to the [Ca²⁺] inside of it; thereby after the sudden rise of [Ca²⁺] at sarcomere surface, we have to further consider the time needed for this concentration to diffuse deeply into the sarcomere and get uniform. We denote this time as τ_c.

The chemical diffusion process of [Ca²⁺] can be modeled according to the geometric features of sarcomeres. Sarcomeres are cylindrical, and terminal cisterna is located between successive T-tubules. Considering that myofibril is composed of periodically patterned sarcomeres, only the part between the T-tubules of a sarcomere (half-sarcomere) needs to be investigated, as shown in Figure 2.5a. Ca²⁺ channels and Ca²⁺ pumps concentrate on the terminal cisterna [20], while SR distributes sparsely at the central region of a sarcomere; thus, we can take 1/3 of the cylinder at both ends in Figure 2.5a as the regions where Ca²⁺ comes in and out. Furthermore, actually we do not have to calculate the concentration change in the whole volume, due to the symmetric characteristics of the cylinder, the boundary condition, and initial condition at its wall. No current exists at the φ direction, so the calculation of concentration change can be

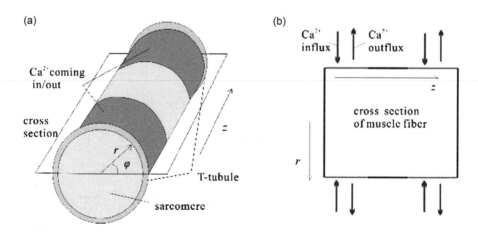

FIGURE 2.5   (a) The model of calculation region of [Ca²⁺]; (b) the cross section for calculating [Ca²⁺].

carried out with a cross section passing through the cylinder axis, as shown in Figure 2.5b. The diffusion equation of $[Ca^{2+}]$ is

$$\frac{\partial n_{Ca}}{\partial t} = \nabla^2 (D_{Ca} n_{Ca}), \tag{2.10}$$

where n_{Ca} denotes $[Ca^{2+}]$ and D_{Ca} is the diffusion coefficient, the calculation of which is similar to D_K, and $D_{Ca} = \sim 1.177 \times 10^{-8}$. The simulation results show that the $[Ca^{2+}]$ inside the sarcomere gets uniform after at least 0.6 ms, which implies that $\tau_c = 0.6$ ms, as shown in Figure 2.6a. Figure 2.6b shows the distribution of $[Ca^{2+}]$ in the sarcomere schematically, and the depth of the yellow color represents the corresponding $[Ca^{2+}]$ value. This implies that the delay time for $[Ca^{2+}]$ in a sarcomere to reach the peak value $(10^{-2}$ mmol/L) from the resting value is τ_c, which is also the time for a sarcomere to be completely stimulated. Besides, the lasting time of the peak value is related to the duration of APs, as has been discussed; this time is about 1.8 ms.

The efficiency of Ca^{2+} pumps should be identified when investigating the characters when $[Ca^{2+}]$ decreases. From physiological data, 20 Ca^{2+} can be delivered by a pump every second, and nearly 90% of the SR surface is occupied by Ca-ATP enzymes; thus, given the area of a single pump on SR and the total area of Ca^{2+} exchange region (Figure 2.5a), we can get the total Ca^{2+} current pumped back into SR as

$$I_{Ca} = \frac{0.9 A_c}{A_0} \times 20, \tag{2.11}$$

where A_c is the area of Ca^{2+} exchange, whose value is $\sim 3.1414 \times 10^{-12} m^2$ due to the geometric feature of sarcomere. A_0 is the area of a single pump, which can be approximated by a circle with the diameter of 4 nm [21], so $A_0 = 1.2567 \times 10^{-17} m^2$, and $I_{Ca} = 7.4744 \times 10^{-18}$ mol/s. At the end of APs, Ca^{2+} channels are closed, and the Ca^{2+} outflux produced by Ca^{2+} pumps will dominate; therefore, the $[Ca^{2+}]$ in a sarcomere can be described by the following continuity equation:

$$\frac{\partial n_{Ca}}{\partial t} = -\frac{I_{Ca}}{V_s}, \tag{2.12}$$

where V_s characterizes the volume of the cylinder in Figure 2.5a and $V_s = 1.7671 \times 10^{-18} m^3$. From Eq. (2.12) it can be seen that it costs ~ 2.3 ms for $[Ca^{2+}]$ to drop back to the resting value from the

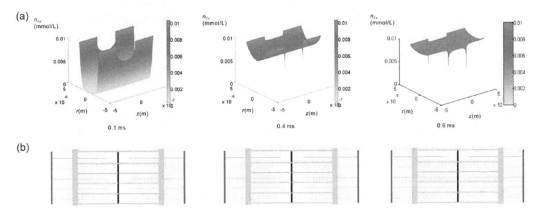

FIGURE 2.6   (a) The simulation of $[Ca^{2+}]$ diffusion process in a sarcomere; (b) scheme of the diffusion process.

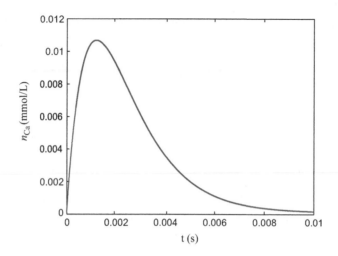

FIGURE 2.7 [Ca²⁺] variation process in a sarcomere during a single AP.

peak value. Based on the above discussion, the [Ca²⁺] variation process caused by a single AP can be obtained, as shown in Figure 2.7, and it can be fitted with the following function:

$$n_{Ca} = \frac{t}{a_3}\exp\left(-t/b_3\right) + c_3, \tag{2.13}$$

where $a_3 = 0.0422$, $b_3 = 0.00121$, and $c_3 = 1 \times 10^{-4}$. From Figure 2.7 we see that the shape of n_{Ca} is very similar to that of an AP and n_{Ca} approximately follows it, with the delay time of τ_c.

2.1.1.3 Regulation of [Ca²⁺] Inside Sarcomeres by AP

The so-called "all or none" property exists when APs burst [22]; i.e., their amplitudes are nearly constant and almost do not vary with stimulation intensity. This property holds for the APs on sarcolemma, so the [Ca²⁺] inside sarcomeres can only be modulated via frequency; i.e., the APs are variable-frequency control signals. On the other hand, [Ca²⁺] is directly related to muscle fiber tension, and this is the reason why [Ca²⁺] is equivalent to the drive signal.

If the frequency of APs is very low (e.g., less than 2 Hz), a single sarcomere will exhibit "twitch" behavior, which means that obvious contraction–relaxation cycles appear. When the frequency rises to some extent, the [Ca²⁺] during unit time becomes uniform, and the originally independent twitches will be so dense as to perform like a constant force. Thus, instantaneous [Ca²⁺] can be approximated by the average [Ca²⁺] during unit time interval, and this is similar to the conception of equivalent power of alternating current, as shown in Figure 2.8. Besides, due to the not less than 2.2 ms absolute refractory period of Na⁺ channel [23], the maximum frequency of APs cannot exceed 450 Hz, and there is almost no intersection among the potentials. It is obvious that the higher the frequency, the higher the temporal mean of [Ca²⁺]. Such regulation behavior implies the following: (1) Under isometric tensions (the two ends of a sarcomere is fixed), the tension provided by the sarcomere is determined by the number of working molecular motors, because the maximum tension a single motor can generate is nearly constant, while the higher the average [Ca²⁺], the more motors are stimulated and, as a result, the larger the tension of the sarcomere. (2) When the load is smaller than the maximum tension a sarcomere can provide, i.e., the sarcomere is able to produce contraction displacement and speed (e.g., isotonic tension), the temporal mean of [Ca²⁺] actually determines the power of the sarcomere, for the reason that the average [Ca²⁺] is decided by the number of stimulations of the sarcomere during the unit time (Figure 2.8).

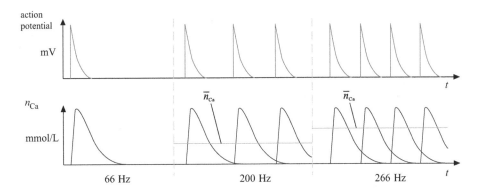

FIGURE 2.8   The regulation of [Ca²⁺] by APs.

From the results of Eq. (2.9) and Eq. (2.13), it is not difficult to calculate the relation between frequency of APs and average [Ca²⁺], and actually this can be done via calculating the temporal mean of neighboring [Ca²⁺] waves in one period. Figure 2.9a shows the simulation result, and the curve obviously exhibits sigmoidal features; indeed, it can be fitted well with the sigmoid function

$$\overline{n_{Ca}} = \frac{a_4}{1 + \exp(-b_4 f)} + c_4, \tag{2.14}$$

where f is the frequency of APs, $a_4 = 2.009 \times 10^{-2}$, $b_4 = 7.702 \times 10^{-3}$, and $c_4 = -1.008 \times 10^{-2}$. As mentioned, the average [Ca²⁺] determines the amount of stimulated myosin during isometric tension, so it should be positively correlated to the isometric tension, and because of the fixed number of molecular motors in a sarcomere, there should be a saturation value of the contraction force. The contraction force of muscles can be stated as

$$F = \beta \cdot F_{\max}, \tag{2.15}$$

where $F_{\max}$ denotes the maximum tension of a muscle and is related to the factors such as the cross-sectional area of the muscle, the load, [ATP], etc. The stimulation level of the muscle is characterized by β, which can be expressed as

$$\beta = \frac{\left[Ca^{2+}\right]^2}{\left[Ca^{2+}\right]^2 + K_2\left[Ca^{2+}\right] + K_1 K_2}, \tag{2.16}$$

where K_1 and K_2 denote the ratios of the separation rate to the binding rate of Ca²⁺ during two stages and their values are 8.72 and 0.194 μM [24], respectively. Combining Eq. (2.14) and Eq. (2.16), it is easy to obtain the relation between muscle tension and the frequency of APs, as shown in Figure 2.9b. Note that the tension in the figure is expressed as normalized force ($F/F_{\max}$). On the other hand, relevant experiments indeed showed that the relation shown in Figure 2.9b does exist [25]. On investigating it in detail, we find that the relation between the contraction force F and the frequency f can also be expressed by the sigmoid function, which is consistent with the experimental results of this section (see Section 2.3). Referring to control theory, Eqs. (2.14) and (2.15) represent two serial links during the drive process of muscle fibers. Moreover, we know that many types of skeletal muscles exist [25], and due to the assumption that the K⁺ channel density is very high on T-tubules during our modeling, the result shown in Figure 2.9a is closer to the characteristics of fast-type muscle fibers, while it may be different to some extent for slow-type ones.

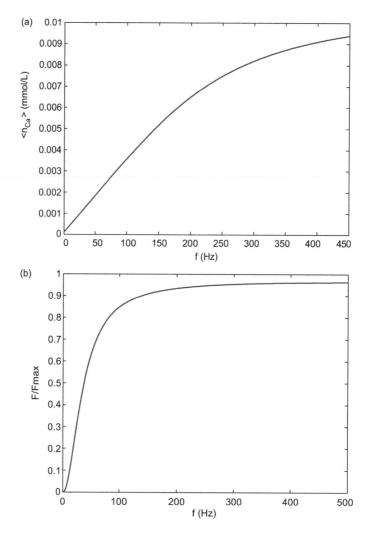

FIGURE 2.9 (a) The relation between average [Ca²⁺] and frequency of APs; (b) the relation between normalized tension and frequency of APs.

Actually the relation in Figure 2.9a is obtained under steady state; i.e., the muscle fiber is stimulated by steady series of APs, while for the understanding of the control of muscle contraction, it is equally important to investigate the transient response of the average [Ca²⁺] to the variation of AP frequency (e.g., the frequency jumps to 400 Hz from zero), because during the normal operations of muscle, the frequency of APs changes all the time, which leads to the variation of muscle power affected by sarcomere [Ca²⁺]. Therefore, the dynamic regulation mode of average [Ca²⁺] by APs is variable-frequency control, and the transfer function from frequency to [Ca²⁺] can be obtained via system identification as

$$G(s) = \frac{B_1 s^2 + B_2 s + B_3}{s^3 + A_1 s^2 + A_2 s + A_3}, \tag{2.17}$$

where the coefficients are $B_1 = -0.2794$, $B_2 = -609$, $B_3 = 1.934 \times 10^5$, $A_1 = 3.887 \times 10^3$, $A_2 = 9.385 \times 10^6$, and $A_3 = 8.674 \times 10^9$. Equation (2.17) shows that this is a third-order system, which is apparently composed of an inertia link originating from the chemical diffusion of Ca²⁺ and a

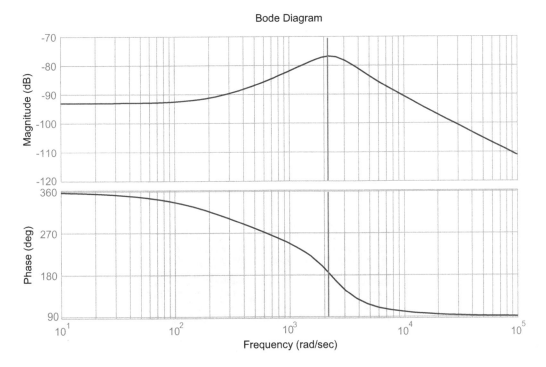

FIGURE 2.10   The frequency-domain characteristics of the drive signal of muscle fibers.

second-order vibration link coming from the wave features of APs. The system $G(s)$ has two zeros, one positive and the other negative, and three poles whose real parts are negative. Despite of being an open-loop system, it is stable against step input and ramp input. From the discussion above, we know that sarcomere $[Ca^{2+}]$ changes frequently when a muscle performs reciprocal motion, and the corresponding frequency of APs also varies up and down at this moment, so the frequency-domain properties of the system in Eq. (2.17) need to be investigated. The Bode diagram of the system is shown in Figure 2.10. It should be noted that the physical meaning of the horizontal axis in the figure is "frequency of the frequency", i.e., the variation frequency of the frequency of APs, and it corresponds to the variation frequency of sarcomere $[Ca^{2+}]$, which characterizes muscle contraction power. It can be seen from Figure 2.10 that the amplitudes of the system at low frequencies are almost constant and reach the maximum at mediate frequencies, while at high frequencies inhibition appears, which is similar to the behavior of a low-pass filter. On the other hand, it has been mentioned that the maximum frequency of APs is ~450 Hz; thus its variation frequency must be lower than this value, which is marked by a vertical red line located near the maximum amplitude in the figure. This indicates that within the range of variable frequency, muscle power increases with the frequency of contraction cycles, while it hardly changes at low frequencies. Moreover, the operation-frequency domain of muscle fibers does not enter the low-pass filter region.

2.1.1.4   The Application of the Variable-Frequency Regulation Model in Muscle Force Estimation

We took experiments on human rectus femoris of thigh to verify the steady relation between the isometric tension of muscle and the frequency of APs. Rectus femoris is located at the front of thighs, and it connects the tendons of the knee joint and hip joint; thus its contraction will raise the thigh or the leg. The experimental apparatus is shown in Figure 2.11, and tension signals and electromyogram (EMG) signals were collected with the lower-limb exoskeleton robot designed by our research group. EMG signals are formed by the superposition of massive APs of muscle fibers

(a)

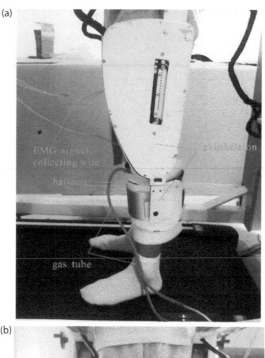

(b)

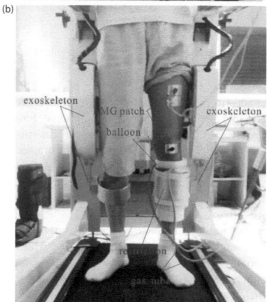

FIGURE 2.11   (a) Side view of the experimental apparatus; (b) front view of the experimental apparatus.

in a muscle, and the analysis of EMG can be used to diagnose muscle diseases [26] or identify the motion pattern of muscles [27], while here we judged the stimulation level of rectus femoris via the characteristic frequency of EMG.

The exoskeleton has two degrees of freedom, and it can fix the thigh and leg of the experimental subject. During our experiment, the left leg of the subject was bound to the exoskeleton; also bound was his hip joint, so his thigh was not able to move. A balloon used as the pressure transducer connecting with gas tubes was bound to the leg, and both the balloon and the leg were bound to the exoskeleton by the restriction. EMG patches (electrodes) were located at the middle of rectus femoris to monitor its stimulation level. When the experiment started, the balloon was firstly charged with gas, and then the subject slowly extended his leg out. The rectus femoris contracted during this motion, and its stimulation intensity was recorded by EMG signals. Due to the fixed position of the restriction, actually no displacement of the leg occurred, while the force that the leg exerted on the balloon varied in the process; thus the pressure of the balloon always changed, and the tension of rectus femoris could be characterized by this pressure. Therefore, EMG signals under different contraction conditions of the rectus femoris could be obtained. The sampling rates of EMG signal and tension signal were both 2,000 Hz, so one datum was recorded every 400 sampling intervals; i.e., the data recording period was $\Delta T = 0.2$ s. In the experiment, the EMG signals during every ΔT were dealt with Fourier transform, and the characteristic frequency was extracted in real time. The formula of the characteristic frequency is

$$f_{ch} = \frac{\sum_{i=1}^{N} A_i n_i}{\sum_{i=1}^{N} A_i} \cdot \xi, \tag{2.18}$$

where A_i denotes the amplitudes of the points on the half-Fourier spectrum, n_i is the position of the point, and N denotes total number of sampling points. For the reason that the ranges of EMG frequency and AP frequency of a single muscle fiber are different, an adjustment coefficient ξ was introduced, and it matched the experimental EMG frequency with the AP frequency of muscle fibers so as to better verify the relation between tension and AP frequency. As mentioned, the frequency range of APs is ~450 Hz, while the range of EMG frequencies in the experiment was ~60 Hz, so we took $\xi = 1/8$. The characteristic frequency f_{ch} was also output in real time, as well as the mean force during ΔT.

One group of original data of balloon pressure and f_{ch} of EMG are shown in Figure 2.12a, from which we see that these two quantities approximately follow each other, i.e., the higher the EMG frequency, the larger the force (the tension of rectus femoris). Note that when f_{ch} reaches the peak value and does not change with time (the region between the dashed lines in the figure), the force remains growing for a while. This is because the number of stimulated muscle fibers is increasing under the same stimulation level. Figure 2.12b shows four groups of successively processed experimental data, which have already been expressed as the relation between the pressure and EMG frequency. The subject had a rest of 4–5 min between groups; still it is obvious that the contraction force at the same frequency became larger in later sets of data; i.e., the number of muscle fibers stimulated by APs of the same frequency would increase. This phenomenon is called "activity-dependent potentiation" [28], after which fatigue happens.

To avoid the effect of fatigue, we fitted the data in the first and the second groups in Figure 2.12b. The experimental data and the fitted curve are shown in Figure 2.13a, and the fitting process is based on the sigmoidal feature of the data. The resulting function is written as

$$F = \frac{a_5}{1 + \exp\left(-b_5\left(f + c_5\right)\right)} + d_5, \tag{2.19}$$

where F and f are the pressure and the EMG frequency, respectively. The parameters are $a_5 = 1{,}734$, $b_5 = 5.503 \times 10^{-3}$, $c_5 = -318$, and $d_5 = -256.724$. The fitted curve represents the realistic steady relation between muscle contraction force and AP frequency, and Figure 2.13b compares the normalized experimental relation expressed in Eq. (19) with the theoretical relation (Figure 2.9b). From the figure, we see that the changing trend of the theoretical curve is basically consistent with that of the experimental one, and that the slopes of the curves match during the stage of the normalized force increasing with the frequency, while the theoretical curve falls behind the experimental one near the saturation stage, and after that the experimental curve always leads. This is due to the slow approaching to infinity process of the force reaching the maximum value, according to

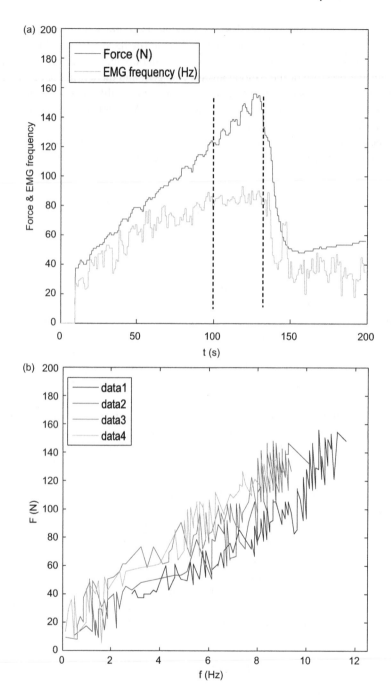

FIGURE 2.12   (a) Real-time data of pressure and EMG frequency; (b) four successive groups of experimental data.

the theoretical results. On the other hand, Hill and Kesar et al. measured the muscle forces of the subjects *in vivo* with the method of functional electric stimulation (FES) [29,30]. Their researches aimed at the fatigue process of human muscles, and the frequency of FES was able to reach 100 Hz. On the contrary, in our experiment the subject provided force actively while EMG frequency was measured. Although the input and output were reversed in these two kinds of experiments, the corresponding relation should hold, and indeed, such consistence is also shown in Figure 2.13b.

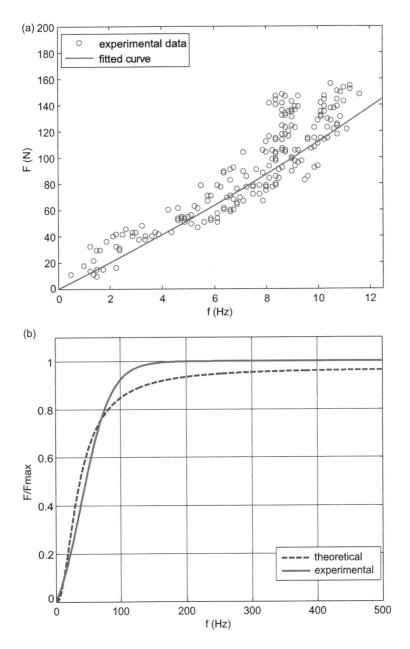

FIGURE 2.13 (a) The fitted curve of the experimental data; (b) comparison between the experimental and theoretical curves.

When discussing $[Ca^{2+}]$, we calculated the time τ_c for it to reach the peak value, and this time interval is regarded as a characteristic constant and holds special significance, because it represents the minimum time for muscle fibers to contract after the control signal happens. This time constant is similar to the electromechanical time constant in mechatronic control and is decided by the physical properties of muscle fibers. For the reason that τ_c is the time constant of skeletal muscle and APs are electric signals, we name it as "electromuscular time constant", without losing representativeness. When elucidating how $[Ca^{2+}]$ is controlled by APs, we proposed two indications of the regulation mechanism, which play a key role in the understanding of motion intention. From the indications, we know that although the final representation of motion intention is muscle force (contraction speed and displacement are also dominated by the force), motion intention cannot be quantified by measuring the contraction force. This is because when the same APs are applied to different motor units, the tension and power produced can differ a lot due to the different numbers of sarcomeres/myosins contained in them. Therefore, the frequency of APs actually represents "intention strength", while the contraction force represents "action strength". Of course the intention strengths for different muscles/people should be different in order to generate the same action strengths. On the other hand, Section 2.1 deduced the theoretical steady relation between AP frequency and muscle force, and we further designed the corresponding experiment to verify the theoretical results. The results show that the experiment well coincides with the theory.

Section 2.1 further elucidated the regulation mode of average $[Ca^{2+}]$ in sarcomeres by AP-variable-frequeny modulation and derived the dynamic response of $[Ca^{2+}]$ to the variation of AP frequency, with the transfer function provided. Besides, with the frequency-domain analysis of the resulting system, we found that the power will gradually increase from the initially constant value with the rise of contraction frequency of muscle fibers; i.e., for some type of skeletal muscle, there exists a contraction frequency at which its power is at maximum, and this frequency is decided by both the highest frequency of APs and frequency-domain characteristics of muscle contraction. There also exists the upper limit of contraction frequency of muscle fibers, while it is only decided by the maximum frequency of APs. When combining the concept of electromuscular time constant with the regulation and control mechanism of sarcomere contraction, it is not difficult to tell that the theoretical results of Section 2.1 actually provide the first forward-transfer function of skeletal muscle control links, although deduced with the sarcomere closest to the sarcolemma. Thus, based on these results, the control characteristics of a muscle fiber can be obtained with the distributions of APs and sarcomeres. Furthermore, the control model of the whole muscle can also be obtained because a single piece of muscle is composed of massive muscle fibers in series and in parallel; then the unification of microscopic and macroscopic models for skeletal muscles can be completed. While Section 2.1 has provided the regulation mechanism and properties of sarcomere contraction, it does not mean that the whole control model has formed because the real muscle operation process is in a closed-loop system fed back via biologic neural network. In this section, only the open-loop characteristics of muscle fibers are discussed; thus in future studies, the information feedback features of skeletal muscle motion should be further explored based on the mechanism presented here. Finally the complete transfer function of skeletal muscle control can be obtained.

2.2   MODELING THE FORCE-PRODUCING MECHANISM OF SKELETAL MUSCLE

2.2.1   CLASSICAL MODELS

2.2.1.1   Hill-Type Model

The prototype of Hill-type model was obtained by Hill in 1938 via measuring the heat released by a small muscle bundle under isotonic contraction. In each experimental trial, the load is maintained constant, while for different trials, the load can be set as needed so that even the stretch under activation state can be accomplished. During the experiments, the muscle was first stimulated tetanically and then released under a certain load. As the core of Hill-type model, Hill's equation is deduced according to the following facts:

- Under isometric contractions, the released heat is minimum, while when muscle shortens, the heat begins to increase and is proportional to the shortening distance, as shown in Figure 2.14.
- For different shortening distances, the heat release rate is almost always constant and is nearly the same as the initial stage of isometric contraction (Figure 2.14a).

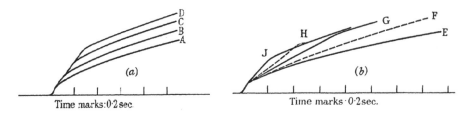

FIGURE 2.14 (a) Heat release under isotonic contraction, where curve A denotes isometric contraction; (b) heat release of the shortening under different loads, where curve E denotes isometric contraction [1].

- During isotonic contractions, the heat release rate is negatively correlated to the load, i.e., the larger the load, the slower the heat release (Figure 2.14b).
- Only if the final shortening distances are the same, the final released heat would also be the same, and the heat release rate would be the same as that under isometric contraction once the shortening is ceased (Figure 2.14b, curve E).

It is worth noting that during isometric contraction, curve E shows clearly a hump release rate at the initial phase, which is due to the residue motion of myosin motors, while the motors reach the real rigor state at the flection point of curve E, where the elastic components of sarcomeres have been stretched to the maximum extent.

Based on the above features, Hill classified the extra heat (relative to that of isometric contraction) during shortening into two types: shortening heat and mechanical work. Thus, the total energy can be denoted as

$$E = (P + a)x,$$ (2.20)

where x is the shortening distance, P is the load, and the parameter a is a constant with the dimension of force. This parameter depends on the cross-sectional area of the muscle bundle and the stimulus intensity (featured by the maximum force P_0), so for a specific muscle, a/P_0 is also a constant. According to Eq. (2.20), the energy release rate is

$$\dot{E} = (P + a)\dot{x} = (P + a)v,$$ (2.21)

where v is the shortening velocity. Moreover, the experiments show that the energy release rate is a linear function of load, as shown in Figure 2.15a, so we have

$$(P + a)v = b(P_0 - P), \text{ or}$$

$$(P + a)(v + b) = (P + a)b = \text{const.},$$ (2.22)

where b is also a constant with the dimension of velocity. Equation (2.22) is the widely recognized Hill's equation that represents the relationship between the contractile force P and the shortening velocity v (P–v relation). It is actually a hyperbola with the asymptotes of $P = -a$ and $v = -b$, as shown in Figure 2.15b.

The P–v relation provided by Hill's equation is actually quasi-static; i.e., it can only describe the properties of muscle under a constant load and a stable shortening state. Consequently, Hill's equation is not a dynamical equation and cannot describe the general contraction properties under a varying load, neither can it explain the behavior of accelerating contraction or decelerating contraction. On the other hand, the phenomena concluded by Hill's equation is limited to the situation of tetanic stimulation, not including the influence of dynamically varying stimulus intensity

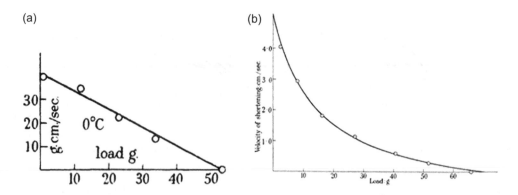

FIGURE 2.15   (a) The relation between energy release rate and load; (b) the relation between load and shortening velocity [1].

(AP's frequency) on the contraction behavior. Thus, Hill's equation cannot be applied directly to the cybernetic modeling of muscular contraction. For these reasons, Hill's equation is not applicable to the twitch behavior of muscle under the excitation of a single AP either.

Based on the above achievements, Hill further proposed the three-element model of skeletal muscle, as shown in Figure 2.16. To describe the mechanical properties of muscle, this model assumes that muscle is composed of a contractile element (CE), a series element (SE), and a parallel elastic element (PE). In fact, CE corresponds to the collective working behavior of myosin motors and is responsible for producing the active force, so it is also called "active element". SE is generally considered as the elastic behavior of thin filament, while PE corresponds to the elasticity of titin. Therefore, SE and PE are named as a whole as "passive elements". Hill's three-element model has been widely applied to the fields of biomechanics, biomedical engineering, and bionics. However, its defects are also evident. For instance, it does not take into account the damping feature of muscle, which is actually ubiquitous in biological tissues, and damping is also the major limiting factor for the unloaded shortening velocity of muscle. Besides, this model oversimplifies the dynamic properties of passive elements, while the academia has recognized the remarkable nonlinear viscosity of PE. This leads to the discrepancies between the results of three-element model and the mechanical behavior of resting muscle.

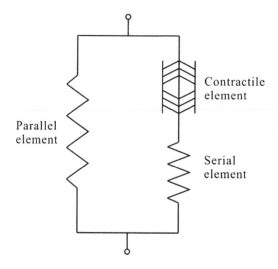

FIGURE 2.16   Hill's three-element model.

2.2.1.2 Conformational Change Model

The earliest widely accepted conformational change model is the cross-bridge model [29] proposed by Huxley, and cross-bridge refers to the structure formed by the strong binding of thin filament and myosin motor's head. Huxley proposed that such structures enhance the stiffness of the sarcomere, and the force is attributed to the rotation of the motor head, which generates the relative sliding between thin and thick filaments. As a groundbreaking work, the cross-bridge model provides a preliminary explanation toward the experimental phenomena, while the model is not very elaborate as it only provides a qualitative explanation. Single-molecule experiments are always promoting the research of the working mechanism of molecular motor. Kaya et al. [30] tested that a myosin motor is able to move a distance of 8 nm during one power stroke, and the nonlinear elastic features of the motor neck make great impacts on the motor force. Sellers et al. [31] observed directly the reversibility of molecular motor's power stroke with laser trap technology. On the other hand, Spudich proposed the swinging cross-bridge model or lever arm model [31] based on microscopic experiments. As the improvement of cross-bridge model, lever arm model not only specifies the key effects of the molecular loops of motor head on the binding of the motor with the thin filament and ATP, but also identifies that the motor domain of myosin motor is near the connection region between motor head and neck, as shown in Figure 2.17a. The lever refers to the neck of myosin motor, which amplifies the deformation caused by the conformational change in the motor domain, making the neck rotate for about 70°. As the second-generation conformational change model, lever arm model is still being used today and serves as the blueprint for more meticulous experiments in the future. It should be noted that the Osaka group in Japan has made important contributions to the single-molecule experimental research of molecular motor, as they combined the technologies of optical tweezers and fluorescence microscopy for the first time and observed quantitatively the dynamic motion of the motor and the stiffness change of the system during the hydrolysis of a single ATP [32]. Furthermore, they found that when the myosin motor is in the optimal direction, it can move a distance of about 15 nm, consisting of several substeps of 5.5 nm length.

The physical source of conformational change model is the interactions between molecular groups, involving quantum mechanics (QM) and molecular mechanics (MM). Most of such type of studies are based on single-molecule experiments or molecular dynamics simulation, aiming at investigating what changes of which groups have led to the deformation of the motor. Recently, a QM/MM hybrid method has been applied to this field. In this hybrid method, QM is responsible for computing the interactions at atomic level, while MM is used to study the interactions between molecular groups, so that a good balance can be attained between the computation speed and precision. With the improvements of QM/MM hybrid method, it has made great success in studying the structure and the reactions of biological large molecules [33–36].

Most of the current conformational change models originate from Huxley's cross-bridge model, which assumed that several states of myosin motor exist during its binding with the thin filament, and Markov kinetics is used to describe the transitions among these states. Despite the fact

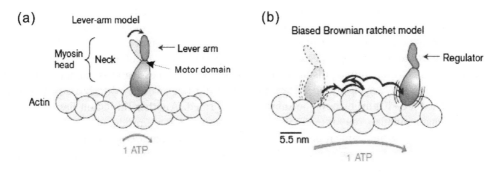

FIGURE 2.17 (a) Conformational change model; (b) Brownian ratchet model [32].

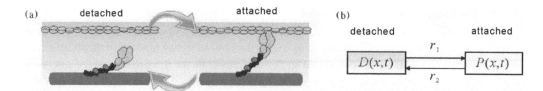

FIGURE 2.18 (a) State transitions in two-state cross-bridge model; (b) Markov model for the transition process.

that models with different numbers of states have been proposed, the most basic and widely used paradigm is still the two-state (attached and detached states) model, as shown in Figure 2.18a. The corresponding Markov model describing the transition process is shown in Figure 2.18b. $P(x, t)$ denotes the probability density of a motor binding to the position x (relative to the equilibrium position) at time t, and $D(x, t)$ denotes the probability density of a motor detaching from the position x at time t. The forward and backward transition rates between the two states are r_1 and r_2, respectively. The Markov kinetics can be expressed as

$$\begin{cases} D(x,t) = 1 - P(x,t) \\ \left.\dfrac{\partial P(x,t)}{\partial t}\right|_x = r_1 - (r_2 + r_1)P(x,t) - v\left.\dfrac{\partial P(x,t)}{\partial t}\right|_t \end{cases}. \tag{2.23}$$

In effect, Eq. (23) describes the evolution process of the single-motor mean displacement with time. In cross-bridge model, Huxley assumed that the contractile force of sarcomere comes from the neck stiffness k_m of the motor, which would produce force when a deformation of x is imposed at the attached state. Thus, the force produced by the active element (F_{AE}) can be denoted as

$$F_{AE} = G(L)N_0 \left(\frac{1}{R} \int_R P(x,t)(k_m x)\, dx \right), \tag{2.24}$$

where $G(L)$ represents the overlap degree of the thin and thick filaments, depending on the sarcomere length L, and N_0 can be regarded as the total number of myosin motors available for work or the "force capacity". R denotes the allowed range for the deformation x, which is usually the distance of adjacent binding sites on the thin filament. In Eq. (2.24), the integral term in the bracket represents the average force produced by a motor, and F_{AE} is the active force produced by a sarcomere. It should be noted that the transition rates r_1 and r_2 in Eq. (2.23) are usually not constants but may hold complex forms in multi-state detailed models. For example, r_1 may depend on the cytoplasmic [Ca^{2+}] and the binding position x, while r_2 may depend simultaneously on [ATP] and x. It can be seen that the transition rates are also time-varying quantities that are coupled with x or force. Thus, numerical methods are commonly applied for solving Eq. (2.23).

In essence, the descriptive paradigm of conformational change model or Huxley's cross-bridge model is statistical. It starts from the microscopic working mechanism of molecular motor, so the precision is higher than that of Hill-type model, and conformational change models have been widely used in explaining the optical-tweezer-based experimental data of a single motor. However, the major challenge is the moving distance of the motor, because these models cannot explain why a motor is able to move such a long distance of 15 nm during an ATP hydrolysis cycle (current prediction is about 5–10 nm) or how the substeps are formed. Another limitation lies in that conformational change models only provide the explanation of the force-producing mechanism of the active element, but the mechanical properties of the passive element are not included. In addition, the description of a single sarcomere cannot be applied directly to the behavior prediction of a whole macroscopic muscle. Therefore, conformational change model does not unify the descriptions of microscopic and macroscopic scales, largely limiting its engineering value.

2.2.1.3   Statistical Thermodynamical Model

In the biomechanical research domain of skeletal muscle, the most widely studied statistical thermodynamical model is Brownian ratchet model. The earliest concept of Brownian ratchet was proposed by Feynman [37], who modeled a microscopic ratchet making the diffusion of the particles in some direction easier (with a gradual potential well) while that in the opposite direction more difficult (with a steep potential well). The larger diffusion probability of the particles in a specific direction makes possible the macroscopic directional transport of mass. In practical physical applications, this imagined ratchet is equivalent to an asymmetric potential distribution, which is referred to as ratchet potential. The Brownian ratchet model of molecular motor treats the myosin head as a Brownian particle diffusing in the cytoplasm, and the periodic ratchet potential originates from the periodically distributed binding sites on the thin filament. As for the cause of the asymmetry of the potential, diverse opinions exist, such as the asymmetry of the motor head structure or the ATP's binding [38]. Brownian ratchet model proposes that myosin motor surfs forward under the effect of ratchet potential to produce displacement or force. Although there are occasional backward movements, the net effect is a forward movement in a statistical sense, as shown in Figure 2.17b. The core mechanism of Brownian ratchet model is described by Langevin equation, in which the inertia force is often neglected due to the tiny mass of the motor and the overdamped solution environment. The detailed descriptive paradigms [39] include fluctuating force, fluctuating potential, and fluctuating between states. For the fluctuating-force mode, myosin motor is located in a ratchet potential $W(x)$ and feels a fluctuating force that does not obey the fluctuation–dissipation theorem. The dynamics of the motor is described by the Langevin equation:

$$\xi \dot{x} = -\partial_x W(x) + F(t), \tag{2.25}$$

where ξ is the friction coefficient (constant), x is the position of motor, and the fluctuating force $F(x)$ has a zero mean value: $\langle F(x) \rangle = 0$, but it has a more complicated correlation function than Gaussian white noise. Under the fluctuating-potential mode, the ratchet potential is assumed to be time-varying:

$$\xi \dot{x} = -\partial_x W(x,t) + f(t), \tag{2.26}$$

where ξ, x, and W have the same meanings as those in Eq. (2.25), while W becomes dependent on time, and the stochastic force $f(t)$ is Gaussian white noise that satisfies the fluctuation–dissipation theorem:

$$\langle f(t) \rangle = 0, \quad \langle f(t) f(t') \rangle = 2\xi T \delta (t - t'). \tag{2.27}$$

Under the fluctuating-between-states mode, the dynamics of myosin motor is still described by Langevin equation for each state:

$$\xi_i \dot{x} = -\partial_x W_i(x) + f_i(t), \tag{2.28}$$

where i is the number of the state, $i = 1, \ldots, N$, and $f_i(t)$ still satisfies the fluctuation–dissipation theorem:

$$\langle f_i(t) \rangle = 0, \quad \langle f_i(t) f_j(t') \rangle = 2\xi_i T \delta (t - t') \delta_{ij}. \tag{2.29}$$

In most cases, the transitions among states are described using Fokker–Planck paradigm (see Section 2.2.3). Taking the two-state ratchet model as an example, the working process of a myosin motor is shown in Figure 2.19a, where q denotes the distance between adjacent motors on the thick filament, y_n denotes the binding position of the motor's tail part on the thick filament, and x_n is the position of

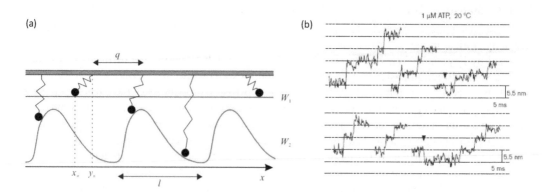

FIGURE 2.19 (a) Two-state Brownian ratchet model; (b) substeps of the myosin motor during a single power stroke [32].

the motor's head. The periods of the two states' potentials W_1 and W_2 are both l, and W_1 is the ratchet potential. The molecular motor fluctuates between W_1 and W_2, making the whole thick filament move leftward [40]. When the motor is in the near equilibrium state, the correlation between energy transformation and particle transport is often expressed by the Onsager relationship [41].

As shown in Figure 2.19b, during single-molecule experiments, the data indicates that in one ATP hydrolysis cycle, a myosin motor can move a distance of 15 nm composed of several substeps of 5.5 nm [42]. The Osaka group conducting this experiment inferred that the substep size is consistent with the interval of G-actins and proposed that the movement of myosin motor is attributed to Brownian ratchet mechanism. However, it is hard to imagine that the motor is even able to work effectively if it detaches from the thin filament frequently during a power cycle. Besides, if we view the data in Figure 2.19b, the motor actually did not detach from the thin filament, because the substeps happened in a manner of continuous jumps. Consequently, the approximate size of the 5.5 nm substep and the distance between neighboring G-actins might be just a coincidence, while for the power stroke of myosin motors, the explanation of conformational change in the head region seems more reasonable; i.e., the substeps are generated by the periodic release of the energy produced by the hydrolysis of ATP, indicating four to five energy levels in the molecular structure of the motor. The transition mechanism among these energy levels needs to be analyzed from the perspective of free energy combining the QM/MM method. Currently, when applying Brownian ratchet model, people have paid too much attention to its functionality and have neglected some basic questions; thus one needs to treat Brownian ratchet model properly via assembling and unifying the physical meaning of the model and the object being considered.

2.2.2 COUPLING MECHANISM OF MULTI-FORCE INTERACTIONS OF A SINGLE MYOSIN MOTOR

This section discusses the motion principles of a molecular motor under the coupling effect of vdW force, Casimir force, electrostatic force, and Brownian force and demonstrates the application of Monte Carlo method in dynamical simulation aiming at analyzing the stochastic features of the microscopic environment. Finally the influence of each force on the motion of the motor is concluded.

Does the Casimir force play a role in the myosin motor system? The forces normally associated with protein–protein interactions include electrostatic force, vdW force, and the solvent force [43]. There are similarities and differences between the Casimir force and the vdW force [44]. Based on quantum electrodynamics, the vdW and Casimir forces can be unified. At two points, the correlation of the quantized electromagnetic field in vacuum is not equal to zero.

The interaction of two macroscopic particles at large distances is reduced due to the finite speed of light, and this phenomenon is called the retardation effect. The Casimir force is often referred to as the retarded vdW force. Compared with the vdW force, the Casimir force is a relatively long-distance force. In vacuum, the Casimir effect emerges at a separation distance larger than 5 nm, although this distance may be shorter in solvent. It is well known that the vdW force (dispersion force) plays an important role in proteins and in complex biological systems. We suggest here that the Casimir force also plays a role in these systems.

Which forces are involved in binding the myosin motor to the actin filaments? X-ray crystallography studies on the structure of the myosin–actin system have shown that the myosin head has positively charged segments, and the actin has negatively charged segments, indicating that electrostatic interactions are important in the binding process [45]. Myosin is a large protein with a high molecular weight, and the vdW force is likely to play a crucial role in their interactions. When the distance between the myosin and actin is large, the Casimir effect should be considered. Recent progress in experimental techniques has allowed the accurate measurement of the Casimir force. Lifshitz [46] was the first to extend the Casimir effect to ordinary dielectric particles. Later, Guo and Zhao analyzed and compared the influence of vdW and Casimir forces on electrostatic torsional actuators in static equilibrium [47]. Recently, a repulsive Casimir force has been verified and measured in a fluid by Munday and coworkers. This force could make nanomachines work better with less or more friction as needed [48].

It is, therefore, important to analyze the influence of the Casimir and vdW forces on the dynamics of the myosin motor in nanoscale in the solvent. We will begin by discussing some of the factors that affect the vdW and Casimir forces.

Temperature and surface roughness: Under normal temperature ($T = 300$ K) conditions, the influence of temperature on the vdW and Casimir forces can be neglected. When the diameter of the particle is 1–2 μm with a roughness of 4–7 nm, the roughness correction to the Casimir interaction is usually computed using atomic force microscopy (AFM) images of the surfaces [49]. For the myosin motor, the diameter is only several nanometers with atom-scale roughness. Therefore, we neglect the roughness influence on the interactions when the distance of the surfaces is larger than a nanometer scale and calculate the forces assuming a smooth surface.

Media: The interactions between molecules in a solvent are different from their interactions in vacuum. The forces involved can be changed from attractive to repulsive by varying the nature of the interacting materials in the solvent. Considering the dielectric permittivities of the material ε_1, ε_2, and ε_0, the interaction of material 1 with material 2 across medium 0 is a summation of terms with differences in material permittivity. When the material permittivity qualifies $\varepsilon_1 = \varepsilon_2$, $\varepsilon_2 \leq \varepsilon_1 \leq \varepsilon_0$, $\varepsilon_1 \leq \varepsilon_2 \leq \varepsilon_0$, the forces are always attractive; however, when the dielectric permittivity ε_0 of the medium is between that of the two interacting particles ε_1, ε_2, the forces are repulsive. For proteins in water, the dielectric permittivity of the proteins is smaller than that of water, and the forces between myosin and actin are attractive. The dielectric permittivities of the medium and proteins have some influence on these forces, and this will be discussed later in this section.

We calculated the magnitude of the vdW and Casimir forces based on the Hamaker approach, taking advantage of its applicability and simplicity and ignoring, for now, its several shortcomings.

2.2.2.1 Forces Involved in the Approaching Process

As shown in Figure 2.19, actin is composed of two coiled-coil helical fibrous proteins of diameter 6–7 nm and length 1.6 μm. Myosin II contains a head domain, a neck domain, and a C-terminal tail domain. The myosin subfragments 1(S1) are 16.5 nm long and 6.5 nm wide. Each of the myosin heads is capable of binding to actin [43].

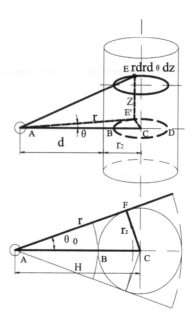

FIGURE 2.20 The interaction between atom A and a cylinder. The radius of the cylinder is r_2; E' is the projection point E in the cross-sectional plane BCD; $AE' = r$; the distance between an atom at a point A and a differential volume element at point E in the cylinder is $(r^2 + z^2)^{1/2}$; $EE' = z$; and $\theta = \arccos((r^2 + H^2 - r^2)/2rH)$.

The structure of the myosin motor can be simply represented as an ellipsoid particle (with a long axis c and a short axis a). Because its length, L, is much larger than its radius, r_2 ($L \gg r_2$), the actin is shown as an infinitely long cylindrical particle. The interaction potential between myosin and actin is equivalent to the attractive potential between the ellipsoid and cylindrical particle.

   i. vdW force and Casimir force: The vdW and Casimir potentials between myosin and actin can be calculated by summing the interactions over all the atoms involved. The calculation was carried out in steps as outlined below.

   Step 1: The potential of two atoms separated by a distance, r, was expressed as

$$U = -\frac{C}{r^m}, \tag{2.30}$$

   where C represents the potential coefficient related to the well-known Hamaker constant and m depends on the model used for the intermolecular potential; for the vdW potential $m = 6$ and for the Casimir potential $m = 7$.

   Step 2: The attractive potential between an atom A and a cylinder is the sum of the interactions between atom A and all of the atoms in the cylinder (Figure 2.20):

$$U_1 = n_1 \int_{H-r_2}^{H+r_2} \int_{-\theta_0}^{\theta_0} d\theta \int_{-\infty}^{\infty} \frac{C}{\left(r^2 + z^2\right)^{m/2}} r \, dr \, dz, \tag{2.31}$$

   where n_1 is the number density of the atoms in the cylinder

   Step 3: The interaction potential of the myosin motor and the actin filaments is the total interaction between a sphere and a cylinder and is given by (Figure 2.21)

$$U_{21} = n_2 \int_0^{2c} U_1 \frac{a^2}{c^2} \pi (2c - \alpha) \alpha \, d\alpha, \tag{2.32}$$

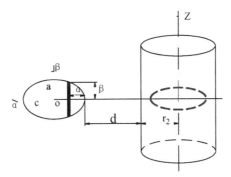

FIGURE 2.21 The interaction between an ellipsoid and a cylinder, where d represents the distance between the surfaces of the two particles. Considering a disk of cross-sectional area $\pi\beta^2$ and thickness $d\alpha$ in the ellipsoid, the total number of atoms in the disk is $\pi n_2\beta^2 d\alpha$. A point in the ellipse satisfies the equation $(c-\alpha)^2/c^2 + \beta^2/a^2 = 1$, because all atoms in the thin disk are at the same separation distance $(\alpha+d)$ from the surface of the cylinder, and the overall interaction potential between this element and the cylinder is $n_2U_1(a^2/c^2)\pi(2c-\alpha)\alpha d\alpha$.

where n_2 is the atom density of atoms in the ellipsoid particle.

When the surface distance d between the myosin and actin filaments is small, $m = 6$, from Eq. (2.32) the vdW potential can be simplified as

$$U_{vdW} \approx \frac{\pi a^2}{8c^2} A_{102}$$

$$\left\{ \begin{array}{l} \left[\dfrac{c^2-(d+c+2r_2)^2}{2(d+2c+2r_2)^2} + \dfrac{(c+d)^2-c^2}{2(d+2c)^2} + \dfrac{2(c+d+2r_2)}{(d+2c+2r_2)} - \dfrac{2(c+d)}{(d+2c)} + \ln\left(\dfrac{d+2c+2r_2}{d+2c}\right) \right] \\[4mm] -\left[\dfrac{c^2-(d+c+2r_2)^2}{2(d+2r_2)^2} + \dfrac{(c+d)^2-c^2}{2(d)^2} + \dfrac{2(c+d+2r_2)}{(d+2r_2)} - \dfrac{2(c+d)}{(d)} + \ln\left(\dfrac{d+2r_2}{d}\right) \right] \end{array} \right\}.$$

$$(2.33)$$

When the distance d is larger, the retardation effect should be considered ($m = 7$), and the Casimir potential is given by

$$U_{cl} \approx \frac{2\pi a^2 B_{102}}{c^2}$$

$$\left\{ \begin{array}{l} \left[\dfrac{(c+d)^2-c^2}{3(d+2c)^3} - \dfrac{(c+d+2r_2)^2-c^2}{3(d+2c+2r_2)^3} - \dfrac{c+d}{(d+2c)^2} + \dfrac{c+d+2r_2}{(d+2c+2r_2)^2} + \dfrac{1}{(d+2c)} - \dfrac{1}{(d+2c+2r_2)} \right] \\[4mm] -\left[\dfrac{(c+d)^2-c^2}{3d^3} - \dfrac{(c+d+2r_2)^2-c^2}{3(d+2r_2)^3} - \dfrac{c+d}{d^2} + \dfrac{c+d+2r_2}{(d+2r_2)^2} + \dfrac{1}{d} - \dfrac{1}{(d+2r_2)} \right] \end{array} \right\},$$

$$(2.34)$$

where the non-retarded Hamaker constant is defined as $A_{102} = \pi^2 n_1 n_2 C vdW$, the retarded Hamaker constant is defined as $B_{102} = 0.1\pi n_1 n_2 Ccl$, the vdW force $F_{vdW} = -\partial U_{vdW}/\partial d$, and the Casimir force $Fcl = -\partial U_{cl}/\partial d$.

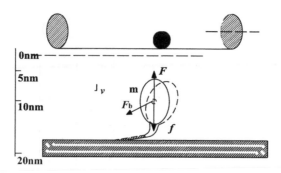

FIGURE 2.22 The dynamical process of the attachment of the myosin motor to the actin filaments.

ii. Electrostatic force: The electrostatic force is also involved in the interaction between the myosin motor and the binding site of actin. Because of the different structure and components of myosin and actin, this force cannot be calculated directly using the electrostatic double layer force formula. Based on Coulomb's law, the potential energy can be expressed as

$$U_e(r) = \frac{q_1 q_2}{4\pi\varepsilon_0\varepsilon d},$$ (2.35)

where ε_0 represents the dielectric permittivity of the solvent water, ε is the permittivity of a vacuum, and q_1 and q_2 are the charges on myosin and the binding site of actin, respectively.

iii. Brownian force and friction: The myosin motor has remarkable stochastic features due to thermal fluctuations of the surrounding medium. Using the fluctuation–dissipation theorem, the stochastic Brownian force is represented as $F_b = \sqrt{2\gamma kT\varepsilon_d(t)}$, in which the thermal noise $\varepsilon_d(t)$ is Gaussian white noise which satisfies $\langle\varepsilon_d(t),\varepsilon_d(t')\rangle = \delta(t-t'), \langle\varepsilon_d(t)\rangle = 0$, k is the Boltzmann constant, and T is the temperature. The solvent viscosity acts on the motor as friction $f = \gamma v$, where v is the velocity of the motor and γ is the friction coefficient of the motor.

iv. Solvent force: Solvent forces that include hydration forces and hydrophobic forces may exist between the water and protein molecules with hydrophilic and hydrophobic residues. The physical mechanisms that underlie solvent force are debated. Empirically, the potential energy is $U_s = U_0 e^{-d/\lambda_0}$ (where λ_0 represents the attenuation length and U_0 is the interaction energy per unit area). Because there are, as yet, no experimental parameters for the myosin motor, the influence of solvent forces on the molecular motor is not taken into account in the present study.

2.2.2.2 Calculation of the Main Interaction Force

Based on the above discussion, we assume that during the binding process between myosin and the actin filaments, the active potential energy consists of electrostatic potential energy, and vdW and Casimir potential energies, as shown in Figure 2.22.

The active potential energy can be written as

$$U(d) = U_e + U_{vdW} + U_{cl}.$$ (2.36)

The Langevin equation for the myosin motor in the solvent is given by

$$m_1\ddot{d}(t) + \gamma\dot{d}(t) = -\frac{\partial U(d,t)}{\partial d} + \sqrt{2\gamma kT}\,\varepsilon_d(t),$$ (2.37)

where m_1 is the mass of the motor and $m_1/\gamma \ll 1$. Neglecting inertia effects, we get the following overdamped Langevin equation for the dynamics of the motor in the solvent:

$$\gamma \dot{d}(t) = -\frac{\partial U(d,t)}{\partial d} + \sqrt{2\gamma kT} \varepsilon_d(t). \tag{2.38}$$

The active force is $F(d) = -\dfrac{\partial U(d)}{\partial d}$, and $\dot{d}(t) = \dfrac{F(d)}{\gamma} + \sqrt{\dfrac{2kT}{\gamma}} \varepsilon_d(t)$. The stochastic differential equation is solved using a Monte Carlo method The function $\dot{d}(t) = \dfrac{F(d)}{\gamma} + \sqrt{\dfrac{2kT}{\gamma}} \varepsilon_d(t)$ is expanded using the Taylor expansion [50]:

$$d(t+\Delta t) = d(t) + F\Delta t + \frac{1}{2} FF'\Delta t^2 + \sqrt{2D}Z_1 + F'\sqrt{2D}Z_2 + F''DZ_3. \tag{2.39}$$

Here Δt refers to the integration time step. F' and F'' are first-order differential and second-order differential coefficients of the function F. $D = kT/\gamma$ represents the noise strength. Z_1, Z_2, Z_3 are expressed as

$$Z_1 = \int_t^{t+\Delta t} \xi(t)\,dt = \sqrt{\Delta t}\, Y_1,$$

$$Z_2 = \int_t^{t+\Delta t} Z_1\,dt = {}^{3/2}\sqrt{\Delta t}\left(Y_1/2 + Y_2/2\sqrt{3}\right), \tag{2.40}$$

$$Z_3 = \int_t^{t+\Delta t} Z_2\,dt = \Delta t^2 \left(Y_1{}^2 + Y_3 + 1/2\right)/3,$$

where Y_1, Y_2, Y_3 are three uncorrelated standard Gaussian variables.

We calculate the magnitude of the vdW force, the Casimir force, and the electrostatic force with the feature parameters of myosin motor in Table 2.1.

2.2.2.2.1   The Hamaker Constants A_{102} and B_{102}

Generally, there are two approaches that have been used to calculate the Hamaker constant. The first, based on its definition, depends on the atom densities n_1, n_2 and the potential coefficient C. The second approach, based on the Lifshitz theory, is much more widely used. Taking the dielectric permittivities of two materials as ε_1, ε_2, the non-retarded Hamaker constant A_{12} in vacuum can be written as [51]

$$A_{12} \approx \frac{3hv_c}{8\sqrt{2}} \frac{(\varepsilon_1 - 1)(\varepsilon_2 - 1)}{\left(\sqrt{\varepsilon_1} + 1\right)\left(\sqrt{\varepsilon_2} + 1\right)\left(\sqrt{\varepsilon_1 + 1} + \sqrt{\varepsilon_2 + 1}\right)}, \tag{2.41}$$

where the Planck's constant $h = 6.626 \times 10^{34}$ J, the dielectric permittivity of the protein is 2.5–4 [52], the absorption wavelength $\lambda_c = 125$–280 nm [53], the Hamaker constant in a vacuum is

TABLE 2.1
Feature Parameters of Myosin Motor [19,20]

kT	c	a	L	r_2	γ	m_1	ε_0	q_1	q_2
4.1 pN nm	8.25 nm	3.25 nm	1,600 nm	3.5 nm	75 pN ns/nm	3.65×10^{22} kg	80	$5.5 \times 1.6 \times 10^{19}$ C	$3.5 \times 1.6 \times 10^{19}$ C

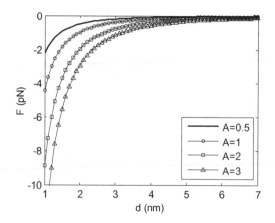

FIGURE 2.23 The vdW force for different values of A_{102} (10^{20} J).

$A_{12} = (3.2–16) \times 10^{-20}$ J. If the proteins are in the solvent, water then the Hamaker constant can be calculated as

$$A_{102} = \left(\sqrt{A_{12}} - \sqrt{A_{00}} \right)^2, \tag{2.42}$$

where A_{00} represents the Hamaker constant of water which is 5.5×10^{20} J.

Therefore, the Hamaker constant of the protein in water is $A_{102} = (0.5–3) \times 10^{20}$ J. Afshar-Rad et al. [54] estimated the Hamaker constant for protein films across water in the range of $(1.0–2.2) \times 10^{20}$ J, and Fernandez-Varea et al. [55] calculated the Hamaker constant of protein as $3.1kT$ (0.74×10^{20} J, $T = 293$ K). Our theoretical result falls within the range of these experimental results. As a consequence, the Hamaker constant is often treated as an adjustable parameter. Figure 2.23 shows the relationship of the vdW force and the distance between the two protein surfaces for different values of A_{102}.

The Casimir effect is likely to occur at relatively large distances. Based on the definitions of A_{102} and B_{102}, the ratio of the retarded Hamaker constant B_{102} and the non-retarded Hamaker constant A_{102} is $B_{102}/A_{102} = 23\lambda_c/60\pi^3$, the absorption wavelength λ_c is in the range of 125–280 nm so that from Eq. (2.34), $B_{102} = (0.075–0.72) \times 10^{28}$ J m. The Casimir force for different values of the retarded Hamaker constant is shown in Figure 2.24.

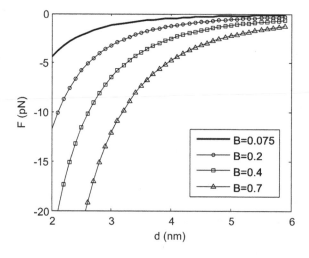

FIGURE 2.24 The Casimir force under different values of B_{102} (10^{28} J m).

2.2.2.3 Monte Carlo Simulation

We have developed a Monte Carlo method to simulate the dynamics of the myosin motor in solution that enables us to analyze the contributions of the vdW force, the Casimir force, and the electrostatic force to the motor motion during thermal fluctuations.

Using a simulation motor number of $N = 100$ and $\Delta t = 0.01$ ns and from a starting state where $d = 6$ nm, we found that the distance of the motor motion reduces from 6 to 3 nm within 1 ns when the Casimir force and electrostatic force are considered (Figure 2.25). The Casimir force and the electrostatic force independently affect the myosin motor. The Casimir force lasts for more than 9 ns, while the electrostatic force acts for only 1.8 ns. Thus, at these distances, the electrostatic force plays a more important role than the Casimir force.

With the simulation number $N = 100$ and $\Delta t = 0.01$ ns and from a starting state where $d = 3$ nm, the interaction forces to be considered include the vdW force and the electrostatic force. As shown in Figure 2.26, the distance between the myosin motor and actin quickly decreases from 3 nm to zero indicating that the myosin has become attached to the binding site of actin. Comparing the contributions of the two forces to the myosin motor, the vdW force acts for nearly 1.8 ns, whereas the electrostatic force lasts for only 0.5 ns, showing that the electrostatic force continues to be the main contributor to the motion of the myosin motor.

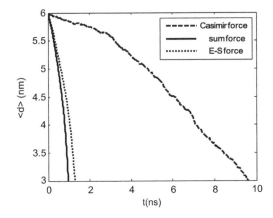

FIGURE 2.25 Dynamics of the myosin motor binding to actin considering the Casimir force and the electrostatic force.

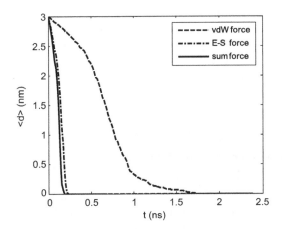

FIGURE 2.26 Dynamics of myosin motor binding to actin considering the vdW force and the electrostatic force.

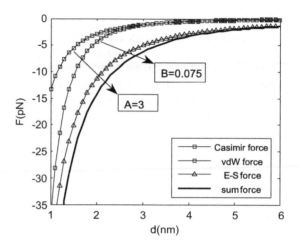

FIGURE 2.27 The interaction forces for myosin and actin.

Figure 2.27 shows the crossover point for the vdW and Casimir forces, when the maximum value of A_{102} is 3 and the minimum value for B_{102} is 0.075. This point indicates the position ($d = 3$ nm) at which the Casimir effect comes into play. If the distance is larger than 3 nm, then the vdW force falls into the Casimir force. When the distance exceeds 3 nm, the Casimir force is lower than 1 pN. The active attractive forces in proteins during the binding process consist of the sum of the vdW force (vdW force), the Casimir force, and the electrostatic force (E-S force) (Figure 2.27). The active forces increase quickly as the distance between the surfaces is reduced. We have shown that when the distance is larger than 3 nm, the attractive forces include both the electrostatic force and the Casimir force and when the distance is smaller than 3 nm, the attractive forces are the electrostatic force and the vdW force. When the distance is smaller than 3 nm, the forces total more than 10 pN. When the distance is between 1 and 3 nm, the forces range from 10 to 35 pN. Nakajima et al. [56] used AFM to measure the interaction force during the binding process and found it to be in the range of (18.4 ± 4–24.7 ± 1.4) pN. Our calculations agree with their experimental data. Although they pointed out that there were other forces besides the electrostatic force involved in this process, they did not discuss this further. In our study, we pay particular attention to the contributions of the vdW and Casimir forces on the binding process. Liu et al. [57] carried out molecular dynamics (MD) simulations of the protein–protein interactions in actin–myosin binding and concluded that, as result of the balance between the favorable vdW and electrostatic interactions and the unfavorable desolvation effect, the overall interaction energy was attractive. They found that the magnitude of the electrostatic interaction was approximately four times larger than the dispersion contribution, dominating the total attractive interactions. We find from our calculations that the electrostatic force is 3–4 times greater than the vdW force, agreeing with the earlier findings. This result supports our choice of Hamaker constants for the vdW and Casimir forces.

2.2.3 The 4M Model of Muscular Contraction

2.2.3.1 Modeling of Sarcomere Activation

2.2.3.1.1 *SR Activated by Action Potential*

When the Ca^{2+} channel is opened by the stimulation of AP on SR, Ca^{2+} is released from SR to sarcoplasmic (SP); meanwhile, the return of Ca^{2+} to SR is controlled by a calcium pump. There are two kinds of Ca^{2+} concentration, one is the concentration in SR, represented as $[Ca^{2+}]_{SR}$, the other is the concentration in SP, represented as $[Ca^{2+}]_{SP}$. The rate of change of $[Ca^{2+}]_{SP}$ mainly as a result of Ca^{2+} release from and return to the SR can be represented as [58]

$$\begin{cases} \dfrac{d\left[Ca^{2+}\right]_{SP}}{dt} = v_{rel} - v_{pump}, \\[3mm] v_{rel} = k_{rel}\left[Ca^{2+}\right]_{SR}, \\[3mm] v_{pump} = \dfrac{f_m\left[Ca^{2+}\right]_{sp}}{\left[Ca^{2+}\right]_{sp} + n_{ca}}, \end{cases} \tag{2.43}$$

where v_{pump} is the calcium pump velocity and v_{rel} is the diffusion velocity, f_m is the maximum pumping velocity, and n_{ca} is the calcium concentration at pumping rate $0.5\,f_m$. k_{rel} represents the diffusion rate of Ca^{2+} from SR, which mainly depends on the AP n_a and stimulation frequency v. The period of AP $T = 1/v$, because all Ca^{2+} channels on SR will be opened by single stimulation; the dwell time is t_0. We define k_{rel} as

$$k_{rel}(t) = \begin{cases} k' & (n_a - 1)T \leq t < (n_a - 1)T + t_0 \\[2mm] 0 & (n_a - 1)T + t_0 \leq t < n_a T \end{cases}, \quad n_a = 1, 2, \ldots \tag{2.44}$$

k_{rel} can be transformed into the function of stimulation frequency:

$$k_{rel}(v) = \begin{cases} k' t_0 v & t_0 \leq T \\[2mm] k' & T < t_0 \end{cases}, \tag{2.45}$$

where k' is the rate constant of Ca^{2+} from SR, which mainly depends on the Ca^{2+}-channel density on SR.

2.2.3.1.2 Ca^{2+} Dynamics

According to the physiological characteristic of skeletal muscle, each Tn has four Ca^{2+} binding sites; after the Tn is attached with two Ca^{2+}, a conformational change takes place on tropomyosin (Tm); myosin motors begin to work and make the sarcomere contract [59]. We use $A \cdot T$, $A \cdot TCa$, $A \cdot TCa_2$ to signify the states of Tn with none, one, and two Ca^{2+} with the probabilities being q_0, q_1, and q_2, respectively. These parameters satisfy the chemical reaction kinetics [25]:

$$\begin{cases} \dot{q}_1 = k_0\left[Ca^{2+}\right]_{sp} q_0 - k_{-0} q_1, \\[2mm] \dot{q}_2 = k_1\left[Ca^{2+}\right]_{sp} q_1 - k_{-1} q_2, \\[2mm] q_0 + q_1 + q_2 = 1, \end{cases} \tag{2.46}$$

where k_0, k_{-0}, k_1, and k_{-1} are the rate constants of Ca^{2+} binding and unbinding to $A \cdot T$, $A \cdot TCa$. The probability q_2 of the state $A \cdot T \cdot Ca_2$ in steady condition can be solved with Eq. (2.4), which is represented as

$$\beta = \frac{\left[Ca^{2+}\right]_{sp}^2}{\left[Ca^{2+}\right]_{sp}^2 + \left[Ca^{2+}\right]_{sp} k_{-1}/k_1 + k_{-0}k_{-1}/k_0 k_1}. \tag{2.47}$$

Sarcomere will contract after two Ca^{2+} bind to Tn. β is described as the activation degree of sarcomere, which is the function of $[Ca^{2+}]_{SP}$. From Eqs. (2.1) and (2.3), we can calculate $[Ca^{2+}]_{SP}$ with a stimulation frequency. So the activation degree β can be calculated with Eq. (2.47).

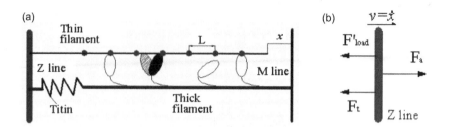

FIGURE 2.28 (a) A simplified structure of half-sarcomere; (b) forces on Z line.

2.2.3.2 Modeling of Sarcomere Contraction

Sarcomere contraction is the cooperative action of myosin motors sliding on actin filaments by hydrolyzing ATP. Here we mainly analyze the influence of active potential on motors' collective behavior. A simple modeling process is illustrated as follows. As shown in Figure 2.28a, a half-sarcomere is analyzed. The total number of myosin motors in a thick filament is n_0; the distance between two binding sites on a thin filament is L. There are N states in a working cycle for a myosin motor; after the sarcomere is activated by AP, Z line is close to M line by the conformational change of myosin motors. Let x be the state variable as the displacement of bound motor along the thin filament and $\rho_i(x, t)$ be the probability density that the mth motor at position x is in occupancy state i at time t. Myosin motor jumps from one binding site to the next with the distance L during each enzymatic cycle.

2.2.3.2.1 Dynamics Model of Z Line

As shown in Figure 2.28b, forces on Z line include the active force F_a produced by the attached motors on thin filament, elasticity force F_t produced by titin, and load F_{load}. In nanoscale, the dynamics of Z line can be described by Langevin equation:

$$m_z \ddot{x}(t) + \gamma_z \dot{x}(t) = F_a - F_t - F'_{load} + \sqrt{2\gamma_z k_B \varepsilon_d(t)}, \qquad (2.48)$$

where m_z is the mass of Z line, γ_z is the drag coefficient which is proportional to the size of Z line, $\gamma_z = 6\pi\eta r_z$, η is viscosity coefficient of water, and r_z is the radius of Z line. k_B is the Boltzmann constant and T is the absolute temperature. $\varepsilon(t)$ is Gaussian white noise. According to the geometrical size of Z line, $m_z/\gamma_z \ll 1$ ns; the Z line is in an overdamped solvent. Considering the size effect in nanoscale, we neglect the influence of inertia; besides, Z lines are connected with each other; Brownian force is also neglected. Equation (2.48) can be simplified as

$$\gamma_z \dot{x}(t) = F_a - F_t - F'_{load}. \qquad (2.49)$$

2.2.3.2.2 Passive Force in Sarcomere System

Because of the nonlinear viscoelastic character of sarcomere, the passive force includes the damping force and elastic force:

$$F_p = A_z \sigma_t + \gamma_z \dot{x} = k_t \Delta x + \gamma_z \dot{x}, \qquad (2.50)$$

where A_z is the cross-sectional area of a sarcomere, σ_t is the nonlinear elasticity stress of titin, k_t is elasticity coefficient of titin, and Δx is the contraction length of sarcomere.

We define the passive stress as

$$\sigma_p = \sigma_t + 6\eta \dot{x}/r_z. \qquad (2.51)$$

2.2.3.2.3 Active Force in Sarcomere System

The active force of sarcomere contraction is the sum of actions of attached motors on the thin filament [11]:

$$F_a = \frac{A_z \alpha \beta n_0 c}{s} \int_0^L x \rho(x,t) \, dx, \tag{2.52}$$

where c is the elasticity coefficient of myosin head, α is the overlap degree between thin and thick filaments. β is activation degree of sarcomere. s is the area of a thick filament and six thin filaments. A_z/s means the number of thick filament in a sarcomere. $\langle x \rangle = \int_0^L x \rho(x,t) \, dx$ is the first-order moment of variable x, meaning the average displacement on the thin filament of all myosin motors in the thick filament. We define the active stress as

$$\sigma_a = \frac{\alpha \beta n_0 c}{s} \langle x \rangle. \tag{2.53}$$

According to non-equilibrium statistical mechanics, $\rho_i(x, t)$ satisfies the Fokker–Planck equation:

$$\frac{\partial \rho_i}{\partial t} = \frac{D}{k_B T} \frac{\partial}{\partial x} \left[\left(\frac{\partial V_i}{\partial x} - F_e \right) \rho_i \right] + D \frac{\partial^2 \rho_i}{\partial x^2} + \sum_{j=1}^N k_{ij} \rho_j.$$

The constraint condition of probability density is given by

$$\rho(0,t) = \rho(L,t) = 0, \quad \int_0^L \rho(x,t) \, dx = 1. \tag{2.54}$$

Equation (2.54) is the rate equation of probability density $\rho_i(x, t)$, where k_{ij} is the transition rate from state i to state j. The diffusion coefficient $D = k_B T/\gamma_m$, γ_m is the radius of motor, and $V_i(x, t)$ is the active potential energy in state i along x direction. Different from the Huxley rate equation, this equation takes into account the load force F_e and reflects N states of working cycle of molecular motor; thereby this model can be used to calculate the active force produced by a sarcomere.

With Eqs. (2.51) and (2.53), the main stress of a sarcomere is given by

$$\sigma = \sigma_a - \sigma_p. \tag{2.55}$$

This equation reflects the active contraction and passive stretch characteristics of a sarcomere. The factors that influence the muscle force include load, [ATP], $[Ca^{2+}]_{SP}$, and the intrinsic elasticity of myosin motor and titin. Because $[Ca^{2+}]_{SP}$ mainly depends on the stimulation frequency and the dwell time of AP, the contraction force is determined by AP with a given load and [ATP].

2.2.3.3 Sarcomere in Series and in Parallel

In order to obtain the macroscopic characteristics of skeletal muscle, the function of sarcomeres arranged in series and in parallel need to be discussed. As is shown in Figure 2.29, muscle fiber is composed of m_p myofibrils in parallel, and each myofibril contains m_q sarcomeres in series.

2.2.3.3.1 Sarcomeres in Series

Each sarcomere has the same length and motors in a myofibril; the force is equal on the section of sarcomere; and the stress is also equivalent:

$$\sigma_1 = \sigma_2 = \cdots \sigma_g \cdots = \sigma_{m_q}. \tag{2.56}$$

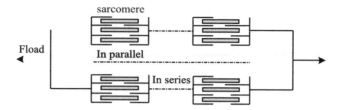

FIGURE 2.29   Sarcomeres in series and in parallel.

1. **Myofibril stretching**: If the force on the myofibril is F'_{load} and the stretching length of a sarcomere is $\Delta x_{\text{g}} = F'_{\text{load}}/k_{\text{t}}$, then the total stretching length of myofibril is equal to $m_{\text{q}}\Delta x_{\text{g}}$ and total elastic stiffness is $k_{\text{q}} = k_{\text{t}}/m_{\text{q}}$.
2. **Myofibril contraction**: If all sarcomeres in a myofibril are activated by pulses under a certain load, then the contraction length of each sarcomere in steady state is $\Delta x_{\text{g}} = \left(F_{\text{a}} - F'_{\text{load}}\right)/k_{\text{t}}$ and total contraction length is $m_{\text{q}}\Delta x_{\text{g}}$. The contraction length and velocity are proportional to the number of sarcomeres in series, while muscle force is constant between each sarcomere.

2.2.3.3.2   Myofibrils in Parallel

The total stress of a muscle fiber is the sum of the stresses of each myofibril:

$$\sigma_{\text{T}} = \sum_{n=1}^{m_{\text{p}}} \sigma_{\text{n}}. \tag{2.57}$$

1. **Muscle fiber stretching**: If each myofibril has the same load, then the passive elastic stiffness of muscle fiber is $k_{\text{m}} = m_{\text{p}}k_{\text{t}}/m_{\text{q}}$.
2. **Muscle fiber contraction**: If all sarcomeres are activated, then load force on muscle fiber in steady state is equal to contraction force $F_{\text{load}} = m_{\text{p}}A_{\text{z}}\sigma_{\text{n}}$. The contraction force, proportional to the cross-sectional area of myofibril in parallel, is m_{p} times larger than single myofibril in muscle fiber.

2.2.3.4   Generalization to the Macroscopic Model

To describe the active contraction and passive stretching characteristics of skeletal muscle, a simplified structure of the muscle model proposed in this section is illustrated in Figure 2.30, which takes into account the influence of load, [ATP], and AP on muscle force. It is basically a variation of the Hill-type model [4], but we consider the actual molecular structure of muscle. The active force F_{a}^{m} is produced by the collective behavior of myosin motors; the passive force F_{p}^{m} is induced by the intrinsic elasticity of titin and water dumping.

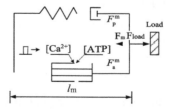

FIGURE 2.30   A simplified structure of skeletal muscle model. The contractile element models the myosin motors working on thin filament; the parallel element models the titin and other connective tissue in the muscle fibers; the muscle length is l_{m}.

2.2.3.4.1   Contraction Force

The contraction force is composed of active force F_a^m and passive force F_p^m. A mechanical model is given by

$$\begin{cases} F_m = F_a^m - F_p^m \\[2mm] F_a^m = \dfrac{A\alpha\beta n_0 c}{s} \displaystyle\int_0^L x\rho(x,t)\,dx, \\[2mm] F_p^m = k_m \Delta l_m + \gamma v \end{cases} \qquad (2.58)$$

where A is the cross sectional area of all muscle fibers, β is the activation degree of muscle, the drag coefficient $\gamma = 6\pi\eta r$, r is the radius of cross section, $A = \pi r^2$, and the elasticity coefficient of muscle $k_m = m_p k_t / m_q$.

2.2.3.4.2   Contraction Velocity

Contraction velocity of sarcomere is the average velocity of Z line related to M line, which mainly depends on the velocity of myosin motors on thin filament:

$$v_s = \frac{d\langle x(t)\rangle}{dt} = \frac{d}{dt}\frac{1}{n_0}\sum_{m=1}^{n_0} x_m(t). \qquad (2.59)$$

Contraction velocity of skeletal muscle is the contraction length divided by contraction time while contraction length is the sum of each sarcomere contraction length:

$$v = \Delta l_m / \Delta t = m_q \Delta x_g / \Delta t = m_q v_s. \qquad (2.60)$$

2.2.3.4.3   Contraction Power

Contraction power is the product of contraction velocity and contraction force.

$$W = F_m v. \qquad (2.61)$$

In sum, we have established a mathematical model for skeletal muscle in the activation and contraction process. Given the elasticity coefficient, [ATP], external force, and other structure parameters, we can calculate the contraction force, velocity, and power with the stimulation frequency of AP.

2.2.3.5   Numerical Analysis and Simulation

A motor unit is a single α-motor neuron combining with all of the corresponding muscle fibers, all of which will be the same type (either fast twitch or slow twitch). When a motor unit is activated, all fibers will contract. Now we study the properties of muscle fibers in a motor unit. The cross-sectional area of muscle fibers is $1\,cm^2$; the length is $5\,cm$; the physical parameters of skeletal muscle are shown in Table 2.2.

2.2.3.5.1   Calcium Ion Concentration in SP

$[Ca^{2+}]_{SR}$ is near $1{,}500\,\mu M$, and $[Ca^{2+}]_{SP}$ is about $0.1\,\mu M$ in the physiological resting state. The duration t_0 of single AP depends on the properties of motor unit. If t_0 is equal to 2 ms, the maximum frequency of AP is 500 Hz. $[Ca^{2+}]_{SP}$ is calculated under a single stimulation in Figure 2.31. Ca^{2+} is released from the SR to SP; $[Ca^{2+}]_{SP}$ increases quickly to the maximum value $1.6\,\mu M$, and if the stimulation stops, Ca^{2+} in SP is pumped back into SR due to closed Ca^{2+} channels. $[Ca^{2+}]_{SP}$ gradually reduces to the resting value.

TABLE 2.2
Parameters of Skeletal Muscle [13,19,20,22]

r_m	γ_m	$k_B T$	s	n_0
3.5 nm	75 pN ns/nm	4.1 pN nm	1.374×10^3 nm^2	150
c	L	D	n_{ca}	k'
0.7 pN/nm	36 nm	5.47×10^7 nm^2/s	2 μM	0.32 μM^{-2}s^{-1}
k_0	k_{-0}	k_1	k_{-1}	f_m
1.77×10^8 M^{-1}s^{-1}	1,544 s^{-1}	0.885×10^8 M^{-1}s^{-1}	17.1 s^{-1}	280 μM^{-1}s^{-1}

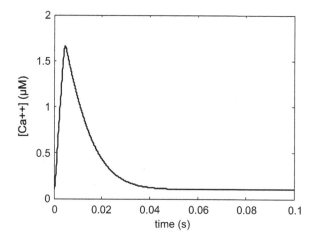

FIGURE 2.31 $[Ca^{2+}]_{SP}$ in single stimulation.

Figure 2.32 shows the change of $[Ca^{2+}]_{SP}$ at different frequencies of AP. With a low frequency of 10 Hz, the change of $[Ca^{2+}]_{SP}$ repeats 10 times in 1 s and reduces to the resting value before the next stimulation. When the frequency is added to 100 Hz, the peak value fluctuates around 2 μM. With a high frequency of 500 Hz, the period of AP is equal to the duration, and Ca^{2+} channels are

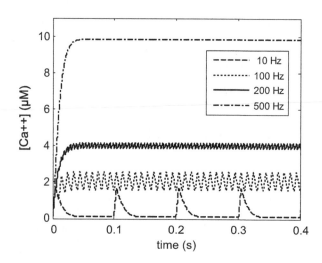

FIGURE 2.32 $[Ca^{2+}]_{SP}$ at different stimulation frequencies (frequencies = 10, 100, 200, and 500 Hz).

always opened. $[Ca^{2+}]_{SP}$ increases quickly into the maximum $10\,\mu M$. The change of $[Ca^{2+}]_{SP}$ from 0.1 to $10\,\mu M$ is the same as the physiological condition, which illuminates the reasonableness of the activation model.

2.2.3.5.2 Contraction Force

Because of the myofibril in parallel, the maximum isometric active force is proportional to the cross-sectional area of muscle fibers. Ikai [60] calculated the isometric contraction muscle strength per unit cross-sectional area in the range of 40–100 N/cm² by means of ultrasonic measurement. 1 cm² muscle fibers contain approximately 7.28×10^{10} thick filaments. When load force on muscle is 22 N, the average load on each molecular motor is about 2 pN if α is equal to one. With Eq. (2.52), we calculate the maximum active force of muscle fibers to be 56.4 N, which is in the range of experimental data. Using the ratio of active force to maximum force F_a/F_{max} as the vertical axis, we obtain the relation of ratio and stimulation frequency, as shown in Figure 2.33. The active force increases with the increasing stimulation frequency and reaches the maximum when frequency is over 400 Hz. This sigmoid curve can be proved in the future.

Active forces at different frequencies are shown in Figure 2.34. A twitch contraction takes place at frequency 1 Hz, the muscle force first increases then decreases to zero. The dwell time is about

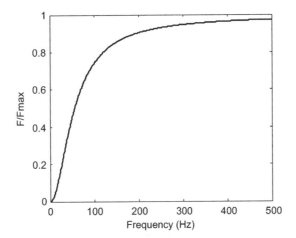

FIGURE 2.33 Active force vs. stimulation frequency.

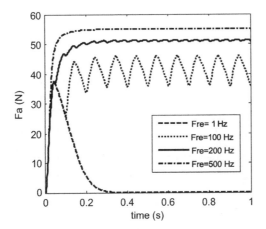

FIGURE 2.34 Four curves representing active forces at different stimulation frequencies (frequencies = 1, 100, 200, and 500 Hz).

50 ms, longer than the time of Ca^{2+} concentration. This phenomenon is due to the process of Ca^{2+} binding to Tn and myosin motors attaching to thin filament. If the frequency continues to increase, summation of muscle contraction will happen. With a high frequency of 500 Hz, the muscle reaches the peak force, resulting in a tetanic contraction.

2.2.3.5.3 Contraction Velocity

Similarly, the relationship between the AP and contraction velocity is shown in Figure 2.35. A sarcomere is 2.5 μm long, which means a 5 cm muscle fiber contains 2×10^4 sarcomeres. Given $F_{load} = 22$ N, [ATP] =10 μM in SR, we can find that the contraction velocity increases rapidly with the increasing frequency. Velocity reaches the max value of about 2.37 cm/s at the frequency 500 Hz. Figure 2.36 shows the change of contraction velocity for different load forces under 500 Hz; contraction velocity decreases with the increasing load force. When the load is greater than 55 N, contraction velocity reduces to zero.

2.2.3.5.4 Contraction Power

The relation between contraction power, stimulation frequency, and load is shown in Figure 2.37. The power reaches the maximum value when the load force is 21 N and reduces to zero when the load reaches the maximum. The power also increases with the increasing of frequency, reaching the peak value at the highest frequency. According to the characteristics of sarcomeres in series and

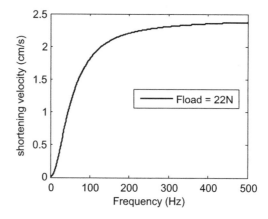

FIGURE 2.35   Contraction velocity vs. stimulation frequency.

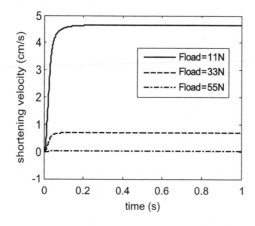

FIGURE 2.36   Velocities for different loads (F_{load} = 11, 33, 55 N).

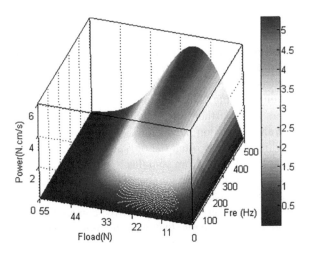

FIGURE 2.37 Contraction power vs. frequency and load.

in parallel, the muscle output power is proportional to its total volume. These features have been confirmed in muscle's physiological experiment [61].

2.2.4 THE NEW SEMIPHENOMENOLOGICAL MODEL OF SARCOMERE

In a general sense, the goals of a biomechanical model for muscular contraction include two aspects. The first aspect is a theoretical explanation of the experimental phenomena or data. The most representative models include Hill's model (heat and energy transformation) [1], Huxley's model (chemical state transition) [3], the Brownian ratchet model (statistical thermodynamics) [39], etc. The second aspect is providing theoretical guidance and a framework for biomechanical or biomedical engineering on the musculoskeletal system, e.g., locomotion, exercise, and rehabilitation [62–64]. According to these aims, an ideal biomechanical model needs to be not only consistent with the experiments but also suitable for practical engineering purposes. The former requirement is rather basic because a model must first yield an acceptable descriptive accuracy, which is exactly the prime topic of most studies in this field.

As is well recognized, muscular contraction is a highly complex mechanochemical process ranging from the generation of APs by a motoneuron and the release of myoplasmic calcium to the final relative sliding of thin and thick filaments. Due to the remarkable nonlinear features of these links, in order to precisely reproduce the corresponding chemical or mechanical responses, nonlinear schemes and partial differential equations are commonly employed in the models. For example, Markov models [65,66] have been applied in the analysis of the open probability of calcium channels dominated by membrane excitation. Very detailed Markov schemes and a multi-compartment model [25] have been proposed to describe the homeostasis of intracellular $[Ca^{2+}]$, taking into account the Ca^{2+} release and uptake by the SR, and the buffering effect of Tn, adenosine triphosphate (ATP), parvalbumin, Ca^{2+} pump, etc. A local control model [11] of the ECC in skeletal muscle was built by formulating the kinetics of ryanodine receptors (RyRs) and dihydropyridine channels (DHPR) with four-state and ten-state models, respectively, as well as the mechanism of calcium-induced calcium release [21]. However, the exploration of working kinetics of the active element or myosin motor has always been a key part of biomechanical modeling of skeletal muscle. Presently, the most prevalent paradigm is the Huxley's cross-bridge scheme, while disputes continue around how many chemical states are exactly involved in the phosphorylation cycle of a myosin motor. Consequently, a variety of models consisting of two states [67], five states [68], or even up to 18 states have been proposed [69], while Zahalak et al. [70] argued that a two-state model is an asymptotic limit of multi-state ones. In spite of the complexity of the states, the transitions among them are further described by partial differential equations of time and the binding position of the motor on the actin filament. With the emphasis on accuracy, the models have become increasingly complicated and contain many internal state variables and parameters, most of which are not observable or measurable. Such complexity has caused great difficulty for these models to be applied to practical engineering, which often requires fast prediction, real-time control, and self-learning of parameters [71]. Furthermore, engineering applications usually require a model to provide the dynamic transfer relation between the stimulus signal and the mechanical output (like force and length), which are very often the only measurable quantities. However, a precise multi-state model for a single link (e.g., from stimulus to myoplasmic [Ca^{2+}]) may cost many minutes and billions of iterations for a desktop computer to generate the objective response of only one second. Thus, it is almost impossible for the aforementioned models to be used in applications such as dynamic force prediction or estimation or the control of exoskeletons for active limb rehabilitation. Furthermore, it is undeniable that even the most detailed model remains unable to precisely describe all the features of a link in muscular contraction because of the highly flexible and time-varying properties of biological systems. For instance, the modeling parameters for a specific muscle would soon deviate from the initial parameters because of fatigue or potentiation after only a few cycles of contractions. Thus, the engineering performance of these models would be severely limited if the possibility exists that they may become inaccurate after a short period of application. Furthermore, the nonlinear reidentification of the parameters is also a costly computation project. That the improvement of a model's accuracy must be based on the cost of its engineering value remains to be an embarrassing situation.

In order to solve the above dilemma, empirical models [72–75] with greatly improved usability have been proposed based on electromechanical approximations. These pioneering works provided significant inspiration for the mechanical abstraction of biological systems; while some of the models are still complicated in computational structure with numerous parameters, others might completely discard the biological mechanisms or become purely phenomenological approximations. As a result, the models are either quasi-static with insufficient capability to account for the smooth transitions among various contraction modes or are too simplified to be satisfactorily accurate. An efficient, dynamic, and comprehensive model for muscular contraction remains to be established. In effect, it is unnecessary for a practical model to pursue very high absolute precision, which is difficult even for detailed biophysical models. Nevertheless, a model competent for engineering applications must be able to correctly reproduce the following aspects of muscle: (1) the activation kinetics, (2) isotonic contraction transients and the force–velocity (F–V) relationship, and (3) the dynamic effect of shortening/lengthening velocity on the force kinetics of myosin motors and the length-control mode responses because it has been verified that the error of Hill's model is the largest during movement [76]. In short, the model must agree well with basic facts and trends of mechanical responses of both active and passive elements under various conditions.

This section introduces a semiphenomenological model aiming at using concise structure, high efficiency, and comprehensive descriptive functions.

2.2.4.1 Modeling Principles

It is recognized that a half-sarcomere can be represented as the combination of an AE and several PEs [58]. Figure 2.38 shows the configuration adopted in this section. The AE characterizes the collective operation of myosin motors, together with their activation kinetics ignited by the stimulus. The PEs include the nonlinear viscoelasticity (P1) of titin [77] and the linear viscous drag (P2) in the cytoplasm. In some models, the elasticity of the thin filament in series with the AE is also considered [58,78,79], while in our scheme, the actin filament is regarded as rigid compared to other elements, referring to the arguments proposed by Huxley [80]. Because the mass of the sarcomere

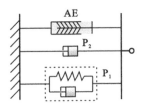

FIGURE 2.38 The mechanical configuration of a half-sarcomere in the semiphenomenological model.

can be neglected [81], the measured external force (F_{ext}), or the total muscle force, is always the summation of active (F_a) and passive (F_p) forces:

$$F_{ext} = F_a + F_p. \tag{2.62}$$

2.2.4.1.1 The AE

For a model aiming at complete descriptions, the working of the AE comprises two aspects: the kinetics of activation degree (β) and the force kinetics of myosin motors influenced by the relative sliding of thin and thick filaments. To facilitate parameter adjustment during application, the forces in the model are all expressed in the normalized form as the fraction of the tetanic plateau force at the optimal (slack) length of the sarcomere. Similar to the formulation in [82], the contractile force of the AE can then be defined as

$$F_a = \beta G(L)(1+\delta), \tag{2.63}$$

where the function $G(L)$ represents the tetanic force–length (L) relationship of the half-sarcomere, ranging from 0 to 1 at different L (see Appendix for the expression) and the variable δ denotes the fluctuation magnitude of F_a induced by sarcomere shortening or lengthening at tetanus state and slack length.

2.2.4.1.1.1 The Activation Kinetics From the perspective of biophysics, the activation degree of a half-sarcomere characterizes the proportion of working myosin motors bound to the actin filament. The influencing factors are abundant, such as the intracellular calcium kinetics and [ATP]. Nonetheless, [ATP] is neglected in this study because presently, neither fatigue nor long-term development are taken into account. Thereby, according to Eq. (2.2), β actually features the variation of the isometric contractile force at slack length under changing stimulus intensity (f), which represents the firing rate of the AP for a half-sarcomere. We define β and f as both normalized quantities ranging from 0 to 1, and β equals unity when the half-sarcomere is tetanized, while f is the ratio of the present stimulus rate and the maximum firing rate. The kinetics of β then characterize the ECC process and can be reflected by the tension development transients of a muscle fiber under end-held stimulation. The activation kinetics demonstrate the evident characteristics of a second-order system [75], as shown in Figure 2.39a. Although under artificial stimulating pulse trains the force transients of a bundle of muscle fibers are sawtooth-shaped (especially at low frequencies), here we only focus on the smoothed trends (dashed curves) because they bear practical engineering significance when large numbers of fibers are voluntarily excited within a muscle [83]. Another important feature is that the relationship between the plateau force, or saturated β (β_{st}), and the firing rate is not linear but can be fitted as an exponential curve as shown in Figure 2.39b:

$$\beta_{st} = 1 - \exp(-pf), \tag{2.64}$$

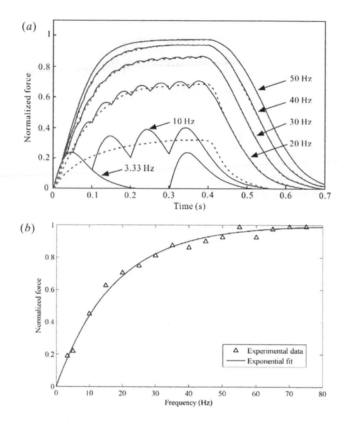

FIGURE 2.39 Activation kinetics represented by the isometric force of muscle. (a) The tension development and relax transients of a muscle under FES (functional electrical stimulation) of various frequencies. The dashed curves represent the smoothed trends; (b) the relationship between the stimulus frequency and the steady-state isometric force. Here, the fitting parameter p is 5.77. The plots of all the experimental data are modified from Ref. [22].

where p is a fitting parameter. Based on the above features, the activation kinetics can be modeled with a mass-spring–damping system (Figure 2.40), whose input "force" $P(f)$ is determined by the equilibrium condition with the steady-state position indicated by Eq. (2.64), and in this scheme, β is represented by the displacement of the mass. Thus, $P(f)$ has the form of

$$P(f) = k_1[1 - \exp(-pf)], \tag{2.65}$$

where k_1 denotes the stiffness of the spring. The transfer function of the system in Figure 2.40 is

$$TF_1 = \frac{Bet}{PF} = \frac{1/m}{s^2 + (b_1/m)s + k_1/m}, \tag{2.66}$$

where b_1 is the damping coefficient of the dashpot. Particularly, if we combine Eqs. (2.65) and (2.66), for the step input of $P(f)$, Bet can be expressed as

$$Bet = [1 - \exp(-pf)]\frac{K_1}{s^2 + B_1 s + K_1} \cdot \frac{1}{s}, \tag{2.67}$$

where $K_1 = k_1/m$, $B_1 = b_1/m$. Therefore, there are only two parameters (K_1 and B_1) left to be identified for the second-order system. According to Eq. (2.67), the transient of β under a specific f step can be written as

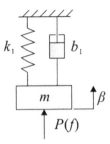

FIGURE 2.40 Schematic representation of the second-order system characterizing the activation kinetics.

$$\beta(t) = [1 - \exp(-pf)] \cdot \left[1 + \frac{T_1}{T_2 - T_1} \exp\left(-\frac{t}{T_1} \right) + \frac{T_2}{T_1 - T_2} \exp\left(-\frac{t}{T_2} \right) \right],$$ (2.68)

where $T_1 = 1 / \left[\omega_n \left(\xi - \sqrt{\xi^2 - 1} \right) \right]$, $T_2 = 1 / \left[\omega_n \left(\xi + \sqrt{\xi^2 - 1} \right) \right]$, $\omega_n = \sqrt{K_1}$, and $\xi = B_1 / \left(2\sqrt{K_1} \right)$.

The identification of T_1 and T_2 (or ξ and ω_n), which is equivalent to that of K_1 and B_1, can be implemented with the experimental data obtained under any f only if the p in Eq. (2.64) is known. Generally, the system parameters could be different during inactivation, or in the case when β declines, while for simplicity, we treat them as the same as those during activations in this study.

2.2.4.1.1.2 The Force Kinetics of the AE Affected by Velocity The AE force kinetics account for the fluctuation of the average motor force, which is caused by the shortening or lengthening of the sarcomere. A truly dynamic biomechanical model of skeletal muscle must be capable of reproducing or predicting the velocity or length transients at the force-control mode, analogous to the force-step experiments used to identify the force–velocity relationship of the muscle. In such cases, first, a muscle fiber is activated tetanically under the end-held condition until the steady-state force F_0 is reached; then, the system jumps to a smaller force ηF_0 ($\eta < 1$), which is maintained afterward. By monitoring the length change, a steady-state velocity is determined corresponding to this force. In the ubiquitous biophysical modeling of myosin motors from the perspective of mechanochemical coupling [68,84], the force kinetics of the AE are described by the evolvement of elastic deformation of the motor's neck region, which determines the magnitude of the force produced by one motor. This deformation is generally described by the probability density of a motor binding to the actin filament (the bound state) at the position x away from the equilibrium position. For multi-state models, other states may correspond to those defined in the Lymn–Taylor cycle [85]. Because a two-state model is an asymptotic limit of multi-state ones [70], here we take a two-state model as a representative case, as shown in Figure 2.41a. One state, $P(x, t)$, denotes the probability density of a motor bound at x at time t, and the other state, $D(x, t)$, stands for the probability of a motor being detached, so we have

$$\begin{cases} D(x,t) = 1 - P(x,t) \\ \left. \frac{\partial P(x,t)}{\partial t} \right|_x = r_1 - (r_2 + r_1) P(x,t) - v \left. \frac{\partial P(x,t)}{\partial x} \right|_t \end{cases},$$ (2.69)

where r_1 and r_2 denote the forward and backward transition rates of the motor between the detached and the attached states, respectively, and v is the relative sliding velocity between the thin and thick filaments (negative for shortening). Similar to Eq. (2.63), the force of the AE (F_{AE}) can be written as

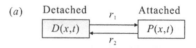

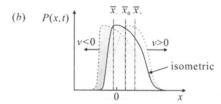

FIGURE 2.41   (a) Schematic representation of the two-state cross-bridge model; (b) the bias of the distribution of $P(x, t)$ and the mean deformation of a myosin motor under various sliding velocities.

$$F_{\mathrm{AE}} = \beta G(L) N_0 \left(\frac{1}{R} \int_R P(x,t)(k_{\mathrm{m}}x)\,dx \right), \tag{2.70}$$

where N_0 is the total number of the available myosin motors and k_{m} is the stiffness of an attached motor. Here, F_{AE} is in the dimension of force. The permitted range of x is denoted by R. The last term in the bracket of Eq. (2.70) represents the mean force of a motor, which is determined by the mean value of attached position $(\bar{x})$ because k_{m} can be regarded as a constant:

$$\bar{x} = \frac{1}{R} \int_R P(x,t)x\,dx \tag{2.71}$$

Another key issue in such models is the form of the transition rates, the definition of which is rather flexible and diverse. However, according to Boltzmann law, a consensual principle is that r_1 declines with the increasing magnitude of x, usually asymmetrically about the equilibrium position; i.e., it is easier for a motor to bind forward. As a result, $P(x, t)$ is often a bell-shaped distribution at the isometric steady state, as shown in Figure 2.41b. Thus, according to the form of the spatial differential term in Eqs. (2.69) and (2.71), the equivalent effect when a velocity v is present is that the distribution of $P(x, t)$ will be biased forward ($v > 0$) or backward ($v < 0$) (Figure 2.41b), leading to an increase or decrease in the mean deformation of the motor, which recovers when v returns to zero. Combining Eqs. (2.70) and (2.71), denoting the mean deformation at the tetanic isometric state as $\bar{x}_0$, the normalized force of the fully activated AE at slack length would be

$$\frac{\bar{x}}{\bar{x}_0} = \frac{\bar{x}_0 + \left(\bar{x} - \bar{x}_0\right)}{\bar{x}_0} = 1 + \delta. \tag{2.72}$$

It can be easily seen that Eq. (2.72) well coincides with Eq. (2.63). Through tetanic step release and stretch experiments, Huxley and Simmons [4] suggest that the AE is composed of two structural elements: an elastic element and a viscoelastic element in series. Palmer et al. [67] further argue that the mechanical behavior of the fully activated AE can be described by a serial spring-dashpot system (Figure 2.42) by sinusoidal analyses. For engineering applications, we are not concerned with the very rapid self-adjustment of the myosin motors (or the transition between weakly and strongly bound states); thus, we adopt the scheme in Figure 2.42 to describe the dynamics of δ under the effect of sliding velocity v. Then, the transfer function of this first-order system is

$$\mathrm{TF}_2 = \frac{\Delta}{V_v} = \frac{1}{s + k_2/b_2} = \frac{1}{s + 1/\tau}, \tag{2.73}$$

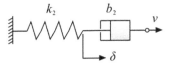

FIGURE 2.42 Schematic representation of the fluctuation kinetics of the AE's force.

where k_2 and b_2 represent the stiffness and damping coefficient, respectively, with τ denoting the time constant. It can be seen that only the identification of τ is necessary in practical applications. In essence, the system expressed by Eq. (2.73) is linear, while the force–velocity relationship of muscle characterized by Hill's equation is hyperbolic for shortening and is recognized as exponential for lengthening (Figure 2.43a):

$$\begin{cases} (F_{ext} + a)(V + b) = (1 + a)b, & V \leq 0 \\ F_{ext} = 1 + A[1 - \exp(-qV)], & V > 0 \end{cases}, \tag{2.74}$$

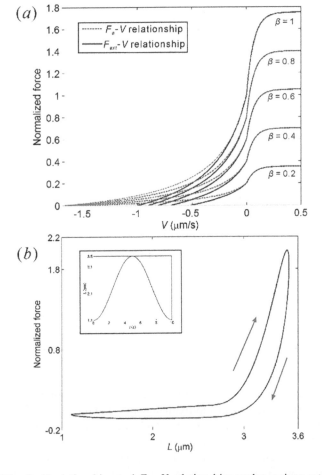

FIGURE 2.43 (a) The F_a–V relationships and F_{ext}–V relationships under various activation degrees. The values of the parameters describing the F_{ext}–V relationship at $\beta = 1$ are $a = 0.333$, $b = -0.333$, $A = 0.75$, $q = 15$, $b_c = 0.1$; (b) the viscoelastic force of P1 under the sinusoidal length change as indicated by the inset. The parameters involved are $c_1 = 0.04$, $c_2 = 2.4$, $c_3 = 2$, $L_1 = 2.6$.

where a, b, A, and q are all fitting parameters. Equation (2.75) accounts for the situation of isokinetic release or stretch of the tetanized half-sarcomere at the slack length.

As mentioned above, such relations are usually obtained by load-controlled step release experiments on muscle fibers. Consequently, to bridge the gap between the proposed linear scheme and the experimental results, we define the measurable velocity of the half-sarcomere as the external velocity (V). Correspondingly, the sliding (input) velocity v in the scheme of Figure 2.42 is defined as the internal velocity. Therefore, a transformation between V and v is needed according to the force–velocity relationship that features the steady-state condition. However, referring to the global mechanical scheme presented in Figure 2.38, the viscous drag force takes effect during the active isokinetic contraction of the sarcomere. Although some existent models [79] might have neglected this drag force, it is, however, the dominating limiting factor of the unloaded or maximum contraction velocity of a muscle fiber [80]. Because we attempt to establish a model compatible with the unloaded contraction mode, this drag force must be taken into account. Without losing generality, it can be regarded as linearly correlated with V during active shortening, while this drag force is assumed to be negligibly small when the muscle is stretched. This comes from the fact that during active lengthening experiments the measured force is recognized as invariant when V is positively large [81]. Then, the drag force F_v can be formulated as

$$F_v = \begin{cases} b_c V, & V \leq 0 \\ 0, & V > 0 \end{cases}, \tag{2.75}$$

where b_c denotes the drag coefficient. In addition, it is worth noting that the viscoelastic force of P1 (Figure 2.38) does not come into play when the sarcomere is at the optimal length [81]. Thus, under the isokinetic condition, we have

$$F_{ext} = F_a + F_v \tag{2.76}$$

Substituting Eq. (2.76) and Eq. (2.63) into Eq. (2.74), and combining the steady-state condition $\delta = v\tau$ of the system in Figure 2.42, the transformation from V to v can be expressed as

$$\begin{cases} v = \dfrac{1}{\tau}\left[(1+a)\left(\dfrac{b}{V+b} - 1\right) - b_c V\right], & V \leq 0 \\ v = \dfrac{A}{\tau_1}(1 - \exp(-qV)), & V > 0 \end{cases}, \tag{2.77}$$

where τ_1 is the time constant in Eq. (2.77) when the muscle is stretched and is often smaller than τ during shortening [86]. For practical convenience, all the velocities in the proposed model are expressed in the unit of μm/s.

Under different activation degrees or cytoplasmic [Ca^{2+}], many studies [87,88] suggest that the force–velocity relationship varies in an approximately linear manner; i.e., β acts like a scaling factor of the force–velocity curves, as shown in Figure 2.43a. Moreover, the maximum shortening velocity has been verified to decrease with smaller β. In our scheme, according to Eq. (12), the internal shortening velocities that make F_a approach zero are the same for different β (Figure 2.43a, dashed curves), while because of the presence of the drag force, the measured unloaded shortening velocities ($F_{ext} = 0$) are indeed positively correlated with β (Figure 2.43a, solid curves). In addition, when β falls to zero, F_a vanishes so that the mechanical property of the sarcomere automatically becomes purely passive.

2.2.4.1.2 The Passive Element

The passive element is composed of P1 and P2 (Figure 2.38), and the mechanical property of P2 has been formulated in the previous section. As for P1, the remarkable nonlinear viscoelastic features have been verified via relaxed sinusoidal stretch experiments [80]. An elaborate dynamic three-element pseudoplastic model for the passive characteristics of the whole fiber was proposed by Meyer et al. [89]. Because P1 does not include the viscoelasticity of the AE, here we adopt the simpler scheme that accounts for the parallel passive force of titin (F_{ve}) proposed by Denoth et al. [81]:

$$F_{ve} = f_1(L)f_2(V), \tag{2.78}$$

$$f_1(L) = \begin{cases} 0, & L < L_0 \\ c_1(L - L_0), & L_0 \le L \le L_1, \\ c_1(L - L_0) + c_2(L - L_1)^3, & L > L_1 \end{cases} \tag{2.79}$$

$$f_2(V) = \frac{2}{\pi}\arctan(c_3 V) + 1, \tag{2.80}$$

where $f_1(L)$ represents the nonlinear elastic response of titin and c_1, c_2, and L_1 are all fitting parameters, with L_0 denoting the slack length of the half-sarcomere (1.1 μm). The nonlinear function $f_2(V)$ characterizes the viscous feature of titin, and c_3 is also a fitting parameter. Equation (2.17) well describes the hysteretic response of a sarcomere under passive sinusoidal stretch–release cycles, as shown in Figure 2.43b. Therefore, at arbitrary conditions, the total passive force is

$$F_p = F_v + F_{ve}. \tag{2.81}$$

2.2.4.1.3 Configuration of Numerical Simulations

All the simulations were implemented in MATLAB® R2010a (The MathWorks, Natick, MA) with a desktop computer (64-bit architecture, dual-core CPU of 3.2 GHz, 2 GB memory). The time step was set to 1×10^{-6} s, which is sufficiently small for applications such as exoskeleton control or rehabilitation exercises. The fourth-order Runge–Kutta method was employed when solving the differential equations such as Eqs. (2.66) and (2.73). It is easy to verify that the whole model is globally stable because linear schemes are used for modeling the activation kinetics and the force kinetics of the AE, and all the possible inputs (f, L, V, or F_{ext}) must be finite values. All the parameter values of the model used during the simulations are listed in Table 2.3, and they were all fitted with relevant experimental data and implemented using the curve-fitting toolbox in MATLAB. The detailed identification processes are elucidated in the following sections.

TABLE 2.3

The values of parameters used in the simulation of the proposed model

Parameter	Value	Parameter	Value
p	5.77	K_1	1132.75
B_1 (s)	79.55	τ (ms)	15.3
τ_1 (ms)	7.6	a	0.33
b (μm/s)	−0.33	A	0.75
q (s/μm)	15	b_c (s/μm)	0.1
c_1 (μm^{-1})	0.04	c_2 (μm^{-3})	2.4
c_3 (μm^{-1})	2.6		

2.3 RESULTS

2.3.1 THE DEVELOPMENT OF ISOMETRIC FORCE

The simulation results of the isometric force transients under the step changes of the stimulus intensity of different magnitudes are demonstrated in Figure 2.44. Here, the involved parameters are fitted using the data at 50 Hz shown in Figure 2.39a, where the maximum stimulus frequency corresponding to $f = 1$ is assumed to be 80 Hz according to Figure 2.39b and the identified values of K_1 and B_1 are listed in Table 2.3. Figure 2.44 shows that during the force development phase, the predicted force transients coincide well with the experimental data. However, when the stimulus is stopped, the discrepancy between the simulated and experimental falling phase of the activation degree is evident, especially when f is large, because of the simplified assumption that the time constant of the deactivation is identical to that of the activation and is independent of the stimulus intensity. In this study, we are more concerned with the activation process, and during practical applications, the kinetic parameters can be easily identified by isometric contraction trials. The time needed for generating one data point during the simulation is approximately 0.58 µs.

2.3.2 ISOTONIC CONTRACTION AND THE FORCE–VELOCITY RELATIONSHIP

Here, we attempt to simulate the load-step experiments for the identification of the F–V relationship to investigate the predictive ability of the proposed model. First, a Hill-type F_{ext}–V curve is assumed (Figure 2.43a), referring to the experimental data of slow-type fibers [90]. The external velocity V is calculated with the instantaneous force equilibrium indicated by Eqs. (2.62) and (2.81), in which a step force of F_{ext} is applied and controlled, and the variation of F_a is computed by Eq. (2.73) with the internal velocity generated by Eq. (2.77) using the resulted V. Therefore, the numerical values of V and F_a are calculated iteratively, and the initial conditions are that the half-sarcomere is at the slack length with $F_{ext} = F_a = 1$ and $\beta \equiv 1$. The time constants τ and τ_1 in Eq. (2.73) are determined according to the force transients obtained by isokinetic release and stretch experiments [86]; hence, we set $V = -1$ µm/s, and it takes approximately 60 ms for the isometric plateau force to decrease by 98% of the steady-state δ. Moreover, when V is positive, it is assumed that $\tau_1 = 0.5\tau$. The length transients of the half-sarcomere under the force step ranging from −0.1 to −1 are illustrated in

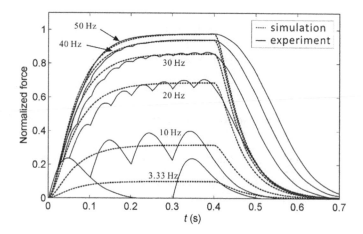

FIGURE 2.44 Simulation of the force transients under the isometric stimulations of various intensities. All the stimuli are applied at the start and stopped at 0.4 s.

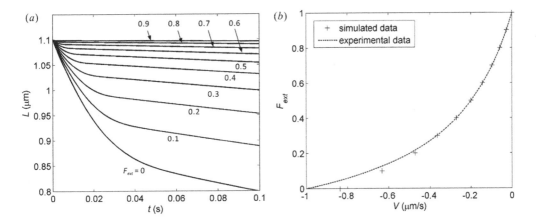

FIGURE 2.45 (a) The length transients of the half-sarcomere under the isotonic contractions with various magnitudes of force steps; (b) the comparison of the F_{ext}–V relationships between the simulated results and the experimental curve.

Figure 2.45a, and the plots of the simulated steady-state F_{ext}–V relation is shown in Figure 2.45b together with the experimental relation. The obtained length transients are consistent with the measured data [90] and the theoretical results deduced by the two-state model of the molecular motor [79]. Figure 2.45b shows that the simulated force–velocity relation agrees well with the experiment except at very small F_{ext} such as 0.1 and 0. This deviation is because under very rapid contractions, the sarcomere length is soon non-optimal and enters the ascending limb of the force–length relation (Figure 2.45b) when the velocity is stabilized. This indicates that it is difficult to precisely measure the force–velocity relation near the unloaded velocity, and such discrepancies are indeed common for experimental data and theoretical fitting. The time needed for a single iteration in the simulation is approximately 3.83 µs.

2.3.3 STEP-LENGTH CHANGE WITH FINITE VELOCITIES DURING ACTIVATION

To verify the numerical stability of the proposed model, successive contractile events were applied during the isometric force development phase, similar to the methods used in [78]. The half-sarcomere is tetanized from the resting state at $t = 0$ and at slack length; then it is stretched at $t = 0.15$ s with a velocity of 1 µm/s for 10 ms. Afterward, the half-sarcomere returns to the isometric state, until $t = 0.25$ s, when it is released with a velocity of -0.3 µm/s for 30 ms. It then returns to the isometric state. The stimulation is cancelled at $t = 0.4$ s. In order to implement the simulation, Eqs. (2.66) and (2.73) should be both involved. During the defined length changes, the force–length relation always stays at the plateau segment; thus, the function $G(L)$ is always unity. The predicted force transients (F_{ext}) are shown in Figure 2.46. The key trends agree well with the results generated by the myocybernetic control model proposed by Hatze [78], while some discrepancies are evident. The recovery processes of the responses after stretch or release are faster in the proposed model, and in our case, the falling phase of the force is also much faster when the stimulus is switched off. These differences originate from the fact that the activation and deactivation time constants are treated as equivalent in this study, and the choices of modeling schemes and time constants for the force kinetics affected by velocity are different. However, during practical predictions, the two models can be equally satisfactory through parameter adjustments, while the computational structure of the proposed model is much simpler. In this simulation, the length of time of a single iteration is approximately 0.69 µs.

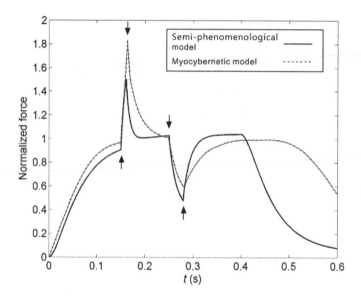

FIGURE 2.46 The force response of the half-sarcomere under the successive stretch and release at constant velocities during activation. The arrows indicate the time when the length ramps are applied or finished. The plot of experimental data is modified from Ref. [24].

2.3.4 Cyclic Contractions under Periodic Burst Activations

From the perspective of physiology, the most ubiquitous form of locomotion in the animal kingdom is cyclic motions of limbs, e.g., running (leg), swimming (fin), or flying (wing). Therefore, a significant contraction behavior of muscle is the cyclic contraction driven by a periodic stimulus, which is usually the burst firing of the AP for mammalians. The mechanical power output for such contractions has been extensively studied [91], showing that the cyclic power is affected by complex factors like cycle frequency, excursion amplitude, and timing of the stimulation. To further test the effectiveness and the robustness of the proposed model, we attempt to reproduce the force responses under sinusoidal length changes and a periodic stimulus and investigate whether the periodic orbit formed by plotting the force against length is consistent with the experimental results. Because all the variables (f, β, F_{ext}, L, and V) are dynamically fluctuating in this case, this simulation is a more comprehensive evaluation of the model.

The frequency of the length cycle is fixed at 1 Hz, and the excursion amplitude is set to be 4% L_0 (0.044 µm), which falls in the reasonable range (2.3%–7.3%) of the amplitudes used in the experiments [92]. The periodic burst-firing stimulus is simulated using a square pulse train of f with a unit pulse height and a pulse width of 100 ms. This corresponds to the effect of 3–4 APs within a burst, which is within the reasonable range for mammalian muscle during cyclic contractions. Here, we define the stimulus phase (P_S) as the ratio between the delay of the time corresponding to the peak activation degree after the time of maximum sarcomere length and the whole cycle period. P_S is expressed as a percentage. Figure 2.47a shows the transients of both force and activation degree of a half-sarcomere with the stimulus train of $P_S = 10.4\%$, and Figure 2.47b shows several force–length orbits with different P_S. It is noteworthy that for each P_S, five stimulus cycles are used in order to let the orbit stabilize and converge. The key features as well as the trend of the variation of the orbits' structure with the changes of the stimulus phase are highly consistent with the experimental results (Figure 2.47c), while the differences between the detailed shapes of simulated and experimental orbits are due to different muscle types or parameters because in [92], the insect flight muscles were used. The time for one iteration in the simulation is approximately 0.73 µs.

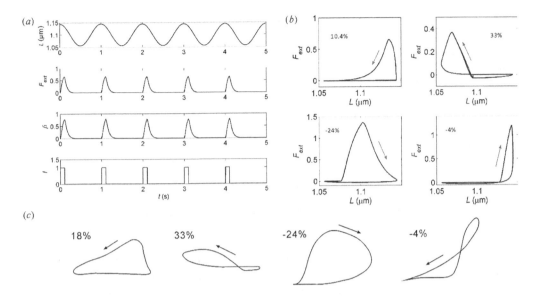

FIGURE 2.47 (a) The transients of f, β, F_{ext}, and L during five cycles of stimulus with the phase of 10.4%; (b) the force–length orbits under the stimulus phase of 10.4%, 33%, −24%, and −4%, respectively; (c) the experimental force–length orbits under the stimulus phase of 18%, 33%, −24%, and −4%. The plots are modified form Ref. [39].

2.4 DISCUSSION

For the purpose of real-time engineering applications such as muscle force prediction, rehabilitation and exoskeleton control, this study proposed a highly efficient semiphenomenological model for a half-sarcomere. To ensure correctness, the model is first based on fundamental experimental facts and the principles of relevant biophysical models. Consequently, the basic linear frames (Figure 2.40 and 2.42) have been extracted from the corresponding experimental phenomena. However, in order to effectively account for the nonlinear features presented in the activation as well as the shortening or lengthening processes of muscle, intermediate inputs (e.g., $P(f)$ and v) are constructed and varied from the originally measurable inputs (e.g., f and V) according to the nonlinear relation between the observable input and the output. Therefore, the model can be sufficiently precise with the carefully identified kinetic parameters, greatly untangling the contradiction between efficacy and complexity of the model.

As shown above, the model is composed of several simple dynamic equations (order ≤ 2), without any partial differential equations or complex integrations. Therefore, the computational structure itself is very concise and efficient. Moreover, only 13 parameters need to be identified in the model, as listed in Table 2.3. All the parameters can be easily identified with normal biomechanical testing of the muscle; i.e., no immeasurable parameter is involved. Here, we systematically conclude the identification processes for these parameters. The parameters p, K_1, and B_1 can be identified with a series of isometric force development experiments (at slack length) of a muscle fiber under different stimulus intensities including the tetanic condition. The time constants τ and τ_1 can be identified by fitting the early phases of force transients induced by isokinetic stretch and release tests starting from slack length. Note that the fiber needs to be tetanized. The parameters a, b, A, and q describing the classic force–velocity relationship can also be identified using isokinetic tests of tetanic fibers, while for the negative half of the velocity range, isotonic tests are adopted. The parameter b_c, which accounts for the drag force, can be approximately determined as follows: first, the fiber is excited and shortened to the minimum length ($L < L_0$); afterward, the stimulus is stopped and isokinetic stretch tests are conducted until the slack length is reached again; then, b_c can be identified with the measured stretch velocity and force in the resting state. Lastly, the parameters c_1, c_2, and c_3 that depict the viscoelasticity of titin can be obtained by sinusoidal stretch and release experiments of relaxed fibers over the slack length.

By investigating the iteration time of the model at different contraction modes, it is clear that the time required would not exceed 4 µs to generate the mechanical response of 1 µs. In practical biomedical/biomechanical engineering applications for skeletal muscle, a time step of several hundreds of µs or even several ms is sufficient for locomotion prediction, as the servo-cycle of an industrial personal computer (IPC) is approximately 400 µs while that of a desktop computer is at least on the order of ms. Therefore, the proposed model can be considered as competent for real-time applications. In particular, this model may also be promising in the numerical investigation of inter-sarcomere dynamics [79], which usually require very complex computations. The cybernetic architecture of the model can be defined, as shown in Figure 2.48, which is aimed at the force-control mode. It can be seen that the cybernetic architecture is also very concise and highly suitable for engineering implementation.

Although this study takes a half-sarcomere as the modeling object, the proposed model can be generalized to describe a larger-scale behavior of muscle with reidentifications of the parameters listed in Table 2.3, and the identification processes are approximately the same as described. However, caution should be exercised when applying the model to a whole muscle because the muscle may be pennate and is usually anisotropic and inhomogeneous, whereas a sarcomere is treated as a one-dimensional system in this study. Therefore, in such cases, the proposed model cannot be applied directly but needs to be embedded into a finite element system or combined with tensor analysis in order to account for issues such as muscle curvature, compression, and tension. This indicates that direct large-scale application of the model is limited to *in vitro* experiments or *in vivo* muscle that is unipennate. In addition, it is worth noting that when the model is applied to a muscle, the stimulus intensity *f* would encompass a more complex meaning than the firing rate; instead, it characterizes the stimulating energy of all the involved motor units, and this usually corresponds to the power of the corresponding electromyography (EMG) signal [93]. Similarly, other parameters will also hold statistical sense because different types of muscle fibers and massive half-sarcomeres with diverse force capacities are fused together. Thus, the model has actually provided a fundamental framework for describing the dynamic elements of a sarcomere. Although not universally applicable for animals, the model can be regarded as generally applicable for most mammals

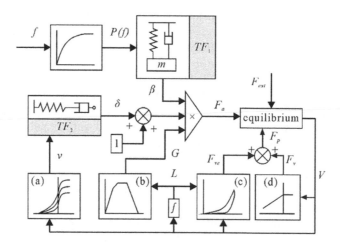

FIGURE 2.48 The cybernetic architecture of the proposed model for the force-control mode, wherein the insets (a), (b), (c), and (d) represent the force–velocity relationship, the force–length relationship, the passive force of titin, and the response of drag force, respectively.

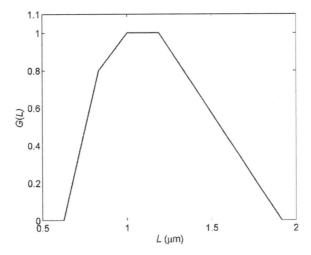

FIGURE 2.49 The form of $G(L)$ that characterizes the isometric force–length relationship of a half-sarcomere.

because the structure, activation, and contraction mechanisms of fast or slow fibers are almost the same. The biggest variation exhibited in the detailed dynamic features of contractile behavior of different kinds of muscles may be that of the time constant and amplitude of the response, which can be reproduced by careful identifications and adjustments of the parameters. In conclusion, we anticipate that the proposed model will be able to meet the requirements posed by real-time engineering applications. Furthermore, it provides a promising scheme for the self-adaption of the model in force prediction and cybernetics, due to its concise structure, few parameters, and easy identification processes.

As shown in Figure 2.49, the isometric force–length relation denoted by $G(L)$ is formulated based on the form in [94]. The only adjustment is that the length needs to be scaled in order to account for the force–length relation of a half-sarcomere. The expression of $G(L)$ is

$$G(L) = \begin{cases} 3.846L - 2.404, & 0.625 \leq L < 0.833 \\ 1.197L - 0.197, & 0.833 \leq L < 1 \\ 1, & 1 \leq L < 1.187 \\ -1.371L + 2.628, & 1.187 \leq L \leq 1.916 \\ 0, & \text{otherwise} \end{cases}.$$

REFERENCES

1. Hill A V. The heat of shortening and the dynamic constants of muscle. *Proc. R. Soc. Lond. B*, 1938, 126: 136–195.
2. Zajac F E. Muscle and tendon: Properties, models, scaling, and application to biomechanics and motor control. *Crit. Rev. Biomed. Eng.*, 1989, 17: 359–411.
3. Huxley H E, Hanson J. Changes in the cross-striations of muscle during contractions and stretch and their structural interpretation. *Nature*, 1954, 173: 973–976.
4. Huxley A F, Simmons R M. Proposed mechanism of force generation in striated muscle. *Nature*, 1971, 233: 533–538.
5. Uyeda T Q, Abramson P D, Spudich J A. The neck region of the myosin motor domain acts as a lever arm to generate movement. *Proc. Natl. Acad. Sci. USA*, 1996, 93: 4459–4464.
6. Piazzesi G, Reconditi M, Linari M, et al. Mechanism of force generation by myosin heads in skeletal muscle. *Nature*, 2002, 415: 659–662.
7. Hernandez-Gascon B, Grasa J, Calvo B, et al. A 3d electro-mechanical continuum model for simulating skeletal muscle contraction. *J. Theor. Biol.*, 2013, 335: 108–118.

8. MacIntosh B R, Gardiner P F, McComas A J. *Skeletal Muscle-Form and Function*, Yu Z, Li Q, Xu P, et al., eds. Xi'an: The Fourth Military Medical University Press, 2010.
9. Toyoshima C, Nakasako M, Nomura H, et al. Crystal structure of the calcium pump of sarcoplasmic reticulum at 2.6 Å resolution. *Nature*, 2000, 405: 647–655.
10. Yin C C, D'Cruz L G, Lai F A. Ryanodine receptor arrays: Not just a pretty pattern? *Cell*, 2008, 18: 149–156.
11. Stern M D, Pizzaro G, Rios E. Local control model of excitation-contraction coupling in skeletal muscle. *J. Gen. Physiol.*, 1997, 110: 415–440.
12. Cannel M B, Allen D G. Model of calcium movements during activation in the sarcomere of frog skeletal muscle. *Biophys. J.*, 1984, 45: 913–925.
13. Stuyvers B D, McCulloch A D, Guo J, et al. Effect of stimulation rate, sarcomere length and Ca^{2+} on force generation by mouse cardiac muscle. *J. Physiol.*, 2002, 544(3): 817–830.
14. Edwards R H T, Hill D K, Jones D A. Fatigue of long duration in human skeletal muscle after exercise. *J. Physiol.*, 1977, 272: 769–778.
15. Kandel E R, Schwartz J H, Jessell T M. *Principles of Neural Science*. 4th ed. New York: Elsevier, 2000.
16. Anthony L F, Erickson H P, Rousseau E, et al. Purification and reconstitution of the calcium release channel from skeletal muscle. *Nature*, 1988, 331: 315–319.
17. Fortune E, Lowery M M. Effect of extracellular potassium accumulation on muscle fiber conduction velocity: A simulation study. *Ann. Biomed. Eng.*, 2009, 37(10): 2105–2117.
18. Piitulainen H, Botter A, Merletti R, et al. Muscle fiber conduction velocity is more affected after eccentric than concentric exercise. *Eur. J. App. Physiol.*, 2010, 111(2): 261–273.
19. Jayasinghe I D, Cannell M B, Soeller C. Organization of ryanodine receptors, transverse tubules, and sodium-calcium exchanger in rat myocytes. *Biophys. J.*, 2009, 97(10): 2664–2673.
20. Maxwell M H, Kleeman C R. *Clinical Disorders of Fluid and Electrolyte Metabolism*. New York: McGraw-Hill Companies, 1968: 28.
21. Endo M. Calcium-induced calcium release in skeletal muscle. *Physiol. Rev.*, 2009, 89: 1153–1176.
22. Escobar A L, Monck J R, Fernandez J M, et al. Localization of the site of Ca^{2+} release at the level of a single sarcomere in skeletal muscle fibres. *Nature*, 1994, 367: 739–741.
23. Dux L, Martonosi A. Two-dimensional arrays of proteins in sarcoplasmic reticulum and purified Ca^{2+}-ATPase vesicles treated with vanadate. *J. Biol. Chem.*, 1983, 258: 2599–2603.
24. Allen D C, Arunachalam R, Mills K R. Critical illness myopathy: Further evidence from muscle-fiber excitability studies of an acquired channelopathy. *Muscle Nerve*, 2008, 37: 14–22.
25. Baylo25r S M, Hollingworth S. Calcium indicators and calcium signalling in skeletal muscle fibres during excitation-contraction coupling. *Prog. Biophys. Mol. Biol.*, 2011, 105: 162–179.
26. Wang F, Luo Z. Based on the power-spectrum to classify the pattern of the Surface Electromyograghy. *J. Hongzhou Dianzi University*, 2005, 25(2): 37–40 (in Chinese).
27. Pasquet B, Carpentier A, Duchateau J, et al. Muscle fatigue during concentric and eccentric contractions. *Muscle Nerve*, 2000, 23: 1727–1735.
28. Edwards R H T, Hill D K, Jones D A, et al. Fatigue of long duration in human skeletal muscle after exercise. *J. Physiol.*, 1977, 272: 769–778.
29. Huxley A F. Cross-bridge action: Present views, prospects, and unknowns. *J. Biomech.*, 2000, 33: 1189–1195.
30. Kaya M, Higuchi H. Nonlinear elasticity and an 8-nm working stroke of single myosin molecules in myofilaments. *Science*, 2010, 329: 686–689.
31. Sellers J R, Veigel C. Direct observation of the myosin-Va power stroke and its reversal. *Nat. Struct. Mol. Biol.*, 2010, 17: 590–595.
32. Ishijima A, Kojima H, Funatsu T, et al. Simultaneous observation of individual ATPase and mechanical events by a single myosin molecule during interaction with actin. *Cell*, 1998, 92: 161–171.
33. Yanagida T, Iwaki M, Ishii Y. Single molecule measurements and molecular motors. *Phil. Trans. R. Soc. B*, 2008, 363: 2123–2134.
34. Li G H, Cui Q. Mechanochemical coupling in myosin: A theoretical analysis with molecular dynamics and combined QM/MM reaction path calculations. *J. Phys. Chem. B*, 2004, 108: 3342–3357.
35. Yang Z, Zhao Y P. QM/MM and classical molecular dynamics simulation of His-tagged peptide immobilization on nickel surface. *Mat. Sci. Eng. A Struct.*, 2006, 423: 84–91.
36. Yang Z, Zhao Y P. Adsorption of His-tagged peptide to Ni, Cu and Au (100) surfaces: Molecular dynamics simulation. *Eng. Anal. Bound. Elem.*, 2007, 31: 402–409.
37. Feynman R P, Leighton R B, Sands M. *The Feynman Lectures on Physics*. Chap 46. Cambridge, MA: Addison-Wesley Longman press, 1970.

38. Astumian R D. Thermodynamics and kinetics of a Brownian motor. *Science*, 1997, 276: 917–922.
39. Julicher F, Ajdari A, Prost J. Modeling molecular motors. *Rev. Mod. Phys.*, 1997, 69: 1269–1281.
40. Ai B, Wang X, Liu G. Theoretical study for muscle contraction. *Chinese J. Med. Phys.*, 2003, 20: 107–109.
41. Bao J, Zhuo Y. Bias voltage fluctuation model on one-way ladder jump motion of molecular motor. *Chinese Sci. Bull.*, 1998, 43: 1493–1496 (in Chinese).
42. Esaki S, Ishii Y, Yanagida T. Model describing the biased Brownian movement of myosin. *Proc. Japan Acad.*, 2003, 79: 9–14.
43. Charles M R, Brian L N. Van der Waals interactions involving proteins. *Biophys. J.*, 1996, 2: 977–987.
44. Zhao Y. Severl mechanical problems in nanoelectronic mechanical system. *Chinese Mech. Abstr.*, 2007, 21(4): 1–21 (in Chinese).
45. Parsegian V A. *Van der Waals Forces: A Handbook for Biologists, Chemists, Engineers, and Physicists.* New York: Cambridge University, Press, 2006.
46. Lifshitz E M. The theory of molecular attractive forces between solids. *Sov. Phys. JETP*, 1956, 2: 73–78.
47. Guo J G, Zhao Y P. Influence of van der Waals and Casimir forces on electrostatic torsional actuators. *J. Microelectromech. Syst.*, 2004, 13: 1027–1035.
48. Munday J N, Capasso F, Parsegian V A. Measured long-range repulsive Casimir-Lifshitz forces. *Nature*, 2009, 457(2): 170–173.
49. Klimchitskaya G L, Anushree R. Complete roughness and conductivity corrections for Casimir force measurement. *Phys. Rev. A*, 1999, 60: 3487–3495.
50. Mannella R, Palleschi V. Fast and precise algorithm for computer simulation of stochastic differential equations. *Phys. Rev. A*, 1989, 9: 3381–3385.
51. Ren J, Shen J, Lu S. *Particle Dispersion Science and Technology.* Beijing: Chemical Industry Press, 2005: 66–98 (in Chinese).
52. Gilson M K, Honig B H. The dielectric constant of a folded protein. *Biopolymers*, 1986, 25: 2097–2119.
53. Smith E L, Coy N H. The absorption spectra of immune proteins. *J. Biol. Chem.*, 1946, 164: 367–370.
54. Afshar-Rad T, Bailey A I, Luckham P F, et al. Forces between protein and model polypeptides adsorbed on mica surfaces. *Biochim. Biophys. Acta-Protein Struct. Mol. Enzymol.*, 1987, 915: 101–111.
55. Fernandez-Varea J M, Garcia-Molina R. Hamaker constants of systems involving water obtained from a dielectric function that fulfills the f sum rule. *J. Coll. Interf. Sci.*, 2000, 231: 394–397.
56. Nakajima H, Kunioka Y, Nakano K, et al. Scanning force microscopy of the interaction events between a single molecule of heavy meromyosin and actin. *Biochem. Biophys. Res. Commun.*, 1997, 234: 178–182.
57. Liu Y M, Scolari M, Im W, et al. Protein-protein interactions in actin-myosin binding and structural effects of R405Q mutation: A molecular dynamics study. *Proteins Struct. Funct. Bioinform.*, 2006, 64: 156–166.
58. Dorgan S J, O'Malley M J. A mathematical model for skeletal muscle activated by N-let pulse trains. *IEEE Trans. Rehab. Eng.*, 1998, 6(3): 286–299.
59. Tam B K, Shin J H, Pfeiffer E, et al. Calcium regulation of an actin spring. *Biophys. J.*, 2009,
60. Ikai M, Fukunage T. Calculation of muscle strength per unit cross sectional area of human muscle by means of ultrasonic measurement. *Int. Z. Angew. Physiol.*, 1968, 26: 26–32.
61. Linke W A, Ivemeyer M, Mundel P, et al. Nature of PEVK-titin elasticity in skeletal muscle. *Proc. Natl. Acad. Sci. USA*, 1998, 95: 8052–8057.
62. Fan Y, Yin Y. Active and progressive exoskeleton rehabilitation using multi-source information fusion from EMG and force-position EPP. *IEEE Trans. Biomed. Eng.*, 2013, 60(12): 3314–3321.
63. Neptune R R, Burnfield J M, Mulroy S J. The neuromuscular demands of toe walking: A forward dynamics simulation analysis. *J. Biomech.*, 2007, 40(6): 1293–1300.
64. Yin Y H, Fan Y J, Xu L D. EMG and EPP-integrated human–machine interface between the paralyzed and rehabilitation exoskeleton. *IEEE Trans. Inform. Tech. Biomed.*, 2012, 16(4): 542–549.
65. Chen X, Yin Y. A dynamical system-Markov model for active postsynaptic responses of muscle spindle afferent nerve. *Chinese Sci. Bull.*, 2013, 58(6): 603–612.
66. Destexhe A, Mainen Z F, Sejnowski T J. Synthesis of models for excitable membranes, synaptic transmission and neuromodulation using a common kinetic formalism. *J. Comput. Neurosci.*, 1994, 1(3): 195–230.
67. Palmer B M, Suzuki T, Wang Y, Barnes W D, Miller M S, Maughan D W. Two-state model of acto-myosin attachment-detachment predicts C-process of sinusoidal analysis. *Biophys. J.*, 2007, 93(3): 760–769.
68. Piazzesi G, Lombardi V. A cross-bridge model that is able to explain mechanical and energetic properties of shortening muscle. *Biophys. J.*, 1995, 68(5): 1966–1979.

69. Propp M B. A model of muscle contraction based upon component studies. *Lect. Math. Life Sci.*, 1986, 16: 61–119.

70. Zahalak GI. The two-state cross-bridge model of muscle is an asymptotic limit of multi-state models. *J. Theor. Biol.*, 2000, 204(1), 67–82.

71. Fan Y, Guo Z, Yin Y. Semg-based neuro-fuzzy controller for a parallel ankle exoskeleton with proprioception. *Int. J. Robot. Autom.*, 2011, 26(4): 450.

72. Tsianos G A, Rustin C, Loeb G E. Mammalian muscle model for predicting force and energetics during physiological behaviors. *IEEE Trans. Neural. Syst. Rehabil. Eng.*, 2012, 20(2): 117–133.

73. Iqbal K, Roy A. Stabilizing Pid controllers for a single-link biomechanical model with position, velocity, and force feedback. *J. Biomech. Eng.*, 2004, 126(6): 838–843.

74. Gollee H, Murray-Smith DJ, Jarvis JC. A nonlinear approach to modeling of electrically stimulated skeletal muscle. *IEEE Trans. Biomed. Eng.*, 2001, 48(4): 406–415.

75. Bobet J, Stein R B, Oguztoreli M Nh. A linear time-varying model of force generation in skeletal muscle. *IEEE Trans. Biomed. Eng.*, 1993, 40(10): 1000–1006.

76. Perreault E J, Heckman C J, Sandercock T G. Hill muscle model errors during movement are greatest within the physiologically relevant range of motor unit firing rates. *J. Biomech.*, 2003, 36(2): 211–218.

77. Kellermayer M S, Smith S B, Granzier H L, Bustamante C. Folding-unfolding transitions in single titin molecules characterized with laser tweezers. *Science*, 1997, 276(5315): 1112–6.

78. Hatze H. A myocybernetic control model of skeletal muscle. *Biol. Cybern.*, 1977, 25(2): 103–119.

79. Stoecker U, Telley I A, Stüssi E, Denoth J. A multisegmental cross-bridge kinetics model of the myofibril. *J. Theor. Biol.*, 2009, 259(4): 714–726.

80. Huxley A F. Muscular contraction. *J. Physiol.*, 1974, 243(1): 1–43.

81. Denoth J, Stüssi E, Csucs G, Danuser G. Single muscle fiber contraction is dictated by inter-sarcomere dynamics. *J. Theor. Biol.*, 2002, 216(1): 101–122.

82. Ramírez A, Grasa J, Alonso A, Soteras F, Osta R, Muñoz M, Calvo, B. Active response of skeletal muscle: in vivo experimental results and model formulation. *J. Theor. Biol.*, 2010, 267(4): 546–553.

83. Chen X, Yin Y, Fan Y. Emg oscillator model-based energy kernel method for characterizing muscle intrinsic property under isometric contraction. *Chin. Sci. Bull.*, 2014, 59(14): 1556–1567.

84. Ishii Y, Nishiyama M, Yanagida T. Mechano-chemical coupling of molecular motors revealed by single molecule measurements. *Curr. Protein Pept. Sci.*, 2004, 5(2): 81–87.

85. Lymn R W, Taylor E W. Mechanism of adenosine triphosphate hydrolysis by actomyosin. *Biochemistry*, 1971, 10(25): 4617–4624.

86. Roots H, Offer G, Ranatunga K. Comparison of the tension responses to ramp shortening and lengthening in intact mammalian muscle fibres: crossbridge and non-crossbridge contributions. *J. Muscle Res. Cell. Motil.*, 2007, 28(2–3): 123–139.

87. Julian F J, Moss R L Effects of calcium and ionic strength on shortening velocity and tension development in frog skinned muscle fibres. *J. Physiol.*, 1981, 311(1): 179–199.

88. Julian F. The effect of calcium on the force-velocity relation of briefly glycerinated frog muscle fibres. *J. Physiol.*, 1971, 218(1): 117–145.

89. Meyer G, Lieber R, Mcculloch A. A nonlinear model of passive muscle viscosity. *J. Biomech. Eng.*, 2011, 133(9): 091007.

90. Sun Y B, Hilber K, Irving M. Effect of active shortening on the rate of ATP utilisation by rabbit psoas muscle fibres. *J. Physiol.*, 2001, 531(3): 781–791.

91. Josephson R, Contraction dynamics and power output of skeletal muscle. *Annu. Rev. Physiol.*, 1993, 55(1): 527–546.

92. Josephson R K, Mechanical power output from striated muscle during cyclic contraction. *J. Exp. Biol.*, 1985, 114(1): 493–512.

93. Ko C-Y, Chang Y, Kim S-B, Kim S, Kim G, Ryu J, Mun M, Linear-and nonlinear-electromyographic analysis of supracutaneous vibration stimuli of the forearm using diverse frequencies and considering skin physiological properties. *J. Biomech. Eng.*, 2014, 136(1): 011008.

94. Gordon A M, Huxley A F, Julian F J, The variation in isometric tension with sarcomere length in vertebrate muscle fibres. *J. Physiol.*, 1966, 184(1): 170–192.

3 Estimation of Skeletal Muscle Activation and Contraction Force Based on EMG Signals

Electromyography (EMG) is formed by the action potentials (APs) spreading on the sarcolemma. The APs start from motoneurons and are generated 200 ms prior to muscle contraction. Thus, the EMG signals reflect human motion intention in advance and imply muscle activity information. Because of this feature, EMG signals have been studied by more and more research institutions and have been applied in clinical diagnosis, rehabilitation engineering, and human–machine interaction interface for exoskeleton robot, such as the Hybrid Assistive Limb (HAL) series, the Berkeley Lower Extremity Exoskeleton (BLEEX), and exoskeletons for upper limbs, including the ones of Saga University in Japan and the prosthesis in Shanghai Jiao Tong University. However, the fuzziness of the EMG signals is very large. Distinct EMG signals can be obtained from the same person performing even the same actions. Thus, there is an urgent need to study the EMG signals further to improve the accuracy of motion recognition and prediction and to develop effective EMG-based human–machine interface for stable real-time human–machine coordinate control by integrating the traditional motion information signals that are able to reflect accurate motion conditions, such as angle, force, etc.

The basic physical characteristics and generation mechanism of EMG signals are first introduced in this chapter to make the spreading and motion control mechanism of signals from motorium clear. The relationship between sEMG (surface-EMG) signals and human motion is preliminarily modeled. Then, real-time processing and feature extraction algorithm of sEMG signals are studied based on their time-domain and frequency-domain features, in order to meet the accuracy and real-time requirements in motion intention prediction for rehabilitation applications.

3.1 GENERATION MECHANISM OF sEMG SIGNALS

EMG is generated by the superposition of the APs activated on the sarcolemma. The contraction force is closely related to the number of activated α motoneurons and firing rate. Thus, the EMG signals reflect the motion intention of the motorium system. Although the frequency and the amplitude of the EMG signals are the comprehensive representation of various APs, the statistic characteristics, including the frequency and amplitude, represent physiological features, such as the neural pathway state, muscle contraction state, and contraction force. In consequence, electromyogram has been widely applied in the detection and diagnosis of movement disorders.

Similar to EMG, sEMG is also generated by the superposition of the APs activated on the sarcolemma. But the sEMG signals detected by the patch electrodes are the myoelectric signals after filtering and aliasing by skins. Thus, the sEMG signals reflect the physiological features, including the pathway state, contraction state, and contraction force, of a group of muscles. Different from the detection of the EMG signals, sEMG signals are detected by a set of electrodes stuck to the skin instead of invasive electrodes. Thus, there are no discomforts, such as pains, for users while detecting. Its safety and comfort are relatively higher. Because of these, sEMG has been widely applied in the detection of myoelectric signals, muscle fatigue estimation, behavior prediction, and motion recognition during clinical rehabilitations.

3.2   REAL-TIME FEATURE EXTRACTION AND CONTRACTION FORCE ESTIMATION OF sEMG SIGNALS

Similar to most biosignals, the fuzziness of the EMG signals is very large. Totally different EMG signals can be obtained from the same person performing the same action. Thus, it becomes difficult to accurately process the sEMG signals, and various methods have been applied to gain a deeper understanding [1–4]. The human–machine integrated coordinate control poses higher requirements for real-time motion control. Although there are certain mapping relations between the macroscopic sEMG signals and muscle contraction which have been proved by previous works, the nonlinear mapping relation is still not clear. The sEMG signals are generated by the superposition of the APs activated on the sarcolemma. Theoretically, there are direct mapping relations between the frequency components, which correspond to the firing rate of APs, and muscle contraction. The sEMG signals are typical time-varying signals or non-stationary signals. Traditional processing techniques for time-domain and frequency-domain analyses, including the short-time Fourier transform (STFT), power spectrum estimation (PSE), wavelet transform, etc., have been proved to have certain effects in practical applications. However, accurate real-time analysis is needed in the practical applications of lower-limb rehabilitation. Traditional methods have poor real-time performance and are not able to perform quantitative analysis of signals in a short time; i.e., it is impossible to analyze the components with relatively lower frequency using relatively smaller time window.

To improve the real-time performance and accuracy of feature extraction, differentiated characteristic-frequency algorithm based on periodogram method, Welch method, and autoregressve (AR) spectral estimation algorithm is introduced to perform real-time frequency-domain analysis. The EMG signals with DC components are introduced to reduce the error caused by relatively smaller signal-to-noise ratio (SNR) when the contraction force is small. Comparisons and analyses are given on the accuracy and real-time performance of the proposed method.

3.2.1   TRADITIONAL EXTRACTION METHODS

As the amplitude and frequency of myoelectric signals reflect the contraction force and velocity of skeletal muscle, traditional sEMG signal extraction methods include time-domain, frequency-domain, and time–frequency domain analysis methods.

Among the above, the time-domain feature extraction methods for sEMG signals include the root mean square (RMS), mean value, quadratic sum, etc. as illustrated in Eqs. (3.1)–(3.3). The sEMG signal features such as the amplitude can be obtained through the time-domain analysis methods. For the signals with the length of N, the computing methods are as follows:

$$RMS = \sqrt{\frac{1}{N} \sum_{i=1}^{N} v_i^2}, \tag{3.1}$$

$$AVE = \frac{1}{N} \sum_{i=1}^{N} v_i, \tag{3.2}$$

$$Squ = \frac{1}{N} \sum_{i=1}^{N} v_i^2, \tag{3.3}$$

in which
   N—the number of sampling points,
   v_i—the voltage of the ith sampling point.

In the experiment, the maximal frequency is usually 500 Hz. Thus, the sampling frequency is set as 2 kHz; i.e., the sampling interval is 500 μs.

The PSE is often applied to analyze the frequency distribution feature of sEMG signals. The basic method is Fourier-series-based periodogram method. But as its variance performance is relatively poor, improved-periodogram method was proposed. However, the resolution and variance performance of the traditional Fourier-series–based PSE are still far from satisfactory, and there are also frequency leakages in the process. Thus, the modern PSE method based on parametric model and non-parametric model is proposed.

The relative short windows are applied to meet the real-time performance requirement in the application process. Thus, the time-domain analysis methods which require long time series to analyze the high- and low-frequency characteristics of the series, such as the wavelet transform, are not introduced in this section.

Based on the non-stationary characteristics of sEMG signal and high real-time performance requirement in practical application, the STFT-based periodogram, Welch-method–based improved-periodogram, and AR-model–based PSE methods are selected.

The STFT is illustrated in Eq. (3.4):

$$X_{FFT}\left(e^{j\omega}\right) = \sum_{n=0}^{N-1}\left(x(n) \cdot e^{-j\omega n}\right),$$

$$S_{FFT}(\omega) = \frac{1}{N}\left|X_{FFT}\left(e^{j\omega}\right)\right|^2, \tag{3.4}$$

in which

$x(n)$—sampled signals,
N—signal length; i.e., segment length of the time window is N,
ω—circular frequency, expressed as $2\pi k/N$, $k = 0, 1, ..., N - 1$,
$X_{FFT}(e^{j\omega})$—discrete-time Fourier transform (DTFT) of the sampled series,
$S_{FFT}(\omega)$—the corresponding amplitude of the signal component with the frequency of ω in the sampled signals.

As the variance feature after DTFT is relatively poor, the power spectrum obtained from the periodogram method is filtered by the third-order Butterworth filter.

The Welch-method–based improved-periodogram method divides the sampled series into k segments, which are either independent from each other or overlapped. Get the dot product results of every segment with the selected window function (in this book, the Hamming Window is the data window for the sub-sequences); then perform the discrete Fourier transform (FT), the process of which is illustrated as Eq. (3.5):

$$X_W\left(e^{j\omega}\right) = \sum_{n=0}^{L-1}\omega(n)x(n + iD)e^{-j\omega n},$$

$$S_W(\omega) = \frac{1}{KLU}\sum_{i=0}^{K-1}\left|X_W\left(e^{j\omega}\right)\right|^2, \tag{3.5}$$

in which

$\omega(n)$—Hamming data window,
L—length of the sub-sequences,
$x(n)$—sampling sequence of the sEMG signals,

K—number of the sub-sequences,

D—underlapped data length of adjacent sub-sequences,

$X_W(e^{j\omega})$—DTFT of the sub-sequences,

$S_W(\omega)$—the corresponding amplitude of the signal component with the frequency of ω in the sampled signals,

U—the constant which makes the estimation and can be expressed as Eq. (3.6):

$$U = \frac{1}{N}\sum_{n=0}^{N-1}|\omega(n)|, \tag{3.6}$$

in which N is the length of data window $\omega(n)$.

AR-model–based PSE method takes the signal sequence as a pth-order AR process, as illustrated in Eq. (3.7). It abandons the assumption to window the data sequences

$$x(n) = -\sum_{k=1}^{p}a_k x(n-k) + u(n), \tag{3.7}$$

in which $u(n)$ is the white noise sequence with the mean value of 0 and variance of σ^2. a_k is a parameter in AR model

Based on the AR model of the signal sequence, the transfer function can be expressed as Eq. (3.8):

$$H_{AR}\left(e^{j\omega}\right) = \frac{1}{A\left(e^{j\omega}\right)} = \frac{1}{1 + \sum_{K=1}^{p}a_k e^{-j\omega}}. \tag{3.8}$$

Based on the transfer function and the Burg Algorithm, the system input/output power spectrum is illustrated as Eq. (3.9):

$$S_{AR}\left(e^{j\omega}\right) = \frac{\sigma^2}{\left|A\left(e^{j\omega}\right)\right|^2} = \frac{\sigma^2}{\left|1 + \sum_{K=1}^{p}a_k e^{-j\omega K}\right|^2}. \tag{3.9}$$

Through the STFT-based periodogram, Welch-method–based improved-periodogram, and AR-model–based PSE methods, the power spectrum of the sEMG signal sequence can be obtained respectively. Then the characteristic frequency f can be gotten based on Eq. (3.10):

$$f = \frac{\sum_{i=0}^{N-1}\left(|S(x,\omega_i)| \cdot \omega_i\right)}{\sum_{i=0}^{N-1}|S(x,\omega_i)|}, \tag{3.10}$$

in which

$|S(x,\omega_i)|$—PSE of EMG signals,

ω_i—corresponding frequency,

N—length for PSE.

3.2.2　Differentiated Extraction Method

The frequency-domain distribution of sEMG is approximately between 10 Hz and 500 Hz and is generated 200 ms ahead of muscle contraction. If the sampling frequency of PSE is 2 kHz and the signal length is less than 200 ms, the frequency resolution would be relatively low and power spectrum of the component signal with lower frequency cannot be obtained. On the other hand, if the signal length of the PSE is relatively long, the real-time performance of the signal will be decreased. Meanwhile, the obtained PSE will reflect the frequency distribution of longer time segments, resulting in the inability to perform accurate time-domain analysis of the time-varying signals such as the sEMG.

Thus, discrete PSE based on the traditional PSE is proposed to improve the performance. The linear function of the sampling sequence is the DTFT of the sampling sequence in Eq. (3.4). For the sampling signals x_1 and x_2 with the same start point whose lengths are N and $(N + \Delta N)$, respectively (x_2 can be expressed as ($x_1 + dx$), in which the dx is the incremental signal with the length of ΔN), zero fill the signal x_1 with shorter length at the end so that it has the same length with signal x_2; i.e., the length of $x_2 = (x_1 + dx)$. Based on the linear feature of Fourier series, the relation is as follows:

$$X_d\left(e^{j\omega}\right) = X_2\left(e^{j\omega}\right) - X_1\left(e^{j\omega}\right), \tag{3.11}$$

in which

　　$X_d(e^{j\omega})$—Fourier series of the increment signal dx,
　　$X_1(e^{j\omega})$—Fourier series of the sampling signal x_1,
　　$X_2(e^{j\omega})$—Fourier series of the sampling signal x_2.

That is, Fourier series of the incremental signal can be obtained from Fourier series of the sampling signals x_1 and x_2. Based on the definition of power spectrum, it is the result of Fourier series quadratic sum of signal sequences divided by the signal lengths. Thus, the power spectrum of the incremental signal dx can be calculated through the Fourier series or power spectrum of the sampling signals x_1 and x_2, which is illustrated as

$$S_d(\omega) = \frac{1}{\Delta N}\left|X_d\left(e^{j\omega}\right)\right|^2 = \frac{1}{\Delta N}\left|X_2\left(e^{j\omega}\right) - X_1\left(e^{j\omega}\right)^2\right|. \tag{3.12}$$

Comparing with the ideal power spectrum, the parametric-model–based PSE is unbiased. Thus, the power spectrum obtained from parametric model through Eq. (3.11) can be deemed as unbiased comparing to Fourier series. Similarly, the power spectrum of the incremental signal dx can be calculated based on Eq. (3.12). Process the shorter signal in the same way so that it has the same length with the longer one, resulting in the same length and resolution of the calculated Fourier series and power spectrum. Substitute the results into Eq. (3.10) to compute the characteristic frequency of the incremental signal.

When the muscle is relaxed or the contraction force is small, the SNR is relatively low. The characteristic frequency reflects more of the noise signal than the sEMG signals. In order to reduce the interference from the noise signal in low SNR during the characteristic-frequency-extraction process, signal offset is introduced in the computing process of characteristic frequency. The revised signal based on Eq. (3.13) is

$$x = x_{\text{EMG}} + x_{\text{offset}}, \tag{3.13}$$

in which

　　x—the revised signal after adding the offset,
　　x_{EMG}—sEMG signal,
　　x_{offset}—the added offset.

In practical applications, the sEMG signal amplitude of the activated muscle is approximately 0.1–3 V and that of the noise is about 0–10 mV; thus the offset is added. As the offset is much less than the signals and several times larger than the noise signals, the calculated characteristic frequency is sure to be that of the actual signals when muscle is activated and the characteristic frequency of the offset DC component when the muscle is resting, the value of which is approximately 0. The feature extraction of actual sEMG signals will be done in the next section.

3.2.3   REAL-TIME SIGNAL FEATURE EXTRACTION EXPERIMENT AND EFFECT COMPARISON OF THE DIFFERENT METHODS

3.2.3.1   Artificial Synthesis of Signals

To validate the real-time performance and accuracy of the above algorithm, the artificially synthesized signals are first used. The signals are divided into four groups. The first group is synthesized by one stationary signal with the amplitude of 10 and frequency of 200 Hz and the white noise with the mean value of 0 and variance of 1. The second group is synthesized by two stationary signals with the amplitudes of 10 and 5 and frequencies of 200 Hz and 100 Hz and the above-described white noise. The third group is synthesized by one signal with variable frequency, whose change rule is 200–160–120–80 Hz with the change period of 0.5 s, and the above-described white noise. The last group is synthesized by one signal with variable frequency, whose change rule is 200–160–120–80 Hz with the change period of 0.25 s, and the above-described white noise.

The actual characteristic frequency and the calculated characteristic frequency are obtained by Eq. (3.10), and the relative deviation of the actual characteristic frequency and the calculated one is obtained by Eq. (3.14):

$$\text{RE} = \frac{\left| f(t) - \overline{f}(t) \right|}{\overline{f}(t)}, \qquad (3.14)$$

in which
   f—the calculated characteristic frequency in time t,
   $\overline{f}$—the actual characteristic frequency in time t.

The RMS value of the relative deviation by Eq. (3.2) is the comparison index. The results are illustrated in Table 3.1 and Figure 3.1. Table 3.1 lists the actual characteristic frequencies and the calculated characteristic frequencies of the four groups of artificially synthesized signals obtained through different methods. Figure 3.1 illustrates the time–characteristic frequency curves of the four groups of artificially synthesized signals obtained through different methods.

It can be inferred from Table 3.1 that for the artificially synthesized signals, the RMS value of the relative deviation by the differentiated feature extraction algorithm is 22.86% smaller than that of the conventional algorithm, except for the periodogram method. And the accuracy of the differentiated feature extraction algorithm is also higher. Based on Figure 3.1, for the frequency time varying signals, the differentiated feature extraction algorithm reflects the changing features of the time-varying signals more accurately and is more conducive to analyze the non-stationary signals such as the sEMG signals. On the other hand, the differentiated feature extraction algorithm could estimate the characteristic frequency in advance of the conventional one and thus has better real-time performance.

To further validate the effectiveness of the algorithm, filter the white Gaussian noise with the mean value of 0 and variance of 5 through a fourth-order bandwidth time-varying Butterworth filter [5]. Based on the distribution of the main frequencies of sEMG signals, the initial cutoff frequency of this band-pass filter is 90–200 Hz. The cutoff frequency then decreases linearly with

TABLE 3.1

The Actual Characteristic Frequencies and the Calculated Characteristic Frequencies of the Four Groups of Artificially Synthesized Signals Obtained through Different Methods

	Error of Signals with 200 Hz (Hz)	Error of Signals with 200 Hz + 100 Hz (Hz)	Error of Low-Frequency Time-Varying Signals (Hz)	Error of High-Frequency Time-Varying Signals (Hz)
AR model	2.16e–08	3.6249	8.5352	12.6786
Differentiated AR model	1.82e–08	2.9251	6.0696	9.1026
Improved-periodogram method	0.1021	13.0889	6.5241	9.7846
Differentiated improved-periodogram method	0.1039	13.3745	1.8637	2.3870
Periodogram method	1.40e–10	8.28e–11	29.9483	44.9917
Differentiated periodogram method	3.01e–10	1.65e–10	97.3618	109.3405

time to 45–100 Hz, and increases back to 90–200 Hz, generating a group of artificially synthesized signals with time-varying bandwidth. In the experiment, ten groups of time-varying signals are generated. Conventional AR model, improved-periodogram method, periodogram method, and differentiated feature extraction method are applied to calculate the feature frequency at every moment. The mean characteristic frequencies of the ten groups are used as the calculated values. The results are illustrated in Figure 3.2, displaying the time–characteristic frequency curves from different methods. It can be inferred from the figure that the curve of the differentiated feature extraction method is on the left of the conventional algorithm, indicating that differentiated feature extraction method possesses better real-time performance in the calculation of characteristic frequencies.

Figure 3.3 illustrates square, variance, and relative deviation of the mean error between the calculated characteristic frequency and the actual characteristic frequency of the bandwidth time-varying artificially synthesized signals. Table 3.2 lists the corresponding statistics. The computing process is illustrated in Eqs. (3.15)–(3.17):

$$\text{Bias}^2 = \left[\frac{1}{l} \sum_{n=1}^{l} \left(f(t) - \overline{f}(t) \right) \right]^2, \tag{3.15}$$

$$\text{Var} = \frac{1}{l} \sum_{n=1}^{l} \left(f(t) - \overline{f}(t) \right)^2, \tag{3.16}$$

$$\text{RE} = \frac{1}{l} \sum_{n=1}^{l} \frac{\left| f(t) - \overline{f}(t) \right|}{\overline{f}(t)}, \tag{3.17}$$

in which

l—number of signal segments,

f—the calculated characteristic frequency in time t,

$\overline{f}$—the actual characteristic frequency in time t.

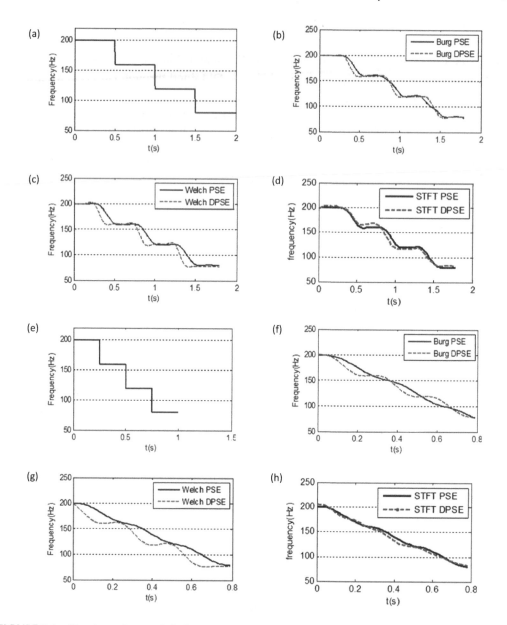

FIGURE 3.1 The time–characteristic frequency curves. Among them, (a) and (e) are the actual frequencies of the synthesized signals; (b) and (f) are the characteristic frequency curves of the AR-model–based conventional method and the differentiated feature extraction method; (c) and (g) are the characteristic frequency curves of the improved-periodogram–based conventional method and the differentiated feature extraction method; (d) and (h) are the characteristic frequency curves of the periodogram-based conventional method and the differentiated feature extraction method.

The experimental results indicate that the statistical error of the differentiated feature extraction methods is smaller than the conventional methods. Thus, the proposed method possesses higher accuracy for the simple synthetized signals or time-varying non-stationary signals. Meanwhile, it has better real-time performance than the conventional methods. Thus, for time-varying non-stationary signals, differentiated feature extraction method has higher accuracy and better real-time performance.

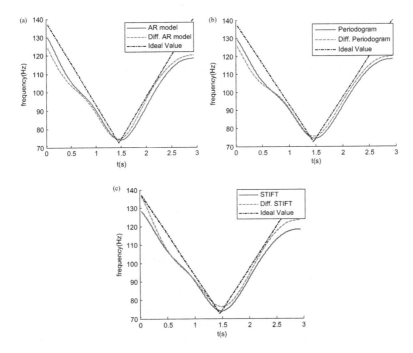

FIGURE 3.2   Time–characteristic frequency curves. Among them, (a), (b), and (c) are the time–characteristic frequency curves based on AR model, improved-periodogram method, and periodogram method. The dash-dotted lines are the actual time–characteristic frequency curves; the solid lines are the time–characteristic frequency curves using conventional algorithm; the dotted lines are the time–characteristic frequency curves using differentiated algorithm.

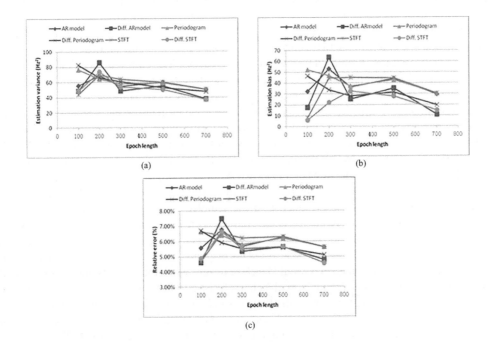

FIGURE 3.3   Statistical curves for the error between the calculated characteristic frequency and the actual characteristic frequency of the bandwidth-time-varying artificially synthesized signals. (a) Mean error; (b) variance; (c) relative error.

TABLE 3.2

Statistical List for the Error between the Calculated Characteristic Frequency and the Actual Characteristic Frequency of the Bandwidth-Time-Varying Artificially Synthesized Signals

	Mean Error (Hz)	Variance (Hz)	Relative Error (Hz)
AR model	36.19 ± 24.32	54.76 ± 30.06	$5.67\% \pm 2.03\%$
Differentiated AR model	25.08 ± 22.53	48.71 ± 24.15	$5.35\% \pm 1.51\%$
Improved-periodogram method	37.19 ± 26.72	57.84 ± 30.67	$5.80\% \pm 2.06\%$
Differentiated improved-periodogram method	27.96 ± 20.16	60.53 ± 25.15	$5.50\% \pm 1.83\%$
Periodogram method	44.94 ± 33.62	63.81 ± 40.64	$6.21\% \pm 2.22\%$
Differentiated periodogram method	32.60 ± 32.84	53.82 ± 37.57	$5.52\% \pm 2.17\%$

3.2.3.2 Real-Time Feature Extraction of sEMG Signals and Comparison of Results

Five healthy male subjects took part in the experiment with the ages of 29, 26, 24, 23, and 22. One of their legs was bound with a leg of the exoskeleton. Biceps muscle and quadriceps muscle of the thigh were two main muscles that related to knee joint movements. Considering the measurability and intensity of the sEMG signals, and in order to trace the knee muscle locations that determined the kinetic characteristics of the human knee, two channels of EMG signals were applied to control the knee flexion and extension: ch1, biceps muscle of the thigh and ch2, quadriceps muscle of the thigh.

In order to avoid the moving influences and perform easy analysis, it was assumed that the experiments were all isometric contraction testing. In the process, the lower limbs of the exoskeleton were fixed, and the joint angle was set to $20°–50°$ randomly so that the subjects were comfortable. The lower limbs of the subjects were bound to the lower limbs of the exoskeleton. First, the subjects were required to perform flexion and extension with 10% of the maximum flexion–extension force and then allowed to relax. The process was repeated for 15 times. Then the subjects were required to perform flexion and extension with the maximum flexion–extension force and allowed to relax. The process was repeated for 15 times. The motion period was 5 s. The data was included in one group sampling signal. Two channels of sEMG signals were collected together with the human–machine interaction force. Each experiment included 30 tests and lasted about 5 min.

The experimental results are illustrated in Figure 3.4 which records the results of one subject completing one flexion–extension experiment. Among them, Figure 3.4a illustrates part of the raw sEMG signals and its characteristic frequency curve of the quadriceps femoris. Theoretically, contraction force is determined by AP frequency and the number of activated motoneurons. Thus, the amplitude and frequency of the sEMG signals would both be high when the contraction force is large. The SNR is very high at the moment. Adding the offset DC components with small amplitude would not affect the characteristic frequency of the sampled signals. On the contrary, the SNR is low when the contraction force is small. As the characteristic frequency of the DC component is 0, adding the offset DC components with amplitude little larger than the noise signal would decrease the characteristic frequency largely, which would correspond to the actual situation of human muscle. Thus, the characteristic frequency would be close to zero when the subjects' muscles relax in the experiments. As illustrated in Figure 3.4b, the characteristic frequency with offset DC components is relatively lower, indicating the contraction force is small, which agrees with the actual contraction force. However, the characteristic frequency without offset DC components is relatively high, and the wave shape is irregular, which does not agree with the actual contraction force. Thus, the offset DC component has better analysis effects when the contraction force is small.

On the other hand, the characteristic frequency curves obtained by AR spectrum estimation and differentiated feature extraction algorithm are illustrated in Figure 3.4c,d.

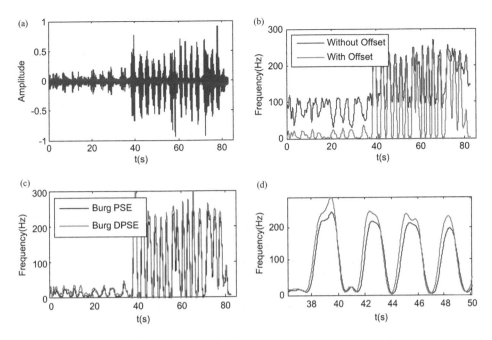

FIGURE 3.4   (a) Raw sEMG signals; (b) time–characteristic frequency with and without offset; (c) time–characteristic frequency curves of the AR-model–based conventional and differentiated algorithm; (d) the partial enlargement of (c).

They have similar trends in the figures. However, the curve of the differentiated feature extraction algorithm is on the left on the conventional one, indicating the judging time is 50 ms ahead, and the maximum value is 10% bigger than that of the conventional algorithm, indicating that the differentiated feature extraction algorithm has better real-time performance than the conventional one in the practical sEMG signal extraction applications, which is similar to that of the artificially synthesized signals. Meanwhile, the maximum value is 10% bigger than that of the conventional algorithm, indicating the average effect caused by the signal with certain length in the signal processing could be reduced, which is also similar to that of the artificially synthesized signals.

3.2.4   PHASE-PORTRAIT–BASED ENERGY KERNEL METHOD FOR FEATURE EXTRACTION AND CONTRACTION FORCE ESTIMATION

Extensive studies have focused on the force estimation of muscle with sEMG [6], and most methods are currently based on the traditional frequency-domain analysis [7–10], including the classic spectrum estimation methods, such as FT and periodogram, and parametric model methods such as AR spectrum estimation. Recently, fractal analysis based on the power spectra of EMG has also been introduced [11]. Aiming at the amplitude–frequency characteristics of the EMG signal, these algorithms are capable of performing asymptotic unbiased estimation against the power spectra density (PSD) and are taking effect in practice. Among these approaches, the RMS and mean power frequency (MPF) are widely used, focusing on the amplitude and frequency features, respectively. Currently, it is recognized that a relatively linear relationship exists between RMS and muscle force [12], while there remain disputations about the effectiveness of MPF, which is regarded as linearly dependent on force only under small percentage of maximum voluntary contraction (MVC) [12,13]. Gabor transform [14], Wigner–Ville transform [15], and wavelets [16,17] can process the signal in time–frequency domain, with a relatively high cost of time and signal resource. As for the motion pattern recognition and classification based on EMG, existent methods include neural networks [18,19], fractal analysis [20], convolution kernel [21], independent component correlation algorithm [22], and so forth [23,24]. The methods introduced above generally start with signal processing theories, with relatively weak associations with the physical origin of EMG. On the other hand, studies aiming at the generation mechanism of EMG or muscle force [25,26] and analyses based on the physical modeling have also been conducted [27,28]. However, due to the extremely high aliasing degree and the typical non-stationarity of the signal, the statistical features differ among individuals, and the same signal can never be attained even when the same motion is performed by the same person. Thus, the methods resulting from the modeling of the source of EMG are difficult to be put into practice, with numerous parameters requiring manual adjustments. It will be greatly helpful if an invariant characterizing the intrinsic property of a muscle can be obtained.

In this section, we did not directly go into traditional signal processing; instead, the aim is to establish a new feasible physical/mathematical model of EMG, which was treated as a kind of abstract motion, and common features were extracted from the phase portraits converted from the raw signals. In this way, we not only avoided the modeling from the source of EMG, but also entrusted the signal reasonable physical meanings. With the analysis on the phase portraits, we hypothesized the EMG signal as a harmonic oscillator and built correspondence between its energy and the momentum/force or the power of the muscle. Another purpose of this study is to find a quantity that characterizes the intrinsic property of muscle. Therefore, the natural frequency of the EMG signal is defined for a muscle based on the oscillator assumption. During the force estimation experiments, we compared the performances of the energy kernel method, RMS, and MPF and made clear whether the natural frequency depends on factors such as different individuals, times, and/or muscles.

3.2.4.1 The Oscillator Model of EMG Signal

EMG is a zero-averaged stochastic wave signal, whose amplitude is featured by the reciprocating motions accompanied by noise [5]. From the perspective of mathematics, such type of behavior can be abstracted as an "oscillator," which can be described by differential equations. Consequently, we take the amplitude of the signal as the variable x and the derivative of x over time as the variable y (velocity). Hence, the vector (x, y) denotes the coordinate of a state point, and the phase portrait of a signal segment can be drawn in the x–y phase plane. Figure 3.5a represents a piece of filtered bipolar EMG signal of human rectus femoris (RF) with the sampling rate of 2,000 Hz, with three rectangular windows placed on the signal. The phase portraits of the signal within each window are drawn, as shown in Figure 3.5b. Figure 3.5b not only labels the state points (circles), but also provides the moving trajectories of these points (line segments). Note that all the portraits within the three windows illustrate elliptic shapes, whose centers of symmetry are located at the proximity of the origin. Besides, the long axes (dashed lines) of the ellipses deviate from the y-axis. Note that the velocity of an oscillator must be zero when it reaches the maximum displacement, and thereby,

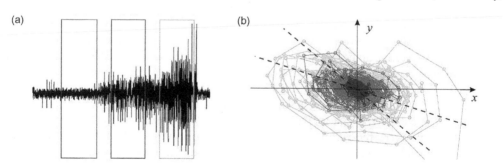

FIGURE 3.5 The phase portrait of the EMG signal within different windows, collected from human RF. (a) Raw EMG signal and (b) the phase portrait of the EMG signal.

theoretically, the long axis should coincide with the y-axis. The deviation here is due to the discretization of the data.

On the other hand, if we assume a harmonic oscillator with mass m and stiffness k and define x and y in the same way, the state of the oscillator can be expressed by the following dynamical system:

$$\begin{cases} \dot{X} = y \\ \dot{y} = -\dfrac{k}{m} X \end{cases} \tag{3.18}$$

The real solutions of the system can be written as

$$x_1(t) = \cos\left(\sqrt{K}t\right)\begin{pmatrix} 1/\sqrt{K} \\ 0 \end{pmatrix} - \sin\left(\sqrt{K}t\right)\begin{pmatrix} 0 \\ 1 \end{pmatrix}, \text{ or}$$

$$x_2(t) = \sin\left(\sqrt{K}t\right)\begin{pmatrix} 1/\sqrt{K} \\ 0 \end{pmatrix} + \cos\left(\sqrt{K}t\right)\begin{pmatrix} 0 \\ 1 \end{pmatrix}. \tag{3.19}$$

If the phase portrait of the two components (x and y) is drawn in Eq. (3.19), it also turns out to be an ellipse. Therefore, we can further approximate the EMG signal within a short time Δt as a kind of harmonic oscillator, which we name as "EMG oscillator". During practical processing, we can rescale the lengths of the long- and short-half axes so as to facilitate the calculation and analysis.

If the phase portrait corresponding to the red window alone is considered (Figure 3.5b), and only the state points are shown, then the elliptic boundary can be sketched out approximately, as shown in Figure 3.6. For that, x and y denote the amplitude and velocity, and for a harmonic oscillator, the quantity x_2 is proportional to the potential energy (with a constant ratio of $k/2$), with y_2 proportional to the kinetic energy (proportional to $m/2$); thus, the total energy of the oscillator can be written as

$$E = \frac{1}{2}kx^2 + \frac{1}{2}my^2. \tag{3.20}$$

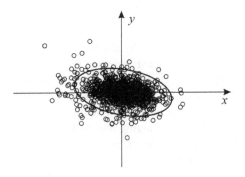

FIGURE 3.6 The energy kernel of EMG oscillator.

Transforming Eq. (3.20) into the elliptic form,

$$\frac{x^2}{2E/k} + \frac{y^2}{2E/m} = 1.\tag{3.21}$$

For an EMG oscillator, neither the stiffness k nor the mass m is known; so, we presume that they are both constants characterizing the intrinsic property of the EMG signal. The area of the ellipse expressed by Eq. (3.21) is

$$S = \frac{2\pi}{\sqrt{km}} E.\tag{3.22}$$

Equation (3.22) shows that the area of the ellipse is proportional to the energy. For this reason, we call the ellipse on the phase portrait as the "energy kernel" (Figure 3.6).

On the other hand, EMG signal is formed by the superposition of the relevant motor unit action potentials (MUAPs) [29,30], which can be considered as propagating waves spreading on muscle fibers [31]. We know that a piece of EMG can be decomposed into a series of harmonic waves. Similarly, MUAP contains different harmonics, each of which takes effect in the EMG signal. Therefore, the energy of the EMG oscillator is actually the summation of the energies of all the harmonic waves; i.e., the energy of the oscillator is determined by that of MUAP, and this is the reason why we say that the EMG signal can be only approximated by a harmonic oscillator within a short time interval Δt. Previously, we have defined the abstract stiffness k and the mass m, and now, we see that these two parameters represent the intrinsic physical properties of the conducting media of MUAP. The mean energy density of a harmonic wave can be expressed as

$$\bar{E} = \frac{1}{2}\rho A^2 \omega^2,\tag{3.23}$$

where ρ is the mass density, A denotes the wave amplitude, and the angular frequency of the vibrating source is characterized by ω. For MUAP, the dominating frequency component corresponds to the firing rate, which we denote as ω_F; so, Eq. (3.23) can be approximated as

$$\bar{E} \cong \frac{1}{2}\rho\left(\sum_i A_i^2\right)\omega_F^2,\tag{3.24}$$

where A_i denotes the amplitude of the ith harmonic. For a particular MU, the amplitude of the AP on the sarcolemma of the fibers is almost constant, and thereby, the energy density mainly varies with the firing rate [32]. With a constant concentration of adenosine triphosphate (ATP), the isometric tension of muscle fiber is approximately proportional to the firing rate at the non-saturated stage of AP firing [33], while for the EMG signal of muscle, the recruitment number of the fibers, represented by the intensity of the signal, also needs to be considered. Referring to Eq. (3.24), both the firing rate and intensity are proportional to the square root of $\bar{E}$. Interestingly, the exact expression of RMS is actually contained in Eq. (3.24), explaining why RMS can be applied to force estimation, while it also tells the reason why RMS cannot be used to extract firing rate [11]. In effect, we have built the relationship between the energy of the control signal (EMG) and that of the output (force or power of muscle), while for isometric contraction, no work is done by the muscle, with only the generation of momentum. Hence, the isometric contraction force is approximately proportional to the square root of $\bar{E}$ within Δt. From this point, when estimating muscle force, we can take a rectangular window of width Δt, let it traverse the signal considered, and then compute the area of the energy kernel S within each window. The force can thus be characterized by $\sqrt{S}$ referring to Eq. (3.22).

The state points in Figure 3.6 fall both inside and outside of the energy kernel; i.e., the moving trajectories of these points show some kind of stochasticity, which can be considered as random walks along the elliptic boundary. As previously noted, the energy level is characterized by the area of the energy kernel. The energy kernel looks like a solid ellipse, while Eq. (3.21) shows that for a non-stochastic harmonic oscillator, the phase portrait consists of a series of concentric hollow ellipses corresponding to different energy levels. This difference sufficiently reflects its statistical characteristics, which originate from two aspects: (1) the noise of the signal and (2) the fluctuation of the firing rate of MUAPs, as well as their random superposition. It is noteworthy that just because of the noise effect, the EMG within Δt can be approximated by a harmonic oscillator, while considering the whole contraction process of the muscle, the oscillator in fact experiences forced oscillation whose energy varies with the that of MUAP. However, the harmonic component is still remarkable since the shape of the energy kernel can be approximated by an ellipse, despite the existence of forced components. As shown in Figure 3.5, during the resting stage of the EMG signal (the blue window), a dense elliptic shape is formed by the state points around the origin. We name this ellipse as the "noise kernel," whose shape and size represent the features of the background noise. Generally, the shape of the noise kernel is different from that of the energy kernel, and during analysis we can certainly remove its area; i.e., only an offset of the area value is produced by the noise kernel, which we will consequently not deal with.

For an oscillator system, there exists a significant physical quantity besides its energy—the natural frequency (f_{nat}). On the other hand, referring to Eq. (3.21), the ratio between the lengths of the short- and long-half axes of the energy kernel can be denoted as

$$\eta = \sqrt{m/k}. \tag{3.25}$$

Thus, f_{nat} can be rewritten as

$$f_{nat} = \frac{1}{2\pi\eta}. \tag{3.26}$$

It can be seen from Eq. (3.26) that f_{nat} can be calculated via the ratio of the short- and long-half axes η, and thereby, after the shape of the energy kernel is determined, the natural frequency can be immediately obtained. Note that the originally unscaled lengths of the half axes should be used when computing f_{nat}. In order to investigate the physical meanings of f_{nat}, the following aspects should be confirmed:

1. Whether the f_{nat} of different skeletal muscles differ from each other for the same subject,
2. Whether the f_{nat} of the same muscle varies with time for the same subject,
3. Whether the f_{nat} of the same type of muscles differ among different subjects,
4. The physical implications that the stiffness k and mass m may have.

3.2.4.2 Algorithm

Now, we need to find a way to identify the elliptic boundary of the energy kernel. For the reason that the state points should be denser inside the kernel and sparser outside, we invented a "linear fencing method" to recognize its boundary. Firstly, we scale the x data and y data into about the same magnitude order so as to facilitate the data processing and the displaying of the energy kernel. Here, we universally reduce the y data thousandfold to avoid the too large magnitude order of y. Next, we take a line L on the phase plane, and let this line approach the origin from infinity; so, L will successively sweep the state points (Figure 3.7a, circle). Now, we set a positive integer N as a threshold of the number of points swept by L and make L stop after N is reached. Then, we change the inclination of the line by the angular step size of $\Delta\theta$ within the interval of $[0, 2\pi]$, repeating the above process, and let $M = (2\pi/\Delta\theta + 1)$; finally, we can get M intercrossing lines from L_1 to L_M enclosing the elliptic shape of the energy kernel, as shown in Figure 3.7a. With the linear fencing method, the line L will rapidly stop when it arrives at the dense region of the state points, making

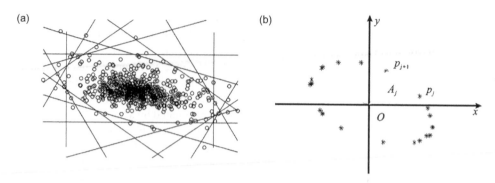

FIGURE 3.7 (a) The linear fencing method for boundary recognition of the energy kernel; (b) computation of the area of the energy kernel.

it possible to retain the reasonable shape of the energy kernel. Now, we choose the points that are closest to the origin from all the intersection points of line L_i ($i = 1, 2, ..., M$) as the boundary points of the kernel. The detailed approach is as follows: judge successively whether the line segment l_{pO} between each intersection point p and the origin is passed by any other line L_i except the lines L_k and L_m that generate point p; if not, p is chosen; otherwise it is abandoned. In this way, we can get the boundary point set U of the energy kernel:

$$U = \left\{ \cup_p : p = L_k \cap L_m, l_{pO} \cap L_i \mid_{i \neq k,m} = \varnothing, i = 1, 2, ..., M \right\}. \tag{3.27}$$

Now, we have converted an EMG segment into a graph. Note that it is critical to select a proper value for N, because if N is too small, a reasonable elliptic shape cannot be produced, or the resultant ellipse is not capable of representing the features of the energy kernels within different windows (low representativeness), while if N is too large, the same problem arises. After many trials, we found that the proper range of N is from 10 to 20, and here, we choose $N = 15$. Moreover, the selection of $\Delta\theta$ owns the same problem: a too large $\Delta\theta$ will result in insufficient boundary points that are inadequate to express the elliptic shape, while an exceedingly small $\Delta\theta$ will unnecessarily raise the computation cost. With the considerations above, we take $\Delta\theta = \pi/10$.

As shown in Figure 3.7b, after the set U (*) is determined, we denote the size of U as P and calculate the area A_j of the triangle $\Delta p_j p_{j+1} O$ generated by two neighboring boundary points p_j, p_{j+1} and the origin; then, the area S of the energy kernel can be approximately obtained via summarizing all the A_j:

$$S = \sum_{j=1}^{P} A_j. \tag{3.28}$$

As mentioned before, the isometric contraction force can be characterized by $\sqrt{S}$; hence, we call $\sqrt{S}$ as the characteristic energy of the EMG oscillator and denote it as E_{ch}.

The set U described previously is also involved in the calculation of the natural frequency of the EMG oscillator [with Eq. (3.22)]. Besides, although the center of the energy kernel should be located at the origin theoretically, due to the inevitable randomness of the linear fencing method, it may slightly deviate from the origin. Thus, in order to compute the lengths of the long- and short-half axes, its center needs to be redefined, and this can be accomplished via calculating the coordinate of the mass center MC of the point set U. Here, we have assumed the unit mass for each point p_j. With the position of MC known, we can choose the longest distance between each point p_j and MC as the length of the long-half axis of the ellipse; meanwhile, the direction of the long axis l_1 can be also determined, as shown in Figure 3.8. Then, we take the direction l_2 that is orthogonal to l_1 as

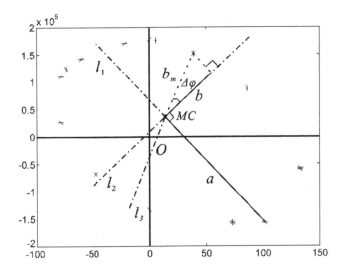

FIGURE 3.8 Calculation of the natural frequency of EMG oscillator.

the direction of the short axis and let the direction of the shortest distance b_m between p_j and MC be l_3; so, the angle $\Delta\varphi$ between l_2 and l_3 can be obtained, and we take the projection length of b_m on l_2 as the length of the short-half axis b. Referring to Eq. (3.26), the natural frequency of the EMG oscillator can be written as

$$f_{\text{nat}} = \frac{a}{2\pi b}. \tag{3.29}$$

For the ease of narration, in the rest part, we sometimes directly call the natural frequency of the EMG signal of a muscle as the natural frequency of this muscle.

3.2.4.3   Extraction Effects' Validation

3.2.4.3.1   Extraction Devices and Methods

Six healthy men, from 23 to 26 years old (mean 24.5), participated in the experiments. The EMG signals were collected from the RF and biceps femoris (BF) of the left thighs of the subjects. Disposable bipolar Ag–AgCl EMG electrodes were applied, with an effective area of 5 mm × 5 mm for each electrode, which was placed on the skin and at approximately the middle part of each muscle, parallel to the assumed muscle fiber orientation with an inter-electrode distance of about 20 mm. The collection of EMG was completed by the self-made data acquisition instrument, with a sampling rate of 2,000 Hz, and the signal successively went through a tenfold pre-amplifier, a 500-fold main amplifier, and an A/D converter.

The forces of RF and BF were registered by the balloons at the front and back side of the leg. The balloons, acting as the force transducers, are installed on an exoskeleton device designed by our research group [34–36]. Contraction of the RF exerts pressure on the front balloon, and the back balloon is compressed when the BF contracts. The gas pressure was transformed into voltage signal to reflect the forces that the balloons experienced. Thereby, the voltage readings from the balloons characterized the isometric contraction force of the corresponding muscle via inverse kinematics. The sampling rate of the gas pressure was also 2,000 Hz.

Figure 3.9 shows the structure of the exoskeleton, which has two degrees of freedom, corresponding to the hip joint and the knee joint, respectively. Right behind the hip joint is a platform used to support the subject, whose hip joint was next to and fixed on that of the exoskeleton; meanwhile, his left thigh and leg were parallel to the upper and lower frames of the

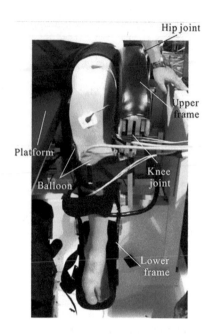

FIGURE 3.9   The EMG signal-acquisition apparatus.

exoskeleton, respectively. The front and back sides of his leg were wrapped by two balloons, which were bound to the lower frame. During experiments, the hip joint and the knee joint of the exoskeleton were locked by servomotors; so, the pose of the thigh and leg was not able to change. As a result, when the subject tried to extend and flex his leg, his RF and BF experienced isometric contraction, making the leg compress the balloons forward and backward. At the same time, the muscle force was fed back via the balloons.

A fourth-order digital Butterworth filter of 10–500 Hz and a notch-rectifier of 50 Hz (used to remove the power noise) were applied to the EMG signal output by the collection instrument, while a third-order digital Butterworth filter of 0.01–1 Hz was applied to the force signal. We denote the EMG and force signals of RF as EMG-RF and F-RF and that of the BF as EMG-BF and F-BF, respectively.

The subject was allowed to extend and flex his leg freely, and each set of experiments lasted about 50 s. A rectangular window with the width of 0.5 s (containing 1,000 sampling points) was applied to EMG-RF and EMG-BF, and linear interpolation was used to compute the temporal derivatives of the signal, denoted as EMG-dR and EMG-dB. The characteristic energies of the EMG, denoted as E_{ch}-RF and E_{ch}-BF, were calculated in a manner of 50% window overlap. Then, E_{ch} RF and F-RF were calibrated with their own maximum values to get E_{ch}-RFC. The same treatment was applied to E_{ch}-BF and F-BF, with the resulting value denoted as E_{ch}-BFC. The difference between f_{nat}-RFC and E_{ch}-BFC, denoted as E_{ch}-rst, characterizes the resultant force of RF and BF. Inverse kinematics was applied to F-RF and F-BF, and the resulting values were subtracted to get the actual resultant force F-rst. Finally, the consistence between E_{ch}-rst and F-rst was investigated.

In order to study the properties of the natural frequency, firstly, for a set of EMG data of the same subject, calculate f_{nat}-RF and f_{nat}-BF of his RF and BF with Eq. (3.29) after the boundary of the energy kernel is determined and check whether f_{nat}-RF and f_{nat}-BF vary with E_{ch}-RFC and E_{ch}-BFC to judge if f_{nat} depends on MU firing rate or not. On the other hand, the problem whether the f_{nat} of a specific muscle of a subject changes with time needs to be investigated, as well as the question whether the f_{nat} of different muscles of the subject differ. Finally, we should compute the f_{nat} of the same type of muscles of different subjects to make sure if the natural frequency of the same muscle differs among individuals.

For the estimation of the muscle force, linear regression analysis was used to evaluate whether linear relationship exists between E_{ch}-rst and F-rst for each subject, as well as the level of the linearity, which can be characterized by the strength of relationship, the r^2 value:

$$r^2 = \frac{\sum_{i=1}^{n}(\hat{x}_i - \bar{x})^2}{\sum_{i=1}^{n}(x_i - \bar{x})^2}, \tag{3.30}$$

where n is the total number of sample points, $\hat{x}$ is the predicted value, and $\bar{x}$ is the mean of measured data. For the estimation of f_{nat}, the analysis of variance (ANOVA) was applied to assess whether the differences among the f_{nat} discussed above are remarkable or not, and the inspecting value F is

$$F = \frac{MS_o}{MS_i}, \tag{3.31}$$

where MS_o and MS_i are the variance between groups and variance within groups, respectively. Here, we choose the significance level α_F as 0.05 and set the null hypothesis as "no remarkable differences exist between groups". The corresponding p value is obtained by substituting F into the F-distribution table, and if $p < \alpha_F$, we accept that the investigated factor has remarkable effect on f_{nat}; otherwise the null hypothesis is accepted.

3.2.4.3.2 Characterization of the Isometric Contraction Force

Figure 3.10 demonstrates a force estimation result for a subject via the energy kernel method. The gray curves correspond to E_{ch}-rst, the estimated values, while the black ones represent F-rst. Here, E_{ch}-rst and F-rst are not normalized; instead, we directly take linear regression between them for better representativeness. Thus, the corresponding r^2 value can be obtained, and the scaled E_{ch}-rst by the resulting fitting parameters and F-rst are further compared. Moreover, for simplicity, all the data are illustrated in the dimensionless form. Figure 3.10a shows the results of relatively fast contractions of RF and BF, while those of slow contractions are shown in Figure 3.10b. In both situations, the subject can freely exert forces on the front or back balloons; i.e., RF and BF can experience all the different intensities of voluntary contraction (VC). We see from Figure 3.10 that E_{ch}-rst faithfully reflects the varying trend of F-rst and even very tiny fluctuations, and the gray curves universally lead the black ones by 50–100 ms, representing the electromechanical delay [37]. However, remarkable undershoots and overshoots appear at some points for the estimated results, due to factors such as filtering distortion, the errors of the force transducers (balloons), or the recruitment of deep layers of the muscle [38].

For each subject (from subject A to F), we took one group of such experiments, with every group containing four sets of data; so, there are totally 24 sets of data registered. The subjects rested for

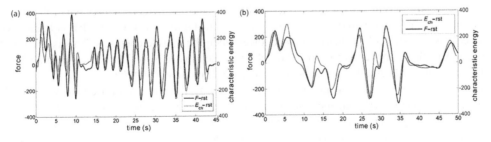

FIGURE 3.10 The force estimation results for one subject. (a) Fast contractions; (b) slow contractions.

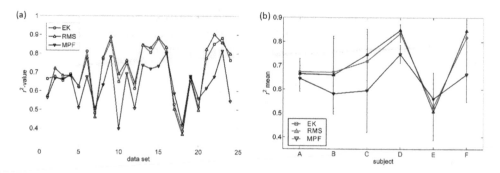

FIGURE 3.11 The r^2 values obtained using EK, RMS, and MPF. (a) The corresponding r^2 values of all the data; (b) the mean of the r^2 values within each group of data.

3–5 min between every two sets of experiments in order to avoid fatigue [39]. For the four sets of data for each subject, we computed their r^2 values, as well as their means and standard deviations (SDs). Aiming at the evaluation of the energy kernel method in force estimation, we further applied the methods of RMS and MPF to the same data, and their r^2 values were obtained in the same way. Figure 3.11a demonstrates the processed results of all the data via these three methods, in which the energy kernel method is abbreviated as EK. Through simple checks, we can find that the consistence of the results estimated by EK with the actual forces may be better than that of both RMS and MPF, or stays in the middle, but hardly falls at the worst position. Figure 3.11b shows the mean of the r^2 values of each group under these three methods, and it is clear that for the data in this paper, the performance of EK is close to that of RMS (p value 0.9046) but is remarkably higher than that of MPF (p value 0.0445). We know that RMS mainly reflects the intensity of the signal (the amplitude-related features) and is able to represent the recruitment level of the fibers to some extent. MPF mainly focuses on the frequency-domain characteristics, and it holds a better correspondence with the firing rate at low levels of VC. The above results indicate that the effect of EK is close to that of RMS when that of MPF is the worst, while the effects of EK and MPF are close to each other when that of RMS falls behind. Consequently, it can be accepted that EK owns the advantages of both RMS and MPF, and this is actually already indicated by Eq. (3.24), which shows that the new method simultaneously reflects the factors of recruitment level and firing rate, making it very robust and stable. We expect that it is especially useful for the applications of force estimation involving large span-VC levels.

3.2.4.3.3 *Natural Frequency of the EMG Oscillator*

To better calculate the natural frequency and to enhance the representativeness of the data, the subjects were asked to make slow flexion or extension motion of their legs so that continuous step force signals lasting for about 5 s could be obtained. Figure 3.12 shows the E_{ch}-RF and the corresponding f_{nat}-RF (dimensionless) of a subject, and f_{nat}-RF is in the unit of Hz. We see that f_{nat}-RF demonstrates a pulse-like pattern, with the width of the pulse matching with the duration of the force. Besides, the variation trends of E_{ch}-RF and f_{nat}-RF approximately complement each other (the variation trend of f_{nat}-RF is indicated by the gray line in Figure 3.12); i.e., f_{nat}-RF is higher when the muscle is at rest, while it turns out to be lower when the muscle contracts. This is because the ellipse on the phase portrait is the noise kernel when the muscle rests. Therefore, the high level of f_{nat}-RF in Figure 3.12 actually corresponds to the natural frequency of "filtered noise" (since the signal has already been filtered), while the low level represents the real natural frequency of the EMG oscillator. This means with our method, the natural frequencies of the noise and the EMG signal can be successfully separated and recognized, with that of the latter to be about 100 Hz, indicated by Figure 3.12. Note that the real natural frequency of noise should be calculated with the raw noise signal. On the other hand, we see that when RF contracts, f_{nat}-RF basically stays constant; i.e., it

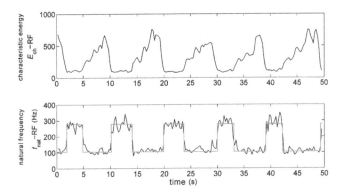

FIGURE 3.12   The correspondence between the characteristic energy and the natural frequency of RF.

does not follow the trend of E_{ch}-RF. This invariance further certifies that a remarkable harmonic component exists, and this fact tells that the natural frequency of EMG is not correlated to the MU firing rate but rather characterizes the intrinsic properties of MUAP or its conducting medium. The conclusions above also apply to BF.

To further investigate whether the natural frequencies of the same type of muscle of different individuals and those of different muscles of the same individual differ or not, ten groups of experiments involving subjects D, E, and F were implemented. In each group, the EMG with the length of ~15 s of the RF and BF of the subjects was collected below 50% MVC, as well as the raw noise signals (collected at rest, ~15 s long) of RF and BF. The first group started at about 10 a.m., and the last one ended at about 7 p.m. within a day, with the interval of ~1 h between two successive groups. Therefore, the experiments were also used to check the time dependence of the natural frequency. The means of the natural frequencies of RF, BF, and their corresponding noises are calculated within each group, denoted as f-RF, f-BF, fn-RF, and fn-BF, respectively. Here, f-RF and f-BF were computed after fn-RF and fn-BF, which were used to define the bandwidth of the notch filters designed to filter the EMG signals before calculating f-RF and f-BF. A digital Butterworth filter of 10–500 Hz was also applied. These quantities of the three subjects are plotted in Figure 3.13, with the x-axis denoting the collection time of each data group.

i. Time factor

Figure 3.13 suggests that not only the f-RF and f-BF, but also the fn-RF and fn-BF of all the subjects vary with time. Table 3.3 lists the p values calculated from the data groups of all the times for each subject and each type of natural frequency. It is obvious that, indeed, all the p values in Table 3.3 are close to zero, smaller than the α_F (0.05); so, we can accept that all these natural frequencies change with time. The time dependence of fn-RF and fn-BF indicates that the frequency-domain stability of the signal can be affected by the environment remarkably, since the natural frequency of the noise may fluctuate by more than 10 Hz at different times, with the range of ~40–50 Hz, which is definitely the range of power frequency. Referring to this fact, we suggest the acquisition of the EMG signal used for frequency-domain analysis to be carried out in the environment with low electromagnetic noise. Moreover, the r^2 values between f-RF and fn-RF, together with those between f-BF and fn-BF, are listed in Table 3.4 for each subject. The r^2 values are all less than 0.5 except those between f-RF and fn-RF of subject E (0.55, denoted by bold style), indicating that normally the natural frequency of muscle does not depend on that of noise, while problems may have occurred during the data acquisition of the RF of subject E, e.g., the deviation of the EMG electrodes from the correct place due to the relatively thick and fat layer of the thigh. Consequently, it is not surprising that the f-RF and f-BF of subjects D

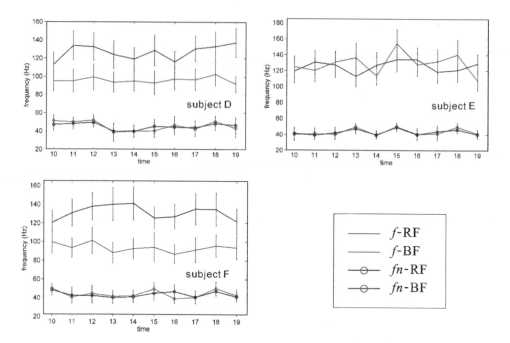

FIGURE 3.13   The mean of the natural frequencies of RF, BF, and the corresponding noises within each group of data.

TABLE 3.3

The p Values against the Time Factor ($\alpha_F = 0.05$) for Each Subject

	Subject D	Subject E	Subject F
f-RF	0.001	5.83×10^{-55}	2.46×10^{-8}
f-BF	1.35×10^{-23}	4.67×10^{-17}	8.07×10^{-20}
fn-RF	4.51×10^{-36}	3.36×10^{-41}	6.15×10^{-25}
fn-BF	1.12×10^{-17}	3.17×10^{-26}	5.76×10^{-20}

TABLE 3.4

The r^2 Values between Natural Frequencies of Muscles and Noises

	Subject D	Subject E	Subject F
f-RF and fn-RF	0.32	**0.55**	0.37
f-BF and fn-BF	0.11	−0.01	0.22

and F and the f-BF of subject E are relatively stable (with a fluctuation less than 20 Hz for different times), while the f-RF of subject E shows remarkable instability.

ii. Muscle-type factor

Referring to Figure 3.13, it is also clear that f-RF and f-BF are distinct from each other for subjects D and F, while the difference is ambiguous for subject E, due to the problem discussed above. The p values between f-RF and f-BF, as well as those between fn-RF and fn-BF for each subject, are listed in Table 3.5, which verifies the facts read from Figure 3.13. The p value between f-RF and f-BF of subject E is also denoted in bold style.

TABLE 3.5
The p Values against the Muscle-Type Factor ($\alpha_F = 0.05$) for Each Subject

	Subject D	Subject E	Subject F
f-RF and f-BF	2.03×10^{-9}	**0.46**	5.52×10^{-11}
fn-RF and fn-BF	0.92	0.86	0.74

Thereby, it can be accepted that the natural frequency depends on muscle type, and f-BF may be generally higher than f-RF for a person. Besides, the p values of the noise are all much greater than α_F, suggesting a reasonable fact that the natural frequency of noise is independent of muscle type.

iii. Individual factor

We show the f-RF and f-BF separately for all the three subjects in Figure 3.14, which indicates the weak distinction of f-BF among individuals, while f-RF differs a lot. The p values of f-RF, f-BF, fn-RF, and fn-BF against individual factors are listed in Table 3.6, from which we can tell that f-BF and the noises do not depend on individuals, while it is not the case for f-RF, represented in bold style. However, the p value of f-RF between subjects D and F can be calculated to be 0.19; hence, if we exclude the abnormal f-RF data of subject E, it can be accepted that the natural frequencies of a specific muscle type are perhaps indistinguishable or at least very close for ordinary people. On the other hand, Table 3.6 also lists the independence of the natural frequency of noise on individuals.

3.2.4.3.4 The EMG Oscillator and the Propagating Wave of MUAP

This chapter constructed a new physical/mathematical model of EMG via the conversion from signal series to portraits and proposed an energy kernel method to characterize the isometric force of skeletal muscle. As illustrated, the phase portrait of a piece of EMG signal demonstrates an elliptic shape carrying stochastic features, and compared with the elliptic phase portrait of a

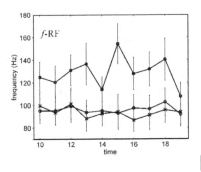
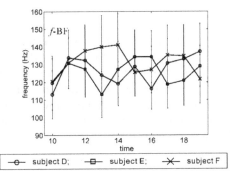

FIGURE 3.14   The mean of the natural frequencies of RF and BF illustrated separately for all the subjects.

TABLE 3.6
The p Values against the Individual Factor ($\alpha_F = 0.05$)[a]

f-RF	f-BF	fn-RF	fn-BF
2.89×10^{-10}	0.21	0.27	0.56

[a] The p value for f-RF excluding subject E is 0.19.

harmonic oscillator, this indicates that harmonic components are dominant in EMG, which can thereby be approximated by the abstract motion of harmonic oscillators. On the other hand, due to the configuration of the measurements by EMG electrodes, the collected signal in effect reflects the time-varying behavior of MUAP at a certain location. As MUAP is a propagating potential wave on sarcolemma, EMG can be regarded as an MUAP observer. The wave source is certainly the neuromuscular junction, and the frequency of the propagating wave should vary with the firing rate; therefore, in a strict sense, the EMG oscillator actually experiences frequency-varying forced oscillations. Considering the effect of noise, we treat the EMG signal in a short-time interval as a harmonic oscillator and characterize the isometric contraction force via the characteristic energy. The results show that there exists good consistence between the force and the characteristic energy, and compared with RMS and MPF, we found that it demonstrates the advantages of both RMS and MPF, with a very high robustness.

3.2.4.3.5 The Natural Frequency

The natural frequency of a specific muscle can also be obtained via the energy kernel method, and f_{nat} is independent of MU firing rate by previous analysis. On one hand, this indicates that f_{nat} indeed represents the intrinsic property of muscle, and on the other hand, it provides strong support for the harmonic-oscillator hypothesis of EMG. Moreover, this provides a new way for detecting the health condition of muscle in biomedical applications. For that, EMG originates from the induced potential oscillations of MUAP waves, f_{nat}, and may be related to the intrinsic electric property of the tissue [40]. For harmonic oscillators, the stiffness k decides the intensity of the restoring force; so, the stiffness of the EMG oscillator may reflect the density ratio between K^+ and Na^+ channels on sarcolemma, or the shape of MUAP, while the mass m of a harmonic oscillator dominates the acceleration; therefore, the mass of the EMG oscillator should represent the capacity of the membrane. Here, we did not discuss the issue of "resonance", which corresponds to the situation that the MU firing rate is equal to f_{nat}. Due to the large damp of the tissue, resonance is not likely to cause destructive effects. The probable case is that the muscle may experience tetanic contraction even under non-saturated firing rate. Moreover, note that it is difficult to accurately measure the f_{nat} of a muscle via surface EMG; so, the results are generally approximations due to the cross talk among different MUs.

3.2.4.3.6 Noise Filtering

When measuring the natural frequency of the muscle, if the noise kernel is treated in the same way as the energy kernel, the natural frequency of the noise can also be calculated (Figure 3.12). Hence, in order to improve the filtering performance of EMG, the natural frequency of raw noise can be computed at first, and then a notch filter can be applied to the signal with the bandwidth obtained from the results. This method actually provides a new approach for the signal–noise recognition and separation, since the real-time dominating frequencies of the noise and signal can be rapidly extracted without traditional FT.

REFERENCES

1. Momen K, Krishnan S, Chau T. Real-time classification of forearm electromyographic signals corresponding to user-selected intentional movements for multifunction prosthesis control. *IEEE Trans. Neural. Syst. Rehabil. Eng.*, 2007, 15(4): 535–542.
2. Lauer R T, Smith B T, Betz R R. Application of a neuro-fuzzy network for gait event detection using electromyography in the child with cerebral palsy. *IEEE Trans. Biomed. Eng.*, 2005, 52(9): 1532–1540.
3. Artemiadis P K, Kyriakopoulos K J. An EMG-based robot control scheme robust to time-varying EMG signal features. *IEEE Trans. Inform. Tech. Biomed.*, 2010, 14(3): 582–588.
4. Choi C, Kwon S, Park W, et al. Real-time pinch force estimation by surface electromyography using an artificial neural network. *Med. Eng. Phys.*, 2010, 32(5): 429–436.
5. Bonato P, Gagliati G, Knaflitz M. Analysis of myoelectric signals recorded during dynamic contractions. *IEEE Eng. Med. Biol. Mag.*, 1996, 15(6): 102–111.

6. Staudenmann D, Roeleveld K, Stegeman D F, et al. Methodological aspects of SEMG recordings for force estimation–A tutorial and review. *J. Electromyopr. Kinesiol.*, 2010, 20: 375–387.

7. Bigland-Ritchie B, Donovan E F, Roussos C S. Conduction velocity and EMG power spectrum changes in fatigue of sustained maximal efforts. *J. Appl. Physiol.*, 1981, 51(5): 1300–1305.

8. Mannion A F, Connolly B, Wood K, et al. The use of surface EMG power spectral analysis in the evaluation of back muscle function. *J. Rehabil. Res. Dev.*, 1997, 34(4): 427–439.

9. Komi P V, Tesch P. EMG frequency spectrum, muscle structure, and fatigue during dynamic contractions in man. *Eur. J. Appl. Physiol. Occup. Physiol.*, 1979, 42(1): 41–50.

10. Güler N F, Koçer S. Classification of EMG signals using PCA and FFT. *J. Med. Syst.*, 2005, 29(3): 241–250.

11. Talebinejad M, Chan A D C, Miri A, et al. Fractal analysis of surface electromyography signals: A novel power spectrum-based method. *J. Electromyopr. Kinesiol.*, 2009, 19: 840–850.

12. Christie A, Inglis G, Kamen G. Relationships between surface EMG variables and motor unit firing rates. *Eur. J. Appl. Physiol.*, 2009, 107: 177–185.

13. Qi L, Wakeling J M, Green A, et al. Spectral properties of electromyographic and mechanomyographic signals during isometric ramp and step contractions in biceps brachii. *J. Electromyopr. Kinesiol.*, 2011, 21(1): 128–135.

14. Gabor D. Theory of communication. *J. Inst. Electr. Eng.*, 1946, 93: 429–457.

15. Claasen T, Mecklenbrauker W. The Wigner distribution–A tool for time-frequency analysis, Part I: Continuous-time signals. *Philips J. Res.*, 1980, 35: 217–250.

16. Wang G, Wang Z Z, Chen W T, et al. Classification of surface EMG signals using optimal wavelet packet method based on Davies-Bouldin criterion. *Med. Bio. Eng. Comput.*, 2006, 44: 865–872.

17. Michele G D, Sello S, Garboncini M C, et al. Cross-correlation time-frequency analysis for multiple EMG signals in Parkinson's disease: A wavelet approach. *Med. Eng. Phys.*, 2003, 25: 361–369.

18. Zhang Q, Luo Z, Ye M. Surface EMG multimode classification based on power spectrum analysis and RBF network. *Mech. Electr. Eng. Mag.*, 2005, 22(11): 35–38 (in Chinese).

19. Kukolj D, Levi E. Identification of complex systems based on neural and Takagi–Sugeno fuzzy model. *IEEE Trans. Syst. Man. Cybern. B*, 2003, 34(1): 272–282.

20. Vineet G, Srikanth S, Narender P R. Fractal analysis of surface EMG signals from the biceps. *Int. J. Med. Inform.*, 1997, 45: 185–192.

21. Holobar A, Zazula D. Multi-channel blind source separation using convolution kernel compensation. *IEEE Trans. Signal Process.*, 2007, 8(55): 4487–4496.

22. Azzerboni B, Finocchio G, Ipsale M, et al. A new approach to detection of muscle activation by independent component analysis and wavelet transform. *Comput. Sci.*, 2002, 2486: 109–116.

23. Nair S S, French R M, Laroche D, et al. The application of machine learning algorithms to the analysis of electromyographic patterns from arthritic patients. *IEEE Trans. Neural. Syst. Rehabil. Eng.*, 2010, 18(2): 174–184.

24. Levi J H, Erik J S, Kevin B E, et al. Multiple binary classifications via linear discriminant analysis for improved controllability of a powered prosthesis. *IEEE Trans. Neural. Syst. Rehabil. Eng.*, 2010, 18(1): 49–57.

25. Guo Z, Fan Y J, Zhang J J, et al. A new 4M model-based human-machine interface for lower extremity exoskeleton robot. *The 5th International Conference on Intelligent Robotics and Applications*, 2012 October 3–5, Canada. Montreal: Springer (Berlin Heidelberg), 2012: 123–130.

26. Gabriel D A, Christie A, Greig Inglis J, et al. Experimental and modeling investigation of surface EMG spike analysis. *Med. Eng. Phys.*, 2011, 33: 427–437.

27. Merletti R, Conte L L, Avignone E, et al. Modeling of surface myoelectric signals–Part I: Model implementation. *IEEE Trans. Biomed. Eng.*, 1999, 46(7): 810–820.

28. Day S J, Hulliger M. Experimental simulation of cat electromyogram: Evidence for algebraic summation of motor-unit action-potential trains. *J. Neurophysiol.*, 2001, 86(5): 2144–2158.

29. Yang J, Yang H. Study on automatic decomposition of EMG signals with overlapping MUAP waveform. *Chinese J. Biomed. Eng.*, 1999, 18(1): 82–88 (in Chinese).

30. McComas A J, Mrozek K, Gardner-Medwin D, et al. Electrical properties of muscle fibre membranes in man. *J. Neurol. Neurosurg. Phychiat.*, 1968, 31: 434–440.

31. Kesar T, Chou L W, Binder-Macleod S A. Effects of stimulation frequency versus pulse duration modulation on muscle fatigue. *J. Electromyopr. Kinesiol.*, 2008, 18: 662–671.

32. Yin Y H, Fan Y J, Xu L D. EMG & EPP-integrated human-machine interface between the paralyzed and rehabilitation exoskeleton. *IEEE Trans. Info. Tech. Biomed.*, 2012, 16(4): 542–549.

33. Yin Y H, Fan Y J, Guo Z. sEMG-based neuro-fuzzy controller for a parallel ankle exoskeleton with proprioception. *Int. J. Robot Autom.*, 2011, 26(4): 450–460.

34. Fan Y J, Yin Y H. Differentiated time-frequency characteristics based real-time human-machine interface for lower extremity rehabilitation exoskeleton robot. *The 5th International Conference on Intelligent Robotics and Applications*, 2012 October 3–5, Canada. Montreal: Springer (Berlin Heidelberg), 2012: 31–40.

35. Zhou S, Lawson D L, Morrison W E. Electromechanical delay in isometric muscle contractions evoked by voluntary, reflex and electrical stimulation. *Eur. J. Appl. Physiol.*, 1995, 70: 138–145.

36. Rasmussen J, Damsgaard M, Voigt M. Muscle recruitment by the min/max criterion-a comparative numerical study. *J. Biomech.*, 2001, 34: 409–415.

37. Zhou Q X, Chen Y H, Ma C, et al. Evaluation model for muscle fatigue of upper limb based on sEMG analysis. *Sci. China Life Sci.*, 2011, 41(8): 608–614.

38. Lowery M M, Stoykov N S, Dewald J P A, et al. Volume conduction in an anatomically based surface EMG model. *IEEE Trans. Biomed. Eng.*, 2004, 51(12): 2138–2147.

39. Yin Y, Guo Z, Chen X, Fan Y. Operation mechanism of molecular motor based biomechanical research progresses on skeletal muscle. *Chinese Sci. Bull.*, 2012, 30: 2794–2805 (in Chinese).

40. Yin Y, Chen X. Bioelectrochemical principle of variable frequency control on skeletal muscle contraction - Operation mechanism of molecular motor based biomechanical mechanism of skeletal muscle (II). *Sci. China Technol. Sci.*, 2012, 42(8): 901–910 (in Chinese).

4 Human–Machine Force Interactive Interface and Exoskeleton Robot Techniques Based on Biomechanical Model of Skeletal Muscle

In the former chapters, studies on biomechanical model of skeletal muscle, as well as surface electromyography (sEMG)-based feature extraction methods for contraction prediction, have been systematically discussed. Both these topics are closely related to rehabilitation exoskeleton robot techniques. Statistical report indicates that stroke incidence in China ranks first all over the world with a total number of 6 million, and it increases by 2 million every year. The nerve injuries caused by stroke or other diseases will result in hemiplegia and even paralysis if not treated in time or treated inappropriately. Slight delay in the treatment will severely affect the reconstruction of human motor function and significantly increase the length of rehabilitation period. For patients with motor function injury such as stroke, early physiotherapy can improve the functional recovery of motion. However, most of the traditional physiotherapies are conducted by physical therapists or medical staffs, and this kind of therapy consumes very much manpower and material resource with very limited effectiveness. Patients often end up with sequelae such as hemiplegia when they are not able to receive effective treatment in time. At present, medication is usually adopted in the early treatment for patients with stroke or spinal injuries. Meanwhile, insufficient attention has been paid to the functional exercise during post treatment. All these contribute to the delay of the best treatment time and the loss of work ability and viability for part of the patients.

Thus, an intelligent rehabilitation system for patients suffering from stroke and sports injury is urgently needed. It is supposed to provide safe and effective rehabilitation treatment and reduce the cost of manpower and medical resource so that more patients are able to receive better treatment. For the fact that two research fields, exoskeleton robot and microelectronic techniques, are closely related to human–machine integrated rehabilitation robot and both are developing rapidly, strong technical supports are available for the advance of a new-generation rehabilitation robot system that integrates biotechnology with electromechanics. For the existent exoskeleton robots, the sEMG-based/myoelectric control methods and human–machine integration have been widely adopted. However, patients are still not able to perform the rehabilitation movement in a natural and instinctive way, resulting in an unsatisfactory rehabilitation efficacy. Thus, challenges remain in the fundamental theories, and technical bottlenecks still exist for developing new-generation devices. Nowadays, there are generally five categories of rehabilitation methods for nerve injury of lower limbs, including standing exercise with standing bed, body-weight–supported treadmill training, functional electrical stimulation (FES), compound rehabilitation, and rehabilitation robot. A brief introduction is as follows:

- **Standing exercise with standing bed**: This exercise aims to provide adaptative training in early treatment. Patient on the standing bed would be able to feel a different proportion of self-weight by adjusting the angle of inclination. It helps the hemiplegic patients in the following aspects: first, it helps patients to do the training exercises from lying down to standing pose when the center of gravity rises so that patients are able to adapt to various standing positions. Second, it helps to enhance the bearing capability of patients' body and lower limbs; maintain the stress load of vertebration, pelvis, and lower limbs; and prevent decalcification of bone, pressure sore, and urinary tract infection. It can also enhance the control ability of neck, chest, waist, and pelvis in the standing position and thus lay the foundation for self-standing and balancing in the future. Third, proprioceptors can be effectively stimulated via the pressing by self-weight on the joint muscle to increase muscular tension, which is relatively low for the patients. Fourth, for other abnormal patterns caused by higher muscular tension of lower limbs, corrected movement can be achieved by long-time tractions with enough strength from self-weight to Achilles tendon. Due to its simplicity and safety, standing bed has been widely used in clinical rehabilitation. However, its efficacy is limited by the relatively onefold function.

- **Body-weight–supported treadmill training**: This training reduces the load of lower limbs from self-weight by a suspension accessory that reduces body weight and conducts the ambulation training with the aid of the accessory. Muscle spasm could be alleviated by reducing the load in this training method. Moreover, patients with insufficient standing ability because of muscle atrophy would also be able to do the ambulation training. It helps to maintain or even recover all of the patients' physiological functions and enforce the central nervous system to be remolded by repetitive training so that normal gait could be achieved. It has been acknowledged that patients' lower-limb motor function, walking velocity, balancing capability, and walking endurance can be improved by repetitive body-weight–supported treadmill training for patients with stroke or spinal injury.

- **Myoelectric feedback and FES**: Myosignals are usually amplified, filtered, bidirectionally rectified, and integrated. The monitor is driven by integral voltage so that the degree of tension can be directly observed. Through the feedback audiovisual signal, patients can contract and relax their muscle voluntarily to improve their motion control abilities and recover motor functions. In the treatment of stroke and hemiplegia, although myoelectric feedback method cannot recover the already damaged brain nerve cells, it can promote the metabolism, open the depressed nerve tract, and maintain the maximum potential of nerve muscle tissue so that physiological functions can also be maintained. FES is used to stimulate one group or multiple groups of muscles by low-frequency current pulse based on a prescribed stimulus program to induce muscular contraction so that the function of the stimulated muscle or muscle groups can be improved or recovered. FES system promotes the refunctioning of brain by making use of the plasticity of central nervous system (CNS), and it plays an important role in the rehabilitation of stroke or hemiplegia patients. In 1961, foot-drop on the hemiplegia side of a chronic stroke patient was successfully rectified using FES by Liberson. It set a precedent for the recovery of motor function for stroke patients after hemiplegia. Afterward, it has been proved that FES could also be used to improve muscle strength, enhance walking ability, improve knee joint coordination, etc. Moreover, FES is recognized as an effective lower-limb rehabilitation technique for stroke patients.

- **Compound rehabilitation**: This improves the rehabilitation efficacy for patients in prognosis of stroke and spinal injury by integrating the existing medical treatment methods with auxiliary rehabilitation technology, such as myoelectric feedback, FES, weight-reduced standing, ambulation exercise, and robot-assisted treatment, to generate effective rehabilitation strategy so that the desired rehabilitation efficacy could be accomplished. For instance, Fields first proposed compound rehabilitation method by integrating myoelectric feedback with FES (myosignal-triggered FES), which achieved satisfactory rehabilitation results. Patients should contract and relax muscle voluntarily to improve their motion control abilities and recover motor functions in the myoelectric feedback method. However, part of the patients with stroke and spinal injury are not able to activate the muscle on the impaired side, leading to weakened rehabilitation efficacy. Although some good results have been obtained in clinical application, FES is a kind of passive treatment rather than active treatment, so the exercise effect is still unsatisfactory in muscle power. When treating stroke patients, there would be spasm in antagonistic muscles because of CNS disorder, which would lead to the failure of muscle power enhancement. Weight-reduced standing, ambulation exercise, and rehabilitation robot help patients move by reducing the body weight or providing assistive power, which is also a kind of passive treatment and thus cannot conduct rehabilitation exercise based on patients' motor intent. In consequence, an effective and active rehabilitation strategy combining existing methods should be developed to shorten rehabilitation cycle and achieve better rehabilitation efficacy.

- **Rehabilitation robot**: Human–machine interaction interface is necessary for rehabilitation robots when performing rehabilitation exercises such as passive training, assistive exercise, and gait training, with the aid of electric motor. The rehabilitation robot could be used in the functional exercise for lower limbs with paralysis after stroke or spinal injury. The Lokomat developed by Swiss researchers is one of the representative exoskeleton robots. It has the entity structure of exoskeleton, balance compensation for human weight, and weight reduction accessories. The indoor rehabilitation exercise of lower limbs can be conducted. However, it is inconvenient to move due to large-space requirement and high price. Erigo rehabilitation training system for early recovery of nerve damage developed by Swiss HOCOMA Company enables the patients in an adjustable heeling position. Moreover, it provides small-movement training for joints of lower extremity to reduce the possibility of complications. The early intensive treatment is achieved by the integration of a continuous adjustable bed with a robotic gait system. However, the joint angle range of the lower extremity is too small, so it can only be used in early rehabilitation. Moreover, it is signal functional and expensive. KineAssist movable rehabilitation robot developed in Chicago aids patients to perform walking. Assistive training of lower limbs is not included in the robot; therefore it is not able to do the rehabilitation exercise. It is worth mentioning that many Chinese research organizations, such as Harbin Institute of Technology, Shenyang Institute of Automation, Beijing University of Aeronautics and Astronautics, National University of Defense Technology, and Shanghai Jiao Tong University, etc. have also contributed a lot to this field, but most of their works are still in the initial stage without mature products.

Rehabilitation robot provides users with effective assistive walking exercise and has become one of the research hotspots around the globe. However, based on the statistical data, natural harmony could hardly be reached between human and machine, and there are still few clinical applications of exoskeleton robots. Hence, there are still great challenges in applying exoskeleton robot; the reasons lie in two main aspects. One is that a fully functional exoskeleton robot system is still under development to overcome the shortcomings of weak stability and insufficient driving force. The second is that human–machine interaction interface and the corresponding control strategy remain to be improved. Exoskeleton robot provides motive force through joint movement; thus interactive force surely exists between human and the exoskeleton robot. However, it still needs to be studied on the generation mechanism of this interactive force. On the other hand, extensive studies have been made on the electromyography (EMG)-based and force-sensing–based human–machine interaction interface. Particularly, the motion capture system, myoelectric apparatus, and force detection equipment have already been applied in the human dynamics and kinematics analysis. Thus, to promote active compliance control of exoskeleton robot, it is a prerequisite to study human–machine interaction interface design and the generation mechanism of interactive force.

4.1 LOWER-EXTREMITY EXOSKELETON ROBOT

In order to recover patients' walking ability as early as possible, rehabilitation exercise is important. Athletic training can promote the spontaneous recovery of neurological function and cerebral functional remodeling so as to accelerate the functional recovery process. With the progress of technology, many kinds of effective cinesiotherapies have been proposed, including myoelectric feedback, FES, body-weight–supported treadmill training, robot-assisted treatment, virtual reality, etc. Rehabilitation robot has been applied in the functional training of patients' lower extremities. Compared with traditional rehabilitation methods, it provides a larger probability to recover the motor function of patients' lower extremities. Exoskeleton is one of the most representative rehabilitation robots that integrate mechanics, electrics, biology, informatics, cybermatics, etc. [1]. With the progress of technology and increase of social needs, great improvements have been made in fundamental theory and applied technology of exoskeleton robot.

4.1.1 STATE OF THE ART

4.1.1.1 Early Exoskeleton Robot

A part of the early exoskeleton robots stayed at the stage of conceptual design and remained unrealized. Only a very small number of these prototypes were physically developed, but unfortunately none of them performed well.

According to the literature, the first exoskeleton structure was mentioned in an American patent that was granted to Yagn [2]. A long arcuate spring was included in the invention and was arranged in parallel with human lower extremity so as to enhance the running and jumping ability. During the gait support phase, the spring was able to deliver self-weight to the ground to reduce the load on leg. During the swing phase, the spring was released so that the lower extremity would be able to bend freely. Although the design proposed by Yagn was supposed to enhance human motor ability, the design has never been developed successfully.

In 1963, Zaroodny in External Ballistics Laboratory of United States Army published a technical report which illustrated the program of active assistive skeleton started in 1951 [3]. The exoskeleton was aimed to enhance the carrying capability of healthy people such as soldiers. Although most of the work was still at the stage of conceptual design, Zaroodny had already proposed the fundamental problems involved in the application of the exoskeleton robot, such as portable power, sensing and control, human–machine interface, and human–machine integrated dynamics. This device was probably the first active force-assistant exoskeleton in history. It had three degrees of freedom (DOFs) actuated by a big cylinder. The exoskeleton started from hip joint and was connected with custom-designed shoes to form the entity of the exoskeleton. However, his proposal was not fully funded to complete the program. Still, this work was the first published one on exoskeleton-related engineering problems.

In the late 1960s, Schenectady, NY, developed a full-body–type active exoskeleton prototype with the cooperation of researchers in Cornell University and financial support from US navy [4,5], and the prototype was called *Hardiman*. The exoskeleton was a huge hydraulic machine with the weight of 680 Kg and 30 DOFs. It could be applied to enhance the upper-body and lower-extremity strength (not including wrist). Compared with many other force-assistant exoskeleton robots, Hardiman program aimed to enhance the strength substantially (approximately 25:1).

Although satisfactory results had been achieved on the force assistance of upper body, there were still unsolved problems in the lower-extremity part, so the full-body–type exoskeleton was not developed successfully, and the Hardiman program ended up being a failure. Regardless of its failure, its significant contribution lies in the discovery of the biggest difficulties in the design and development of exoskeleton robot, such as power and human–machine interface.

In the middle of 1980s, Jeffrey Moore in Los Alamos National laboratory published a paper on the conceptual design of exoskeleton robot to enforce soldiers' strength. It originated from the idea of Heinlein on *Pitman*. However, it didn't give the solution for power supply and design development. The idea did not come true because of the lack of funding, but it did lay the foundation for the exoskeleton development schedule by Defence Advanced Research Project Agency (DARPA)

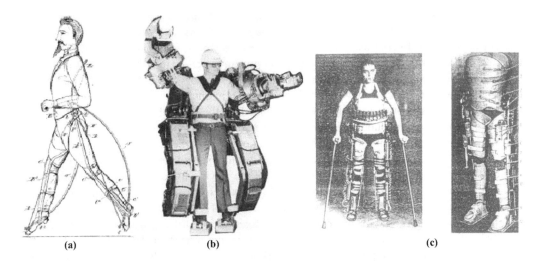

FIGURE 4.1 Mechanical structure of early exoskeleton robots. (a) Yagn's exoskeleton patent; (b) Hardiman exoskeleton developed by GE; (c) structure of early exoskeleton.

10 years later. Besides, an independent researcher named Mark Rosheim further developed the idea of Hardiman and Pitman, bringing in the luffing joint without singular points. Thus, a complete exoskeleton with 26 DOFs (excluding hands) was developed [6]. Figure 4.1 displays the concepts of some early exoskeletons and some mechanical pictures based on these ideas.

4.1.1.2 Exoskeleton Project by DARPA

Exoskeletons for Human Performance Augmentation (EHPA) funded by DARPA greatly promoted the development of robots for performance augmentation. The project aimed to improve individual combat power on the ground [7]. It focused on improving soldier's athletic ability under heavy load and decreasing the corresponding fatigue. The project started in 2001 and was turned over to Program Executive Office (PEO) in 2008. During the period of EHPA, three institutions focused on the development of exoskeleton; others focused on the supporting technologies, such as portable power.

1. **Berkeley Lower Extremity Exoskeleton (BLEEX)**: BLEEX is perhaps the most famous exoskeleton robot in DARPA project. The most notable feature is the portable power, which provides it with great mobility. In fact, its designer defined it as the first exoskeleton robot with the function of carrying, meanwhile having self-sufficient power [8].

   There are three DOFs in the hip joint of BLEEX, one DOF in the knee joint, and three DOFs in the ankle joint. Among them, four are powered, including the flexion–extension in hip joint, pronation–supination in hip joint, flexion–extension in knee joint, and flexion–extension in ankle joint. Three are underactuated, including the plantar flexion and dorsiflexion of the ankle, rotation of hip joint which is connected by spring, and rotation of ankle which is a free joint [9]. Meanwhile, the kinematic and dynamic requirements are set based on the clinical gait analysis of a 75 kg human body.

   The rotary joint of the hip is placed on the back and between the two legs, which share the rotary joint. It meets the kinematic requirements of lower extremity and avoids interference with the wearer's hip joint. Similarly, pronation–supination of the ankle joint is not placed in the same axis of rotation with human joint. The rotation axis is placed on the side of foot in order to greatly simplify the structural design. The other five rotational DOFs are placed in the similar manner as the joints of the wearer [9].

The exoskeleton is driven by a bidirectional linear hydraulic actuator that is specially designed. The power of the hydraulic actuator is 1,143 W, and electric control devices consume 200 W. In contrast, a 75 kg human consumes 165 W during walking [10].

In the control system of BLEEX, the use of human–machine interactive force is reduced to the lowest level. Instead, the information from other sensors of the exoskeleton is applied. Thus, similar to biped robots, the exoskeleton can maintain self-balance autonomously. However, an indicative force has to be provided by the user while walking. The signal acquisition system includes eight encoders and 16 linear accelerometers to determine the velocity, angular velocity, and angular acceleration of the eight powered joints; one plantar pressure distribution sensor to determine contact situation between the foot and the ground; eight one-dimensional force sensors to control the driving force of all the actuators; and one clinometer to determine the direction of backpack relative to that of gravity [9].

In BLEEX, the wearer could walk at the speed of 0.9 m/s with a load of 75 kg and 1.3 m/s without any load. At present, the second-generation BLEEX is under test. When the hydraulic actuators are replaced by electric drivers, the weight can be reduced to half of the original one [11] (approximately 14 kg). Bionics Company is also planning to promote the exoskeleton technique to the market.

2. **Sarcos exoskeleton**: Sarcos research company (Salt Lake City, Utah) attempted to develop a full-body wearable energy self-sufficient robot named WEAR (funded by EHPA of DARPA). Similar to BLEEX, hydraulic actuators are also applied. The difference is that they are not linear but rotary ones to directly drive the joint. Although Sarcos did not make public its power requirements, the company has put a lot of effort on the development of power and servo valves, in order to increase remarkably the efficiency of hydraulic actuators [13].

In the control system of Sarcos exoskeleton, interactive force between human and exoskeleton is used as the control signal. The wearer's feet are connected to exoskeleton via a rigid metal plate containing force sensors. Thus, the wearer's feet can't bend.

Some impressive features can been seen in Sarcos; e.g., the exoskeleton is able to carry the load of 84 kg; the wearer is able to stand on one leg while carrying a person on his back; the wearer is able to walk at the speed of 1.6 m/s or in the mud basin, meanwhile with a load of 68 kg on the back and 23 kg in the hands; it can also perform the activities of twisting and crouch [12]. After the EHPA of DARPA, Sarcos was still funded by the PEO to go on with their research so as to develop it into an individual fighting vehicle. It was put into service to the army in 2008. However, little information about the Sarcos has been unveiled to the public.

3. **Exoskeleton developed by MIT**: In the EHPA project supported by DARPA, MIT proposed the concept of quasi-passive exoskeleton. It aimed to develop a light and effective exoskeleton based on the passive dynamical features during walking.

In the MIT exoskeleton, no active actuator is used to provide power for joints. The design depends completely on effective energy release by the energy storing elements such as springs [13,14]. Selecting and determining the quasi-passive elements such as springs and dampers are based on the dynamic and kinematic features of walking.

There are three DOFs in the hip joint of MIT exoskeleton. There is a spring-loaded joint for flexion and extension, and it stores energy in the process of extension and release in flexion. Wearers are able to swing the joint freely when the springs are appropriately selected and placed. There is also a spring-loaded joint for pronation–supination motion of hip joint, but it is only used to detect the load on the back. A cam mechanism located in the hip joint is used to compensate for the deviation between the length of wearer's legs and that of the exoskeleton caused by the off-centering in joint rotation during the pronation–supination process. Moreover, rotary spring-loaded joints are also added to the hip and ankle joints so as to meet the requirements of motion in the non-sagittal plane.

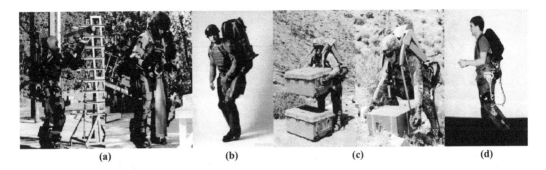

FIGURE 4.2 Exoskeleton robots in the projects of DARPA. (a) SARCOS; (b) BLEEX; (c) HULC; (d) MIT quasi-passive exoskeleton.

The knee joint of MIT exoskeleton includes a magneto-rheological damper (in the direction of flexion and extension) to control the energy consumption during the gait process. As for the ankle, independent springs are applied to control the energy storage and release in the process of plantar flexion and dorsiflexion.

A full-bridge strain gauge placed on the tibia of the exoskeleton and a potentiometer placed on the knee joint provide the necessary information to control the quasi-passive equipment. The human–machine interface in MIT exoskeleton consists of the shoulder harness, waistband, thigh band, and specially designed shoes. When there is no load, the weight of the exoskeleton is only 11.7 kg, and power of only 2 W is consumed to control the variable damper in real time. The quasi-passive exoskeleton makes it possible for wearers to walk at the speed of 1 m/s with the load of 36 kg, and 80% of the load can be transferred to the ground when standing on one leg. However, a wearer's metabolic rate increases by 10% with this load [15]. Although it was not the desired results, the metabolic problem is universal in the exoskeleton-aided walking. In another study, the average metabolic rate increased by 40% with the loads of 20 kg, 40 kg, 55 kg based on the data by Army Natick [16]. To date, there has been no literature proving that the loaded walking assisted by exoskeleton can reduce the metabolic rate effectively. Figure 4.2 illustrates the exoskeletons in the project of DARPA.

4. **Assistive technology**: Oak Ridge National Laboratory developed a plantar force-moment sensor, a control strategy, and a power technique based on the sensor [17]. A special power system was developed by Arthur D. Little, Honeywell, Quointo, and Locust to meet the requirements of the exoskeletons [18]. Boston Dynamics carried out researches on predictive model, and Will Durfe in the University of Minnesota studied human–machine physical interface to reduce the discomfort of the wearers [18]. Besides, the Center for Intelligent Mechatronics at Vanderbilt University developed the unit power system for BLEEX [19].

4.1.1.3 Other Exoskeleton Robots

HAL (Hybrid Assistive Leg): Professor Yoshikuyi Sankai's team in the University of Tsukuba developed the exoskeleton robot HAL, which aims at assistance and rehabilitation [20,21]. As illustrated in Figure 4.3a, the systemic HAL exoskeleton places AC servo motor and harmonic reducer in the knee joint and hip joint to power the joints. The DOF of flexion–extension in ankle is passive. There are a series of connectors in the human–machine interface of exoskeleton for lower extremity, including the shoes equipped with force sensor on shank and thigh, and a waistband. Different from BLEEX, Sarcos, and MIT, HAL does not transfer the load to the ground by the exoskeleton. Instead, it supports the load through the moment of hip, knee, and ankle. There are a lot of sensors in the control system of HAL. Through the surface electrodes placed on the thigh, the sEMG signal

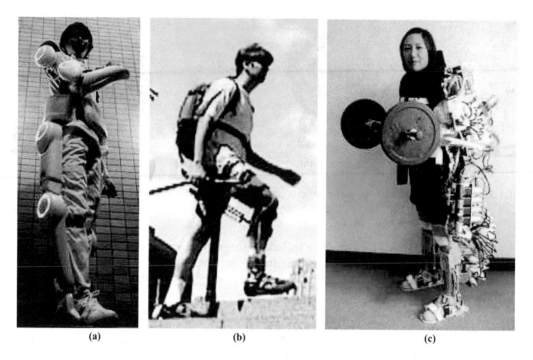

FIGURE 4.3   Other exoskeleton robots (1). (a) HAL-5; (b) RoboKnee; (c) Nurse-Assisting Exoskeleton.

of the wearers can be collected. Joint angle, ground reaction force, and trunk posture are detected through potentiometer, plantar force sensor, and gyroscope and accelerometer, respectively. These sensors are applied in two control systems to decide users' intention and control the structure. The operations of the two systems are based on sEMG signal and mobility pattern, respectively. For a given user, 2 months are needed for the equipment to optimize, demarcate, and calibrate itself and learn the dynamic features of human body.

At present, HAL has been commercialized. Compared to previous versions, the upper part structure has been improved with lighter and more compact power. The battery life is prolonged (the work hours could be as many as 160 min), and the shell is more stylish. The weight of the new generation is 21 kg, and Cyberdyne Company is responsible for the commercialization.

RoboKnee: Yobotics Company (Ohio, Cincinnati) developed a simple force-assistant exoskeleton for knee joint to aid wearers under load to complete the activities of climbing stairs or squats, as illustrated in Figure 4.3b. The series elastic actuator (SEA) in the equipment connects the upper part with the lower part of the knee joint. The equipment has relatively smaller impedance when providing auxiliary power, in order to obtain larger control gain and higher safety. The control system of RoboKnee uses positive feedback. The control information includes the ground reaction force (the vertical direction) and central place of pressure on vertical plane (the fore-and-aft direction). The information is obtained through the force sensors within the shoes.

Nurse-Assistance Exoskeleton: Kanagawa Polytechnic Institute spent more than 10 years to develop an exoskeleton to assist a nurse in taking care of and transporting the patients [21,22]. As illustrated in 4.3c, the directed and actuated pneumatic rotary actuator is included in its lower-extremity part to complete the flexion and extension of hip and knee joints. The power comes from the small air pump placed in each actuator. User's intention is detected by the muscle stiffness sensor. When the knee bends, muscle contracts and the stiffness increases. Meanwhile, a potentiometer is used to detect the joint angle to determine the required joint moment. There are no structures in front of the wearer so that nurses are able to touch the patients. The comfort and safety is then ensured.

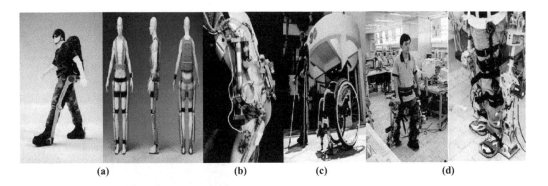

FIGURE 4.4   Other exoskeleton robots (2). (a) Titan; (b) orthosis; (c) ReWalk; (d) exoskeleton by NTU.

Some other representative exoskeleton robots are listed as follows. Titan wearable exoskeleton robot was developed and funded by the French military, as illustrated in Figure 4.4a. It can enhance the users' load capability. It is reported that the exoskeleton robot could walk at the speed of 4 km/h for 20 km with the load of 100 pound; thus it has prospects in a wide range of applications, including helping fireman complete fire mission with load, transporting military goods for special infantry, or providing adjunctive therapy or rehabilitation treatment for disabled patients. Orthosis paralleled knee joint exoskeleton robot was developed by Professor Hommel and his team in Technical University of Berlin. The active muscular contraction force was predicted by the sEMG signal collected from a patient's thigh to calculate the active joint moment so that the active control can be performed, as illustrated in Figure 4.4b. ReWalk exoskeleton robot is developed by Israeli researchers. The robot has a compact structure and concise appearance, but a support structure is needed to maintain its balance during application to help the disabled patients walk, as illustrated in Figure 4.4c. The exoskeleton robot developed by Professor Low Kin Huat and his team in Nanyang Technological University [23,24] is composed of inner exoskeleton and outer exoskeleton. Among them, the outer follows the movement of the inner and is driven directly by the motor to rotate the joint. It is reported that the exoskeleton has been preliminarily used in clinical rehabilitation, as illustrated in Figure 4.4d.

4.1.1.4   Exoskeleton Robot for Rehabilitation

From the perspective of application, the above exoskeletons are mainly used for enhancing the users' strength and endurance or performing assistive walking. The flexibility and mobility of the system are relatively high, but the stability is not satisfactory due to the tandem structure. For a healthy wearer, the system stability can be maintained by his/her own strength. However, for patients with lower-extremity injuries, the stability of the exoskeleton is the most important demand to support patient's trunk in case of falling. Thus, necessary improvement is needed to obtain higher stability and meet the rehabilitation requirements of patients with lower-extremity injuries. It has been recognized by many researchers that the Swiss Lokomat exoskeleton robot is a representative one [25–27]. Its main structure is the exoskeleton robot that is supported by the body-weight–support system to ensure the high stability of the system. Treadmill mechanism is used to do the rehabilitation exercise for disabled patients, while there are still some shortcomings, such as the high price and large floor space demand, as illustrated in Figure 4.5a. The lower-extremity powered exoskeleton (LOPES) gait rehabilitation robot in Netherlands has the similar body-weight–supported system. The joint control is realized by rope-driven mechanism. It has three DOFs, one in knee and two in hip. There are two rehabilitation modes, active and passive, as illustrated in Figure 4.5b. Besides, there are also seat-type and bed-type systems, such as the MotionMaker rehabilitation system with seat [28] (Figure 4.5c) and the bed-type Erigo treatment equipment developed by Swiss HOKOMA Company for early rehabilitation of nerve damage [29] (Figure 4.5d).

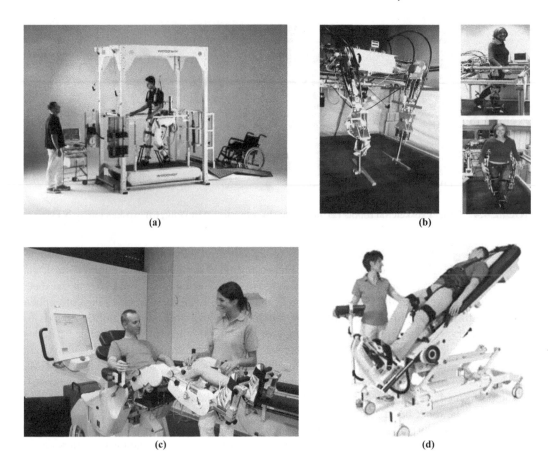

FIGURE 4.5 Exoskeleton robots for rehabilitation. (a) Lokomat; (b) LOPES; (c) MotionMaker; (d) Erigo.

Compared with the extensive research on rehabilitation exoskeleton robot around the globe, the research in China started relatively late, but this domain is getting more attention, and significant progress has been made. Professor Yang Sanjun and his team proposed an intelligent flexible exoskeleton through a deep study on human–machine integration theories, and a series of rehabilitation exoskeleton robots for upper or lower limbs were developed [30–32], among which the one for lower extremity is illustrated in Figure 4.6a. Its main structure is based on a body-weight–supported system. The gait training is performed on the treadmill. Professor Feng Guobiao and his team in Shanghai Jiao Tong University developed the rehabilitation exoskeleton for lower extremity, which has three joints, including the hip, knee, and ankle. There are three DOFs in each lower limb [33], as illustrated in Figure 4.6b. The research group in Hefei Intelligent Machinery Institute of Chinese Academy of Sciences developed an exoskeleton robot for lower extremity with plantar force sensors, as illustrated in Figure 4.5c. Meanwhile, research groups in other Chinese universities, such as Xi'an Jiao Tong University, Harbin Institute of Technology, and Tsinghua University, have also conducted extensive studies on rehabilitation exoskeleton robot for lower extremity and its clinical applications. Fruitful results must be obtained in the near future.

4.1.2 Key Technologies

4.1.2.1 Control System for Exoskeleton

An effective controller for exoskeleton robot is one of the key problems performing active compliance control of human–exoskeleton system and is also a big difficulty for practical application of

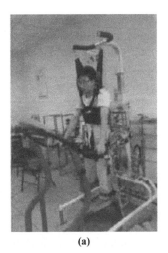
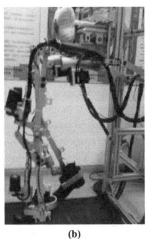
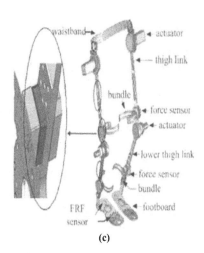

(a)   (b)   (c)

FIGURE 4.6   Exoskeleton robots at home and abroad. (a) Exoskeleton robot developed by Zhejiang University; (b) exoskeleton robot developed by Shanghai University; (c) exoskeleton robot developed by University of Science and Technology of China.

exoskeleton technology. Based on the existing control systems for exoskeleton robots, they can be divided into the following types: the model-based control system, layered control system, physical-parameter–based control system, and application-based control system [34].

4.1.2.1.1   Model-Based Control System

There are mainly two types of control systems based on the model for exoskeleton equipment: the dynamic-model–based control system and muscle-model–based control system [35].

Exoskeleton control system based on dynamic model treats human skeleton as rigid parts, which are connected by revolute pairs, i.e., the joints. Mechanical modeling and calculation are implemented considering the effects of inertial force, gravity, Coriolis force, and centrifugal force [35]. The dynamic model can be developed using three methods: mathematical model, system identification, and artificial intelligence. Theoretical exoskeleton model can be obtained through mathematical models based on the physical features. One typical case applying the control system is BLEEX [9]. No force sensor or moment sensor is used to detect the interactive force in BLEEX. The robot is controlled based on the dynamic model to assist wearer's movement [36,37], with the purpose of developing a system with high flexibility. Thus, an accurate dynamic model is required. To achieve this goal, three different dynamic models, which are determined by different phases in gait cycle, are developed for BLEEX: one-leg–supporting, two-leg–supporting, and two-leg–redundant models. Meanwhile, different control mechanisms are adopted for different dynamic models [38]. System identification is the second method for dynamic modeling. It is usually adopted when no accurate mathematical model can be achieved through theoretical ways. Least square method is introduced by researchers of BLEEX to estimate dynamic model parameters through input and output data in the swing phase [38]. Besides, recursive least square method was adopted by Aguirre–Ollinger to calculate the dynamic model for single-DOF exoskeleton robot [39]. Another method for acquiring dynamic model is the use of artificial intelligence, which has been widely applied in solving nonlinear problems. Wavelet neural network was adopted by Xiuxia to identify the dynamic model of exoskeleton [40]. Inverse dynamics model of the structure was developed by the wavelet neural network to control the virtual joint moment. The inputs were the exoskeleton joint angle, angular velocity, and angular acceleration. The output was the joint moment. The parameters in the net are trained using the input and output data.

Besides the dynamic model, muscle model is also used in the control strategy of the exoskeleton. Different from dynamic model, the muscle model predicts the contraction force of the related muscle by developing the relationship between muscle force (joint dynamics) and motor nerve signal [41]. The input is EMG signal, and the output is the estimated value of contraction force. Muscle models are of two types: parametric and nonparametric. Parametric models are usually based on Hill-type model [41,42]. Parametric muscle model based on Hill-type model is recognized as the biomechanical model for musculoskeletal system of legs and arms. It is composed of three elements: the contractile element (CE), series element (SE), and parallel element (PE) [41]. Besides, its output can be expressed as a function of EMG signal and muscle length. Rosen estimated the active force of elbow joint based on Hill-type model [42] and applied it to the control of the upper-limb exoskeleton robot with two DOFs. Genetic algorithm was integrated into it to search for the optimal parameters of Hill-type model by Cavallaro. Based on the works of Rosen, an upper-limb exoskeleton robot with up to seven DOFs can be controlled [43]. Different from the parametric model, dynamic information of the muscle and joint is unnecessary in the nonparametric model of muscle [44]. Fuzzy neural network (FNN) was applied by Kiguchi to adjust the related parameters between EMG signal and joint output moment [45]. The relationships were illustrated in the muscle model matrix, the parameters of which determine the output of the FNN. The control strategy was applied to the control of the upper-limb exoskeleton robot with seven DOFs. It helped the patients perform the activities such as flexion/extension (F/E) of the shoulder joint in the vertical and horizontal directions, radial/ulnar deviation of shoulder joint, F/E of elbow joint, pronation/supination of forearm, F/E of wrist joint, and radial/ulnar deviation of wrist joint [45].

4.1.2.1.2 Layered Control System

From the perspective of layered theory, the control of exoskeleton can be divided into three layers: task level, high level, and low level. The controller of task level is the highest level in the system and would do coordination control based on the task requirements. The high-level controller controls the human–machine interactive force based on the information provided by the task-level controller. Low-level controller is the bottom controller responsible for controlling the joint angle and torque of the exoskeleton.

4.1.2.1.3 Physical-Parameter–Based Control System

There are three kinds of control strategies for physical-parameter–based control system: the position, torque/force, and interactive force.

Position control mode is usually used to ensure that exoskeleton joints move according to the target angle. The Proportion-differential (PD) controller of ARMin III is a typical example, and the control block diagram is illustrated in Figure 4.7. In practical rehabilitation applications, some exoskeleton joints should be set at fixed positions. For these axes, PD position controller would make the joint angle follow the preset value quickly. Position controller is often used as the low-level controller; e.g., Maryland-Georgetown-Army (MGA) upper-limb exoskeleton robot uses the PD position controller as the low-level controller; RUPERT IV applied the proportional-integral-derivative (PID) position control as the inner control loop; University of Technology Sydney (UTS), HAL, and L-Exos all use PD controller to perform position control [46,47]. Moreover, Aguirre-Ollinger used the linear quadrati (LQ) position controller [48]; Gomes proposed the concept of H∞ controller [49]; Rehab-Robot applied feedback PID controller [48].

Torque/force controller is another form of physical-parameter–based control system. Similarly, it is also often used as a low-level controller; e.g., ARMin III also used the torque/force controller as its low-level controller. The same situation applies for L-Exos, Pnue-Wrex [50], wearable orthosis for tremor as- sessment and suppression (WOTAS) [51], Lokomat [52], LOPES [53], a new active knee rehabilitation orthotic system called (ANdROS) [54], etc.

In addition to position controller and torque/force controller, human–machine interactive force is also often used in exoskeleton robot control and is usually used as high-level controller. The main

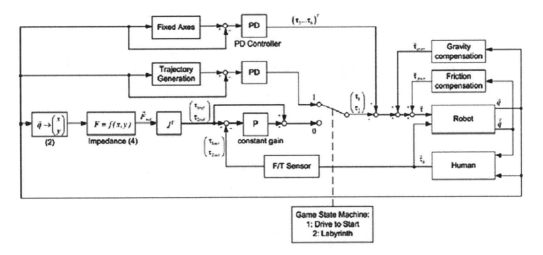

FIGURE 4.7   Control blocks for ARMin III.

aim is to assist the wearer to perform some specific tasks and reduce the interactive force to zero. The human–machine interactive force can be used in the impedance controller or admittance controller. Impedance controller controls force by adjusting position. On the contrary, admittance controller controls the position by adjusting force.

- **Impedance controller** is the extension of position control. It can be used to control not only force and position, but also the relative relationship between force, position, and the interactive force [55]. The structure of impedance controller consists of the impedance model and the torque/force controller. Among them, the impedance model calculates the required force value in the next servo cycle based on the joint position error, while the torque/force controller generates corresponding control torque/force based on the reference force. Similar controllers were applied in SUEFUL-7 [45], Pnue-Wrex [50], WOTAS [51], Lokomat [52], LOPES [53], ANdROS [56], etc.
- **Admittance controller** is composed of the admittance model and the position controller. The admittance model calculates the required control joint angle value in the next servo cycle based on human–machine interactive force. The position controller enables the exoskeleton to reach the corresponding angle based on the reference position. Figure 4.8 illustrates the admittance control model for MGA upper-limb exoskeleton robot. Other cases include the 7 DOF upper limb exoskeleton ((EXO-UL7) [57,58], intelligent pneumatic arm movement (iPAM) [59], UTS [60], one-DOF exoskeleton robot for lower limbs [56,61], etc.

In most cases, the parameters in impedance/admittance model are fixed. However, adjustments should be made to these parameters to adapt to different situations, such as the users with different diseases and different physical conditions. FNN was proposed by Kiguchi to adjust intrinsic parameters in the admittance model [56].

4.1.2.1.4   Application-Based Control System

Exoskeleton control system can also be classified as virtual reality controller, remote manipulation controller, gait controller, etc. based on its application. Most of the exoskeleton robots for upper limbs use virtual reality controller during the rehabilitation process. The controller is able to guide and help patients complete tasks such as grabbing virtual objects, e.g., the RUPERT exoskeleton [62]. Virtual tasks in ARMin include moving virtual objects by the virtual arms, a virtual ball game, and

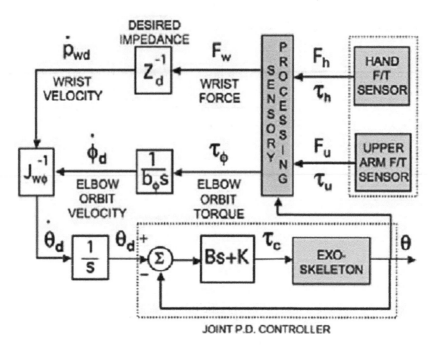

FIGURE 4.8   Control blocks for admittance control of MGA.

a maze game [63,64]. A virtual drawing task on the virtual wall is adopted by MGA [60]. A moving task in a virtual environment is also adopted by L-Exos [65]. In these applications, exoskeleton robots are used as haptic devices.

Virtual reality controller described by ARMin is illustrated in Figure 4.9. Patients need to grasp the rolling virtual balls from the declining virtual tabletop. A reference trajectory will be automatically generated by the virtual controller. When the patients stray away from the trajectory, appropriate assistance will be provided by the system. This kind of controller is a very good supplement for impedance controller as the high-level controller and force controller as the low-level controller [64]. Adaptive reference generator was applied by RUPERT III to increase the accuracy of trajectory generation [62].

Remote manipulation controller is similar to the master–slave controller. The exoskeleton system worn by the manipulator is the master, while the robot being operated is the slave. The slave will follow the move of the master. This kind of controller is adopted by EXOSTATION [66] and European Space Agency (ESA) [67]. The difference between remote manipulation controller and other controllers is that it controls the interactive force between the slave and the environment instead of human–machine interactive force.

Gait controller is often used in the exoskeleton robot of lower extremity. The control system of LOPES is a typical one. Three levels of controllers are included. The first level is the observer to judge patients' gait phase in the virtual model controller (VMC) and to ensure the safety of the patients. The second level is the VMC. The controller is applied in the intervention training through the spring-based impedance controller [53]. The third level is the torque/force controller. The controller ensures that the joint force generated by the exoskeleton is equal to or close to the force generated through the VMC. Transition from one state to another is described by a finite state machine in Vanderbilt exoskeleton robot [68]. To increase the accuracy of gait phase and pattern identification, adaptive identification of the gait pattern is realized using inverse dynamics in Lokomat [52]. Gomes proposed the artificial-neural-network–based gait pattern recognition method.

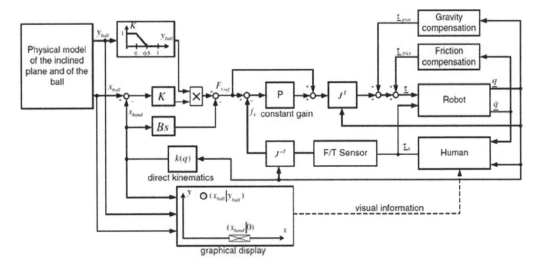

FIGURE 4.9 ARMin III virtual reality controller.

4.1.2.2 Human–Machine Interface Technology

4.1.2.2.1 Multi-Source-Signal–Based Motion Recognition

Quick and effective motion control can be achieved only when there are valid control signal sources for the exoskeleton robot. Exoskeleton robot is essentially an accessory equipment for human motion. As a typical human–machine integrated system, human body should be the control signal source [69].

At present, commonly used control signals include signals from joint inclinometer/angular velocity meter, force/acceleration sensor, etc. These signals are able to accurately feed back the current motion information, such as joint angle/angular velocity, interactive force between human and the exoskeleton, contact force between human/exoskeleton and the ground, force distribution, acceleration, etc. These methods have been applied in the motion control of exoskeleton robots. BLEEX detects the pressure distribution from the human–machine system to the ground using the force sensor placed on pelma based on the dynamic model. The distribution is used to judge the motion condition and is regarded as the control signal source to perform stable control [9].

However, information such as interactive force [70] or joint angle can only reflect motion information which is static and hysteretic. As there are certain mechanical delays in the exoskeleton robot, if the delay of signal acquisition and control accumulates, there will be considerable delay in exoskeleton control in real time, which will produce negative effects on coordinated control of human–exoskeleton system. To solve the problem, some researchers adopted physiological signal as the control signal source and developed real-time control strategies based on related biological models. For example, orthosis exoskeleton developed by Professor Hommel and Professor Kiguchi adopted sEMG signal as the control signal source [69]. Through developing the relationship between sEMG signal with muscle contraction force, joint torque, and angle, the exoskeleton could move freely according to human motor intent [45,71].

However, there is strong fuzziness in human physiological signal, such as sEMG signal. The accuracy and reliability are still relatively low when physiological signal is the only control signal. Thus, some researchers integrated traditional signal with physiological signal and proposed multi-source-signal–based human–machine interaction interface with satisfactory results. Control signal sources, such as sEMG signal, joint angle, plantar pressure distribution, are adopted by HAL exoskeleton robot to perform coordinated control of the human–machine system [72].

4.1.2.2.2   Information Feedback Technology

For a healthy person, force and position information will be detected in real time by sensory organs in muscles and sent to CNS during movement process. However, the perception pathway of the patients with paralysis, stroke, or amputation is often damaged. Thus, related information can be obtained only through the remaining sensing capabilities [73]. Compared to a healthy person, the change in information perception ability will lead to gait disorder and the decrease in balancing capability [74].

Artificial perception feedback technology has been widely applied in fields such as surgical robotics, industrial robotics, virtual reality, video games [75,76], etc. The information feedback mechanism includes vision [77], hearing [78], electrical stimulation [79], and haptic stimulation [79]. Among these methods, electrical and haptic stimulations have proven themselves to be the most effective [79] means. The advantages of electrical stimulation are its high accuracy, strong repeatability, and its better performance in the laboratory-scale sensory feedback [80,81]. However, the surface electrode used in electrical stimulation is easily affected by moisture content in skin and mechanical deformation. This would lead to the feeling of pruritus and burning on skin surface [79]. Implantable neural FES, which will not be affected by changes on skin surface, has also been applied in sensory feedback. It has been proved that FES electrode can be implanted into human body safely. It controls the artificial arm using the myosignal and feeds back the sensory information [82]. However, there would be rejecting reaction because of the biocompatibility when the implanted electrodes are used for a long time and would also lead to impedance effect from surrounding fibrous tissue to electrical stimulation [83]. Moreover, the electrode should be implanted in surgery. If there is position error detected after the surgery, additional minimally invasive surgery is needed to correct it [84]. Owing to these factors, the research on non-implanted sensory feedback method is of great significance to overcome the shortcomings of implantation technology [85].

Thus, researchers proposed some non-implanted methods based on haptic feedback theory, including electric motor drive [86], vibrotactile feedback [79], piezoelectric element drive [87], shape-memory-alloy drive [88], magnetorheological/electrorheological drive [89,90]. These systems stimulate the sensory organs in skin by exerting static or dynamic mechanical deformation on skin surface. The haptic system applies for most of the application fields, but there are still some short-comings; e.g., the adaptive time is long, the output force is low, sensory organs will be damaged after long-time use, or the design is complex and structure is heavy. Facing these challenges, there are still satisfactory developments of vibrotactile feedback system. An energy conversion device is included in all the vibrotactile feedback systems. The vibrotactile feedback system has already been integrated into the artificial-limb systems, providing sensory feedback for lower-extremity-amputation patients [91]. Although the spatial resolution of the vibrotactile feedback system is very high, there are still some negative influences on human sensory organs when stimulated by the external vibration for a long time [86]. Owing to this, vibrotactile feedback systems [77] have not been widely applied in clinical trails. To overcome these defects, non-vibrotactile feedback system is proposed to reduce the damage to human sensory organs. Pneumatic airbag feedback system is one of the methods that are used in robotic surgery to provide haptic feedback. The advantages of airbag feedback system include large output force, close fitting with human, fast response, light weight, good crypticity, etc. [92].

4.1.2.3   IoT-Based Rehabilitation System

The concept of Internet of Things (IoT) was first proposed by K. Ashton [93], the founder of MIT Auto-ID Center, and D. L. Brock [94] in 1999 and 2001, respectively. It was mainly used on the coding of electronic products. Then, IBM introduced the concept and expanded it to the concept of Smart Planet and Smart City [95]. Aiming to develop a network that is ubiquitous, sensible in real time, information interactive, low energy consuming, and highly effective, IoT connects all the public resources in a city and makes the things and things, things and humans, and humans and humans closely connected through the use of wireless communication technology, sensor technology, radio frequency identification technology, portable terminal technology, and global-positioning technology. It makes the *Pervasive Connectivity* possible and has been recognized as the next technological revolution in the near future [96]. Through the real-time intelligence of IoT, effective planning and arrangement of the operation framework and public service of the city or company could be achieved, and it makes quick responses to emergencies. Owing to these advantages, IoT has been applied in industrial scheduling system [97], bus scheduling system [98], etc.

Facing the increasing medical demand and limited medical resources, IoT would effectively increase the availability of medical resources and treatment effect, provide useful technical support for community treatment, and make it possible to solve the problem of limited medical resources. Compared with traditional localized treatment, IoT-based community treatment aims to provide convenient and effective medical service, establish close relationships between patients and doctors, and make the maximum use of medical resource through quick and effective allocation and reconfiguration [99]. Based on this idea, IoT has gradually been applied in medical rehabilitation system [100], and some tentative intelligent medical systems have been developed. BodyMedia, Google Health, and HomeRF are the representative ones. BodyMedia collects physiological data through IoT and develops a huge database of physiological data, providing accurate physiological data and treatment prescriptions for treating obesity and diabetes [101]. Google Health is essentially a recording terminal for individual physiological information. It collects the physiological information and records it in the network terminal through intelligent servers with the function of networking and provides data synchronization and sharing in the process of teletherapy [102]. HomeRF connects the computer, telephone, sound box, and television with one another, making them interoperable and making information sharable through the use of IoT. It provides daily life assistance for inconvenient patients [103]. Although the system has not been widely used, it has drawn much attention. Useful guidance and reference have been provided for future development.

In summary, with the fast development of medical technology, especially the robot techniques, technical supports have been provided to improve traditional rehabilitation treatment and rehabilitation efficacy. Modern rehabilitation method integrating rehabilitation exoskeleton robot has been developed to provide better rehabilitation exercises for patients with lower-limb diseases and to improve their quality of life. However, there are still great challenges on exoskeleton-robot–based rehabilitation techniques. On one hand, exoskeleton robot for rehabilitation is wearable and has high stability to overcome the influence of immobility during usage. On the other hand, coordinated control for human–machine system together with effective human–machine interface should be achieved to collect real-time interacting information between patients and exoskeleton robot. On this basis, active compliance control strategy for exoskeleton robot system is very important. At the same time, developing appropriate rehabilitation strategy based on clinical rehabilitation requirements is necessary to make the system applicable in practice.

4.1.3 Anatomical Structure and Gait Feature of Human Lower Limbs

Human motor system for lower limbs consists of skeletons, joints, and skeletal muscles. Joints of lower extremity include hip joints, knee joints, and ankle joints. The skeletal muscles contract and relax under the control of nervous system. When muscle contracts, the skeleton is dragged to change position with the fulcrum of joints to generate motion. Thus, in the process of motion of lower extremity, skeletal muscle is the source of power, dragging the skeleton's motion around the joints. Human walking, running, jumping, and crouching are achieved through the coordination of many joints. The following knowledge of anatomy concerning lower-extremity joints is from the literature [104] (Figure 4.10).

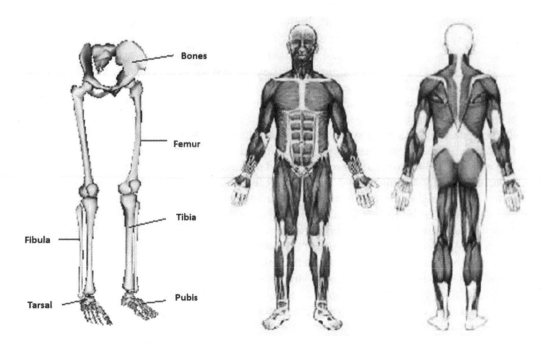

FIGURE 4.10   Skeletons, joints, and muscles of lower extremity.

4.1.3.1   Datum Plane and Datum Axis of Humans

Human motion is usually described by three datum planes which are mutually perpendicular, as illustrated in Figure 4.11. They are the **sagittal plane**, **frontal plane**, and **transverse plane**, and there are three axes: sagittal axis X, frontal axis Y, and frontal axis Z. Among them, the tangent plane, which is along the anteroposterior diameter of the body and is perpendicular to the ground, is the sagittal plane. It divides human body into two parts: the left and right. The tangent plane, which is along the transverse diameter of the body and is perpendicular to ground, is the frontal plane. It divides human body into two parts: the front and rear. The plane which crosses the upright body and is parallel to the ground is the transverse plane. It divides human body into two parts: the upper and lower. Sagittal axis is in the sagittal plane and is perpendicular to frontal plane; it is also the intersecting line of sagittal plane and transverse plane. Frontal axis is in the frontal plane and is perpendicular to sagittal plane; it is also the intersecting line of frontal plane and transverse plane. Transverse axis is in the transverse plane; it is also the intersecting line of frontal plane and sagittal plane.

4.1.3.2   Joints and Muscle Groups of Human Lower Extremity

Hip joint: Hip joint is one of the largest and most stable joints in human body. It consists of caput femoris and acetabulum. There is an aneuros articular capsule, outside of which there are strong muscle groups. The stable structure of joints makes it possible to adjust to the wide range of motion in daily life, such as walking, sitting, and crouching. There are three DOFs in the hip joint, which is able to move in three planes: sagittal plane (extension and flexion), frontal plane (abduction and adduction), and transverse plane (pronation and supination). It has the largest range of motion in sagittal plane with flexion (0°–140°) and extension (0°–15°). The muscles that make the joint move are mainly the lower-extremity girdle muscular group, including the iliopsoas, tensor fascia lata (TF), gluteus maximus, gluteal muscle, gluteus minimus, piriformis, etc. The extension and flexion in sagittal plane are mainly performed in the process of normal walking.

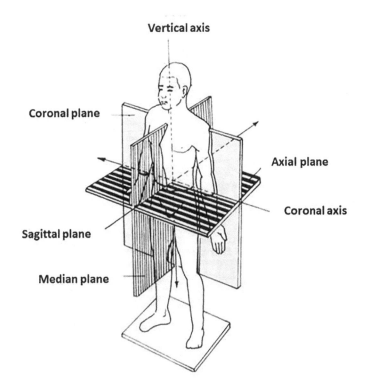

FIGURE 4.11 Datum plane and datum axis of human body.

Knee joint: Knee joint is the largest joint in human body, and it consists of two joint structures, i.e., tibial articular and patellar. Knee joint suffers from heavy load and is located between the longest bones, i.e., femur and tibia, in the human body. It can move in three planes in the tibial articular, where the largest range of movement is in the sagittal plane. From fully extended to fully flexed, the range of motion in sagittal plane is 0°–140°. Thigh muscle group, which is one of the largest muscle groups in human body, is the source of driving force. It includes the quadriceps, sartorius (SR), semitendinosus (ST), semimembranosus (SM), biceps femoris (BF), adductor magnus, gracilis, toe muscle, short adductor muscle, etc.

Ankle joint: Ankle joint is also responsible for the motor function and load-bearing function of the lower extremity. It is a sided-hinge joint, the movement of which is mainly the dorsiflexion and plantar flexion of the foot. In sagittal plane, ankle joint's range of motion is approximately 45°, 10°–20° for dorsiflexion and 25°–35° for plantar flexion. Meanwhile, ankle joint enables foot to do ecstrophy and enstrophe. The muscles that make the joint move are mainly the calf muscles, including the tibialis anterior muscle, extensor digitorum longus, and hallucis longus of the front muscle group; soleus, inner and outer side heads of gastrocnemius, and rear tibial muscle of the rear muscle group; and peroneus longus and peroneus brevis of the side muscle group. The front muscle group flexes the ankle, and the rear extends the ankle. Tibialis anterior muscle and rear tibial muscle are responsible for the enstrophe, and peroneus longus and peroneus brevis are responsible for the ecstrophy (Figures 4.12–4.14).

In sagittal plane, the muscles responsible for joint movement and joints' range of movement are illustrated in Table 4.1.

Referring to the above knowledge, one can see that there are various forms of motion of human lower-extremity joints with complex structure and multiple DOFs. From the perspective of mechanism, realizing multi-DOF motion of all the joints of exoskeleton robot is difficult. Thus, when

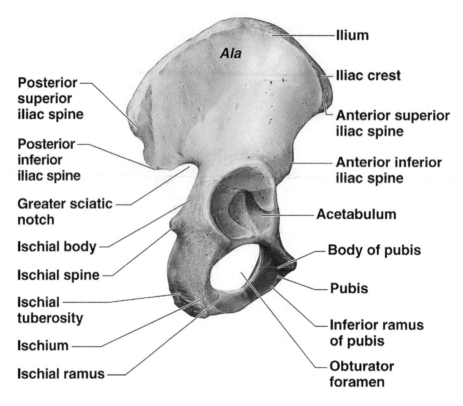

FIGURE 4.12 Hip joint.

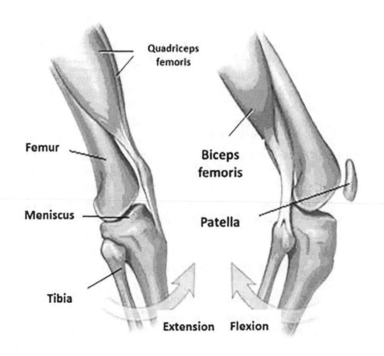

FIGURE 4.13 Knee joint.

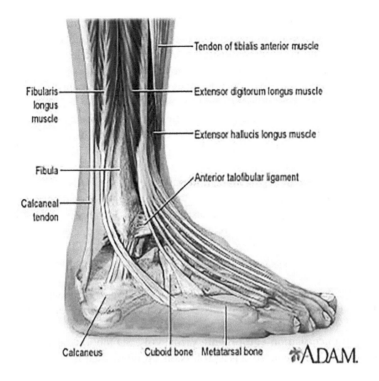

Tendon of tibialis anterior muscle

Extensor digitorum longus muscle

Extensor hallucis longus muscle

Fibularis
longus
muscle

Fibula

Calcaneal
tendon

Anterior talofibular ligament

Calcaneus   Cuboid bone   Metatarsal bone

FIGURE 4.14   Ankle joint.

TABLE 4.1
Range of Motion and Prime Movers

Joint	Motion	Range of Motion	Prime Mover
Hip joint	Antexion	0°–140°	Iliopsoas, RF, SR, etc.
	Extension	0°–15°	Gluteus maximus, ST, SM, etc.
Knee joint	Flexion	0°–140°	BF, ST, SM, etc.
	Extension	0°–140°	Quadriceps (RF, Musculus femoris medius, vastus lateralis muscle, vastus medialis muscle, etc.)
Ankle joint	Dorsiflexion	10°–20°	Tibialis anterior, extensor digitorum longus, hallucis longus, etc.
	Plantar flexion	25°–35°	Soleus, inner and outer side head gastrocnemius, rear tibial muscle, etc.

considering the design of the robot, the spatial arrangement and joint motion requirements, together with the integrity and practicability of the system should be taken into account to achieve the optimal design. When multi-DOF motion of single joint can be achieved by the parallel mechanism, applying such a mechanism in the design would be a good choice. To realize all the required functions with the most compact structure is the basic design principle for optimum exoskeleton design. Meanwhile, joints' range of motion is also one of the references for the structural design of exoskeleton robot.

4.1.3.3   Gait Features of Human Motion

Gait is the motion feature of human walking, which is the most common action in daily life, and is the basis for human living [105]. It is achieved by coordination of the multiple muscles of lower extremity. Walking process and posture include rich information about human motor system and neural control system. Accurate measurement and analysis of the position, velocity, force, and myosignal during walking is the prerequisite for controlling exoskeleton robot of lower extremity. Walking, which mainly depends on the relative movement of two legs, is a complex process. Muscles of the whole body take part in this process, including the shifting of human center of gravity, tilting and rotating of pelvis, F/E and extorsion/intorsion of hip, knee, and ankle joints. Ambulation is the major imitation target for exoskeleton robot of lower extremity. The gait feature of human is also one of the important references for designing exoskeleton robot. Figure 4.15 illustrates the gait features of normal walking.

One gait cycle starts from the time when one leg touches the ground and ends when it touches the ground again. Based on the leg movement in one gait cycle, it is divided into swing phase and stance phase. Stance phase is the phase when feet touches the ground and bears the weight. It takes 60% of the gait cycle. Swing phase is the phase when lower extremity swings forward. It takes 40% of the gait cycle. Also, based on the relative position of the two legs, the whole gait cycle can been divided to single-leg-support phase and two-leg-support phase. Other time/space parameters concerning gait include frequency of stride, length of stride, step length, stride width, etc. [105] (Figure 4.16).

To acquire gait information, 3D gait analyzers can be used to analyze human gait. Motion data and ground reaction force is dynamically detected to acquire the feature data of human joint motion [106].

An example data acquisition equipment: Vicon V612 3D motion capture system and plantar force measurement system. Vicon V612 is a professional product used for motion capture developed

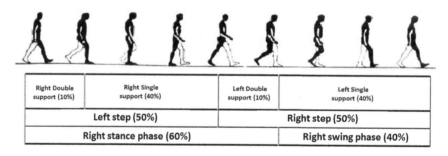

Right Double support (10%)	Right Single support (40%)	Left Double support (10%)	Left Single support (40%)
Left step (50%)		Right step (50%)	
Right stance phase (60%)		Right swing phase (40%)	

FIGURE 4.15   Gait cycle.

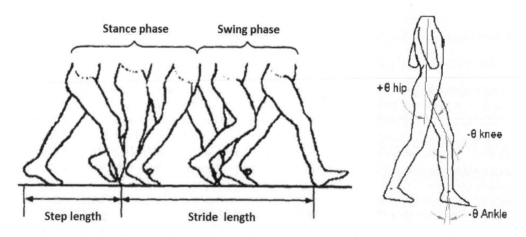

FIGURE 4.16   Gait phase division and definition of joint angle.

by Oxford Metrics Group. The system includes six laser cameras, fluorescence reflection ball, and processing software. It calculates the 3D coordinate of the reflection ball through scanning of the moving reflection ball in the space by different cameras at the same time. Based on the dynamic and kinematic analyses of the coordinates, object position, velocity, and acceleration can be acquired. The reflection balls are placed on human joints when measuring. Acquiring the gait information of normal walking is implemented through capturing the space location of the reflection balls by the camera. Plantar force measurement system is used to get the plantar force. The force plate platform, whose upper surface is parallel to the ground, is located in the center of the lab to measure the plantar force from the ground [106] (Figure 4.17).

Acquisition process:

1. Fix the reflection ball to the marker on the body of the subject. Stick the reflection balls to the corresponding segments of the volunteer. Markers of thigh, calf, and foot are located on the outer side.

   Reflection ball tracking the motion of pelvis is placed on the sacrum.
2. Measure the basic morphological parameters of the volunteer, including height, weight, length of thigh, length of calf, etc.
3. Define the coordinate for the capture system. Define the heading direction as axis x, vertical direction as axis y, and the transverse direction as axis z.
4. Set the sampling frequencies of space marker in the 3D capture system and plantar force measurement platform as 50 HZ and 1,000 HZ, respectively.
5. Collect the static standing data of one leg to build the lower-limb model. The volunteer is required to do normal gait walking exercise with two eyes looking forward to avoid stepping on the force measurement platform on purpose.
6. The volunteer is required to do the gait exercise several times to collect the data of human motion.

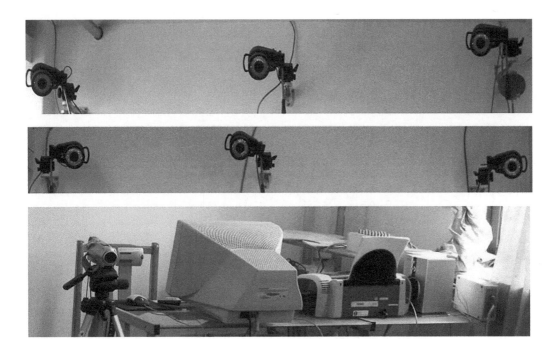

FIGURE 4.17 Gait analysis lab.

Result analysis: Using the Vicon gait analysis system, the dynamic/kinematic features of normal walking can be acquired. When the walking speed is 1.3 m/s, Figures 4.18–4.20 illustrate the rotation angles; joint torque; and power of hip joint, knee joint, and ankle joint, respectively. The unit of joint angle is degree. Joint torque and power are normalized by human weight. The unit of joint torque is Nm/kg and that of power is W/kg. Referring to the figures, the hip joint change in one gait cycle is −20° to 25° in the sagittal plane. When the heel touches the ground at the later stage of the swing phase, the flexion angle of joint is up to 25°. When the heel is off the ground, the extension angle reaches the maximum. The maximum torque generated by the hip joint occurs at the initial stage of swing phase with the value of 55 Nm. The knee joint change in one gait cycle is −20° to 25° in the sagittal plane. From the heel touching the ground as the stance phase starts to toes being off the ground as the stance phase ends, knee joint is near to unbending. In the middle of swing phase, the flexion angle reaches its maximum value of 60°. The largest torque that knee joint bears occurs in the middle of stance phase with the value of 52 Nm when a foot is off the ground. Ankle joint plays a significant role in supporting the motion of human lower limbs. Referring to the Figure 4.20, the range of dorsiflexion/plantar flexion of ankle joint is −20° to 15°. Although dorsiflexion/plantar flexion angle of ankle joint is less than that of hip joint and knee joint, its joint torque and consumed power are much more than those of hip and knee joints. The maximum values are reached at the

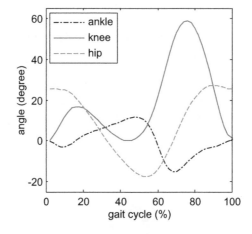

FIGURE 4.18   Joint angles of hip, knee, and ankle in the gait cycle.

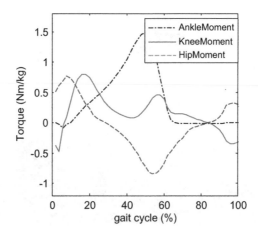

FIGURE 4.19   Joint torques of hip, knee, and ankle in the gait cycle.

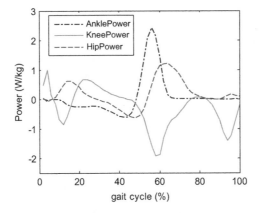

FIGURE 4.20   Joint powers of hip, knee, and ankle in the gait cycle.

later stage of stance phase with the values of 96 Nm and 156 W. Moreover, enstrophe/ecstrophy in the transverse plane is also required in the rehabilitation of ankle joints. The data above can be seen as the reference data for exoskeleton design.

Human gravity center: In the walking process, human gravity center fluctuates up and down. In one gait cycle, the offset change of the gravity center in sagittal plane can be described by sine function. Offset value changes with human height.

The length and mass distribution of lower limb: The length, mass distribution, and centroid position of the segments of human lower limb are important references for the mechanical design of exoskeleton robot and are also the necessary data to do dynamic analysis for the exoskeleton robot. For example, based on the data from Gua Biao (GB) (GB/T 10000-1988, "body dimensions of Chinese adults" [107], and GB/T 17245-1998, "body centroid of adults" [108]), the actual dimensions and mass distribution are illustrated in Table 4.2, which lists the relevant body parameters. The mechanical design will be done based on these standards, which are also part of the evaluation references in the final assessment.

4.1.4   Bionic Design of the Lower-Extremity Exoskeleton Robot

The idea of wearable design is embodied by exoskeleton robots. It integrates many modern techniques at present to do rehabilitation treatment for patients. However, among the existing exoskeleton

TABLE 4.2
Body Parameters of the Reference Object [107,108]

Content	
Height	1.76 m
Length of thigh	0.46 m
Length of calf	0.48 m
Height of feet	0.1 m
Width of feet	0.07 m
Length of feet	0.25 m
Mass of thigh	14.19% of the total weight
Mass of calf	3.67% of the total weight
Mass of feet	1.48% of the total weight
Normal walking speed	95–125 steps/min

robots, there are few exoskeleton systems that meet the requirements of physiological motion and are applied successfully in clinical trials. Many technical difficulties have to be solved, and the robot system needs to be further improved.

Pathological features of the patients with paraplegia and hemiplegia will be analyzed first to determine patients' requirements in this section. Then, the design of the body structure of the exoskeleton robot based on the requirements and lower-extremity gait feature is introduced, and related static and dynamic analyses are implemented to verify whether the structure would be qualified. Next, the design of the various functional modules in the lower-extremity rehabilitation system by integrating the advantages of traditional treatment is introduced. Furthermore, one should complete the hardware design and debug of human–machine integrating interface and motion controller. Meanwhile, it is also necessary to develop corresponding operational system/software and control algorithm. All these will be discussed in detail in the following.

4.1.4.1 Requirements of Lower-Extremity Rehabilitation and Design Key Points

From the perspective of clinical medicine, stroke is the brain disorder caused by the rapid loss of blood supply in the brain. This may be caused by cerebral infarction (tarombokinesis, arterial embolism) or ischemia brought about by hemorrhoea (lack of blood). The consequences are usually temporary or permanent nerve injuries or even death, making the original function of the affected brain regions lost. This would further result in the inability to move one or several limbs, the loss of understanding or linguistic capacity, or even badly affected visual sense and auditory sense. For patients with nerve injuries, rehabilitation time is of equal importance as saving life, because once a nerve cell dies, it cannot be reborn considering the current level of medical science. What can be saved are the nerve cells which are not necrotic or only slightly damaged. There is a time limit for the recovery of nerve cell, 25% within 1 month, 50% in 3 months, and 75% in 6 months. The nerve cells damaged for 6 months to 3 years are almost shaped with little ability to recover.

Thus, 1 month after the stroke is the golden period for rehabilitation treatment. Rehabilitation treatment should be started as soon as possible based on different disease states. Delayed, inappropriate, or even insufficient rehabilitation treatment would largely increase the possibility of lower-limb paralysis and hemiplegia. However, as the aging trend in the world is becoming more and more severe, the incidence of stroke increases gradually. Once it turns into paralysis or hemiplegia, there would be huge impact on patients' daily life, preventing them from walking outside. It will make quite a wound on the patients, not only physically, but also mentally. Meanwhile, taking care of the patients will cause a great burden of life for the patients' family. Thus, the rehabilitation treatment of stroke has attracted more and more attention and has become one of the burning questions.

Based on the Brunnstrom stages for patients with central nervous injuries, it can be divided into three stages. In the early stage (stage I), patients are still in the state of flaccid paralysis and are not able to move. In this stage, physiotherapy means such as massage is needed to improve blood circulation. Meanwhile, the treatment should prevent joint contracture through the passive method and promote the normalization of muscular tension (Bobath). Psychotherapy and medication are also needed. In the middle stages (stages II, III, IV), patients' muscular function has recovered by a small part. Patients now have certain active contraction force, which is still small. Daily activities still cannot be completed. In this stage, active and passive hybrid rehabilitation treatment is needed. High- and low-frequency stimulation should also be conducted to promote neuromuscular facilitation, induce muscle activities, and prevent flaccid paralysis. Combining coordination training, intensive training, and endurance training, patients are expected to perform some easy daily activities. In the later stages (stages V, VI), patients' muscle force recovers to a certain extent. Due to the long-time clinotherapy and equipment-assistant walking and exercises, the motor coordination and balancing ability are still relatively poor. Patients in this stage should receive further muscle force recovery training and endurance training to further strengthen muscular tension. Meanwhile, random motion control training should be conducted to strengthen the balancing capability and motor coordination.

As has been discussed, all kinds of rehabilitation methods have some deficiencies, resulting in the fact that the optimal rehabilitation efficacy cannot be achieved. The structure of standing bed is simple, and it has high stability and safety. Doing standing training with it would help the bedridden patients with stroke or paralysis adapt to their self-weight gradually. It also strengthens muscular tension and stimulates muscle receptors by gravity, but its function is too simple, making it only suitable for early rehabilitation. Body-weight–supported treadmill training helps patients whose lower-extremity muscle atrophies with insufficient support force to do ambulation training to improve their muscular tension and balancing capability so that walking function could be recovered. Yet, it also features a simple function, which is unable to meet the requirements of doing active and passive hybrid training in the middle of rehabilitation. It is also not suitable for the early rehabilitation treatment which focuses on adaptability and safety. Based on the above discussion, design key points of exoskeleton robots are as follows.

First, mechanical structure of exoskeleton robot should meet the joint motion requirements, e.g., joint extension/flexion, normal walking, etc. Universality should also be considered. Owing to differences in stature, the physical dimensions of the limbs are not the same. Thus, the dimensions of the mechanical structure should be adjustable in a certain range to meet the requirements of most people. Also, adjustment of structure height and center-of-gravity height should be realized. Second, mechanical structure of the exoskeleton robot should ensure wearers' safety while taking rehabilitation training. Thus, the prosthetic body of the exoskeleton robot should be combined with auxiliary supporting mechanism. Third, the masses of exoskeleton robot and the wearer should all be supported by the exoskeleton robot; thus, necessary stiffness and intensity of the mechanical structure should both be guaranteed. Fourth, the security of the user in the rehabilitation process should also be considered. No matter whether the system is properly functioning or in the failure condition, personal safety of the wearer should be of the highest priority. Necessary safety devices should be placed on the main motion joints, including the mechanical limits and electrical limits. Finally, hodegetics should be fully considered, and the optimal design should be carried out based on doctors' advices.

Driving method selection: Traditional driving methods include hydraulic drive, pneumatic drive, and electrical drive. They are all applied in the existent exoskeleton robots. BLEEX of UC Berkeley adopts hydraulic drive, which provides larger driving force. However, it is inconvenient to carry if the hydraulic source has a large size. The noise of hydraulic drive is also big. It is originally designed for military use and has its limitations in clinical application. Pneumatic drive also has its applications, such as the Power-assisted Wear developed by Kanagawa Institute of Technology. Its main shortcomings include high system complexity and low control accuracy. The mainstream is the application of electric motor drive. Considering the compact requirements of the structure and the big torque to drive human joint motion, AC servo motor is commonly used.

4.1.4.2 Configuration Design for Exoskeleton Robot

Referring to the motion feature of lower extremity, joint motion is realized by skeletal muscle, the function of which is the same as linear actuation. Thus, linear actuation is usually applied to simulate muscle contraction. In the design scheme in the following example, slider-crank mechanism is applied on the hip and knee joints of the exoskeleton robot to realize the F/E of the two joints in the sagittal plane. Electric actuator is responsible for the rectilinear motion of this mechanism. Besides, compared with serial mechanism, parallel mechanism has the advantages of high stiffness and high integration degree, which are more suitable for exoskeleton robot design. Thus, the parallel mechanism of 3-RPS (Revolution Prismatic Spherics) is selected in the ankle joint. The two rotational DOFs are responsible for the dorsiflexion/plantar flexion and ecstrophy/enstrophe of the ankle. The linear DOF along axis Z is responsible for adjusting the length of the exoskeleton limbs to suit it to people with different heights [109]. The configuration designs of hip, knee, and ankle joints of the exoskeleton robot are illustrated in Figure 4.21.

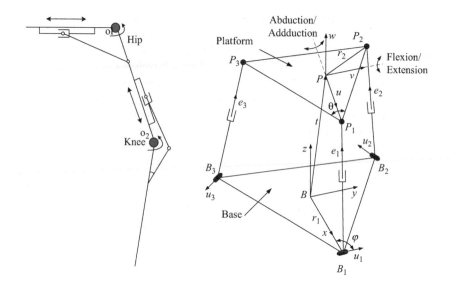

FIGURE 4.21   Configuration design for hip, knee, and ankle joints.

Exoskeleton robot is mainly used in F/E and walking rehabilitation treatment of lower extremity for patients with paraplegia or lack of muscle strength. Based on the feature that patient is weak in the supporting ability of lower limb, the following features have to be realized by the exoskeleton robot. First, high security of exoskeleton in use should be guaranteed, reducing the risk of fall to the lowest level. Thus, the system is composed of exoskeletal prosthesis and auxiliary supporting system. Second, the masses of exoskeleton robot and the wearer should all be supported by the system; thus, necessary stiffness and intensity of the mechanical structure should all be guaranteed. Third, exoskeleton robot should be applied for various patients with paraplegia, lack of muscle force, or others. Thus, the different auxiliary supporting systems, including the bed type, standing type and seat type, can be developed based on the same exoskeleton prosthesis. This aims at meeting various motion requirements, such as F/E, normal walking, etc.

Referring to the above analyses, lower extremity of exoskeleton robot and auxiliary supporting system are included in the exoskeleton design in this section. The lower extremity is built with two eudipleural lower-extremity structures with two main DOFs of knee joint and hip joint and one DOF of passive mechanism composed of link mechanism on the calf to meet the requirements of patients with different body features. When the link mechanism is compact with large stiffness, it can be applied as the transmission device. The servo motors placed on the trunk and the ball screw are connected through the coupling at the hip joint. It transforms motor rotation into rectilinear motion of ball screw, driving the slider to move back and forth. The rotation of hip joint is then realized by the four-bar linkage connecting the trunk and the thigh of exoskeleton robot. Timing pulley connects the servo motors placed on the thigh and ball screw, transforming rotation of motor into translational motion of screw nut. It drives the slider to move back and forth and rotates the knee joint by the four-bar linkage connecting the calf and thigh of the exoskeleton robot. The mechanical model is illustrated in Figure 4.22 (one leg).

Based on the average statistical data, the critical dimensions are determined as follows: $L_1 = 70\,\text{mm}$, $L_2 = 108\,\text{mm}$, $L_3 = 60\,\text{mm}$, $L_4 = 95.5\,\text{mm}$, $L_5 = 350\text{–}450\,\text{mm}$, $L_6 = L_5/2$, $L_8 = 400\,\text{mm}$, $L_7 = L_8/2$, $h_1 = 9.5\,\text{mm}$, $h_2 = 38\,\text{mm}$. The dimensions correspond to the parameters in Figure 4.23.

Based on the different requirements from various patients, the research group developed auxiliary supporting system of several kinds, such as the bed type, the standing type, and the seat type. The mechanical models are illustrated in Figure 4.24. Among them, the bed-type exoskeleton combines the standing bed with lower extremity of exoskeleton, enabling the rehabilitation-robot-assisted

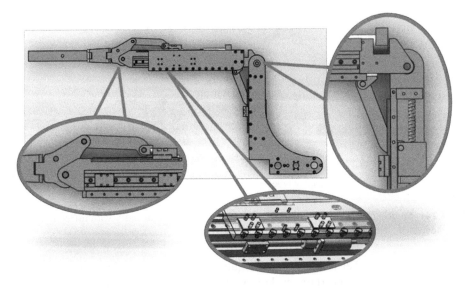

FIGURE 4.22   Mechanical model for one leg of exoskeleton.

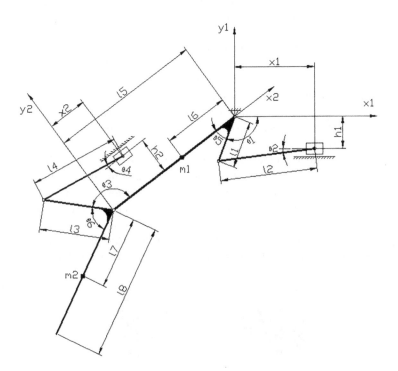

FIGURE 4.23   The schematic diagram for exoskeleton robot of lower extremity.

treatment and rehabilitation training to be connected with standing bed. Thus, patients are able to adapt to self-weight from lying to standing while taking step-by-step trainings. While lying relaxed and being labor-saving, the bed type is suitable for patients with weak muscle force, older age, or severe diseases. Standing-type exoskeleton integrates weight-reducing gait training device with treadmill and lower extremity of exoskeleton, enabling the patients to do self-conscious and safe gait training with the aid of the rehabilitation system.

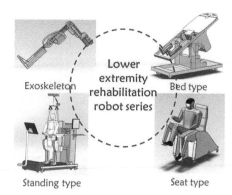

FIGURE 4.24   Models of exoskeleton rehabilitation robots of lower extremity with different auxiliary supporting systems.

As standing-type exoskeleton has higher requirements on muscle force of lower extremity, it is suitable for patients with a certain level of muscle force, slight abnormal gait, and younger age. Seat-type rehabilitation robot integrates seat with exoskeleton for lower extremity, enabling patients to do rehabilitation training in the sitting pose to improve the degree of comfort. Meanwhile, the seat back is able to incline, making it possible to do the rehabilitation exercise in seated position, semi-supine position, or prone position. Its function lies between the bed type and standing type.

The prototypes of exoskeleton rehabilitation robots of lower extremity with different auxiliary supporting systems were developed and illustrated in Figure 4.25. The mechanical design process is illustrated as follows with the example of standing exoskeleton.

Mechanism of exoskeleton robot: As illustrated in Figure 4.26, mechanism of exoskeleton robot includes exoskeletal prosthesis joints, body supporting mechanism, mobile platform, suspension frame, and protection casing. Suspension frame is located on the mobile platform. The skeletal joints and suspension frame are connected together to form the exoskeleton robot. The control system is located in the control cabinet. The design ideas of each module are illustrated as follows.

Hip/knee joint: For human body, joint motion is motivated by the coordinated contraction of inside and outside antagonistic muscle groups. As discussed before, extension/flexion of the knee joint is realized by a couple of antagonistic muscles (quadriceps femoris (QF) and BF). Thus, in the embodiment design of the exoskeleton, the mechanism of crank-slider is applied, transforming the rectilinear motion of screw nut to rotation along the joint center through the inbuilt servo motor and ball screw. The skeletons of thigh and calf are mainly driven by connection rods. Slide optimization

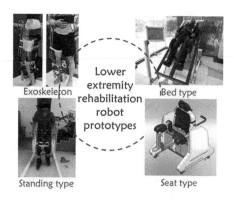

FIGURE 4.25   Prototypes of exoskeleton rehabilitation robots of lower extremity with different auxiliary supporting systems.

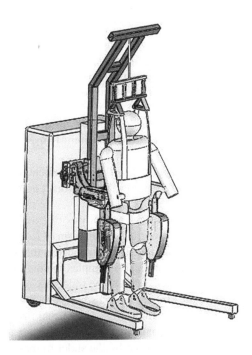

FIGURE 4.26   3D diagram of exoskeleton robot.

is also done to make the exoskeleton a compact structure with large range of rotation. The swing range of knee is 0°–110° and that of hip is −26° to 56°, both of which meet the motion requirements. The length of every limb can be adjusted through fixing the pin to meet the requirements of patients with different limb lengths (Figure 4.27).

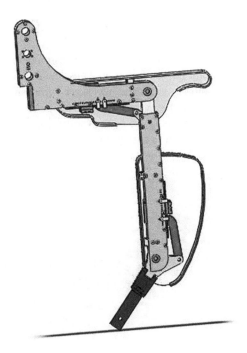

FIGURE 4.27   Hip and knee joint of exoskeleton.

Ankle joint: From the perspective of joint motion, muscles that drive the joint motion are in parallel. It is of bionic significance to design the exoskeleton joint in the parallel form. The ankle joint simulation of the exoskeleton is implemented by a parallel mechanism of three DOFs and three RPSs. The joint mechanism is a compact structure with the ability to rotate around a specific point in two DOFs with high stiffness. Thus, the ankle joint can well perform the dorsiflexion/plantar flexion and ecstrophy/enstrophe with heavy load. The mechanical design and its physical picture are illustrated in Figure 4.28. As the designed ankle joint is large in size, it should be used separately with the hip/knee joint. It is mainly used in the rehabilitation training of the ankle.

Orthosis: Developing the orthosis should meet the requirements of doctors. The orthosis connects with the inner side of exoskeleton robot. It is used to protect human lower extremity and drive joint motion,

Body supporting mechanism: Referring to the analysis of existing exoskeleton robots, shock absorbing spring is applied in the body supporting mechanism of Lokomat to act as a buffer for the vertical displacement deviation during walking. The deficiency is that the required spring should be of great stiffness and the mechanical design is also complex. Human lower limbs should passively adjust to exoskeleton lower limbs. To better simulate the trajectory of body center of gravity, linear servo motor is applied here to drive the exoskeleton prosthesis and the slider of the electric motor to move at the same time and adjust human center of gravity in real time. Meanwhile, the suspender placed on the body supporting system is connected with the orthosis to support the upper part of body. The height of suspension frame is adjusted by the slider to make it suitable for patients with different heights. Active adjustment of body center of gravity is done to meet the fluctuation features with gait alternation while doing gait rehabilitation exercises. The suspender on the suspension frame is used to support the human body to prevent patient it from falling. On the lumbar part, there are screw threads to adjust the width of exoskeleton with hand shank so as to meet the requirements of patients with different statures.

Vehicle platform: The vehicle platform is driven by electric motor with gradeability and acceptable velocity. Moving the exoskeleton prosthesis by controlling the vehicle wheels aims at meeting the requirement of walking trainings. Besides, treadmill can also be placed on the bottom to adjust human walking speed with the velocity of the treadmill to do the gait rehabilitation exercises (Figure 4.29).

Safety limit: The joint range of motion is limited, so the design of exoskeleton joints should protect the patients by meeting the joint range of motion. Thus, the exoskeleton joint range of motion should be consistent with that of human joint, and necessary limits should be added to restrict the activity of exoskeleton joints to prevent them from hurting the patients because of misoperation or system failure. In addition to the limits set in the control software, mechanical and electrical limits are also applied in the exoskeleton design to ensure patients' safety.

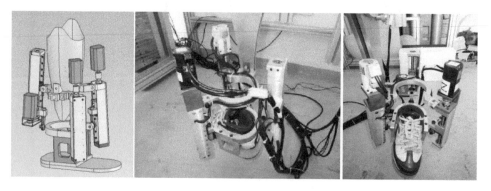

FIGURE 4.28 The mechanical design and its physical picture.

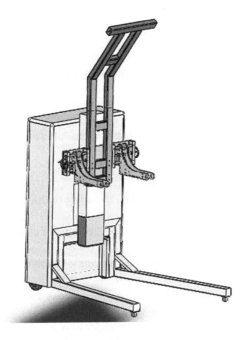

FIGURE 4.29 Vehicle platform and body support mechanism.

4.1.4.3 Static/Dynamic Analysis of Exoskeleton

4.1.4.3.1 System Simplification and Coordinate Definition

We still take the standing-type rehabilitation robot as an example and develop the system model for the exoskeleton robot (not including the parallel structure of ankle joint), i.e., the static and dynamic analyses. It is not only the verification of exoskeleton mechanical design and actuator selection, but also a necessary procedure for exoskeleton control. Referring to the above discussion, when the vehicle stays still, the system has five DOFs, including the hip joint and knee joints on both sides and the prismatic pair to adjust center of gravity. The simplified model is illustrated in Figure 4.30.

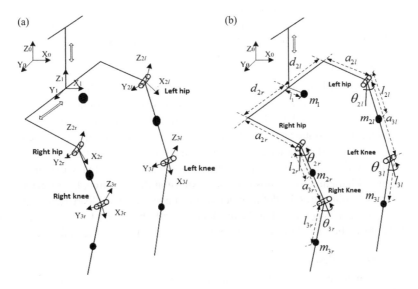

FIGURE 4.30 (a) Coordinate definition; (b) parameter definition.

Coordinate definitions:

Base coordinate: O-X_0-Y_0-Z_0. It is set on the vehicle platform and does not move relative to the ground.

Prismatic coordinate: O-X_1-Y_1-Z_1. It is the prismatic pair of the body supporting mechanism relative to vehicle platform.

Revolute coordinate: O-X_{ir}-Y_{ir}-Z_{ir}, $i = 2, 3$. It is the revolute pair of hip and knee joints on the right.

Revolute coordinate: O-X_{il}-Y_{il}-Z_{il}, $i = 2, 3$. It is the revolute pair of hip and knee joints on the left.

Parameter definitions for the mechanism:

θ_{2r}: rotation angle of hip joint on the right, i.e., the angle of thigh bone relative to vertical axis Z_{2r} in the sagittal plane.

θ_{3r}: rotation angle of knee joint on the right, i.e., the angle of calf bone relative to exoskeleton for thigh in the sagittal plane.

θ_{2l}: rotation angle of hip joint on the left, i.e., the angle of thigh bone relative to vertical axis Z_{2r} in the sagittal plane.

θ_{3l}: rotation angle of knee joint on the left, i.e., the angle of calf bone relative to exoskeleton for thigh in the sagittal plane.

a_{2r}: distance from right hip joint axis Y_2 to the slider axis Y_1.

a_{3r}: distance from right hip joint axis Y_2 to right knee joint axis Y_3.

a_{2l}: distance from left hip joint axis Y_2 to the slider axis Y_1.

a_{3l}: distance from left hip joint axis Y_2 to left knee joint axis Y_3.

d_{2r}: distance from slider to the right side of exoskeleton.

d_{2l}: distance from slider to the left side of exoskeleton.

m_1: mass of joint supporting system.

m_{2r}: mass of the right thigh of the exoskeleton.

m_{3r}: mass of the right calf of the exoskeleton.

m_{2l}: mass of the left thigh of the exoskeleton.

m_{3l}: mass of the left calf of the exoskeleton.

l_1: distance from the center of gravity of the supporting system to vehicle platform.

l_{2r}: distance from the center of gravity of right thigh of the exoskeleton to hip joint axis.

l_{3r}: distance from the center of gravity of right calf of the exoskeleton to knee joint axis.

l_{2l}: distance from the center of gravity of left thigh of the exoskeleton to hip joint axis.

l_{3l}: distance from the center of gravity of left calf of the exoskeleton to knee joint axis.

4.1.4.3.2 Static Analysis

As discussed above, the exoskeleton rehabilitation robot is used to do rehabilitation exercises for patients with motor function injuries. It bears the self-weight and the patient's weight. Thus, the requirements for the mechanism's strength is relatively high. The research group did static analysis using ANSYS. The external loadings in the static analysis of exoskeleton lower limbs are illustrated in Figure 4.31. A is fixed with the structure body in practical application and is regarded as a fixed point during analysis. B, C, and D are located on the lower extremity of human and are connected with bandages. Based on the statistic weight of human lower limbs and joint extension/flexion force, the external load force is set as 90 N. Figure 4.32 illustrates the deformation results under the preset load. Referring to the figure, the big deformation happens at the end of the mechanism with the value of 1 mm. In the rehabilitation application, the deformation is relatively small and acceptable for clinical rehabilitation.

4.1.4.3.3 Dynamic Analysis

D–H method is adopted to do the dynamic analysis of the robot. The coordinate is illustrated in Figure 4.30. Calculate the 4×4 homogeneous transformation matrix for every coordinate and set

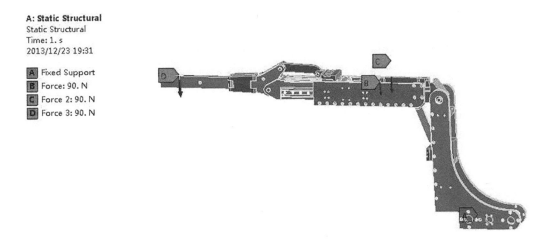

A: Static Structural
Static Structural
Time: 1. s
2013/12/23 19:31

A Fixed Support
B Force: 90. N
C Force 2: 90. N
D Force 3: 90. N

FIGURE 4.31 External load forces in the static analysis of exoskeleton lower limbs.

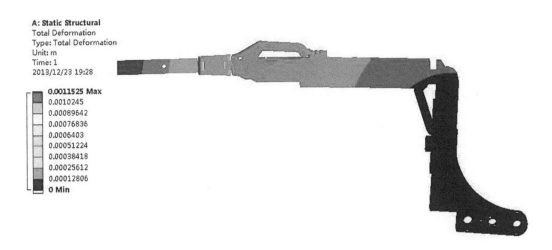

A: Static Structural
Total Deformation
Type: Total Deformation
Unit: m
Time: 1
2013/12/23 19:28

0.0011525 Max
0.0010245
0.00089642
0.00076836
0.0006403
0.00051224
0.00038418
0.00025612
0.00012806
0 Min

FIGURE 4.32 Deformation results of the exoskeleton under the preset load.

the calf skeleton as the system end. As the two sides of exoskeleton are symmetrically distributed, we can take the right leg as an instance. Table 4.3 lists the coordinate parameters for the elements of the robot. The computation and solving of robot dynamics are based on these parameters.

When calculating the transformation matrix using D–H method, the definition of each parameter corresponding to the predefined ones should be noticed. The details are as follows [110]:

θ_i: Joint angle rotating from axis X_{i-1} to axis X_i along axis Y_{i-1} (based on the right hand rule), in which the subscripts 2 and 3 stand for hip joint angle and knee joint angle, respectively.

a_i: The shortened distance between axis Y_{i-1} and Y_i.

d_i: Distance from the origin of the $(i-1)$th coordinate to the intersection of axis X_i and axis Y_{i-1} along axis Y_{i-1}.

Based on the definition of the coordinates and parameters, the transformation matrix between every joint coordinate can be determined. The transformation matrixes of adjacent coordinates are as follows.

Note: c is the abbreviation of cos, and s is the abbreviation of sin.

TABLE 4.3

Coordinate Parameters for Elements of Exoskeleton Robot

	Elements' Parameters			
Joint i (1, 2, 3)	θ_i	a_i	d_i	Range
Slider 1	0	$a_1 = 0$	$d_1 = 0$	0
Right hip $2r$	$90° - \theta_{2r}$	$a_{2r} = 11$	$d_{2r} = 11$	$-30°$ to $50°$
Right knee $3r$	θ_{3r}	$a_{3r} = 111$	0	$-120°$ to $0°$
Left hip $2l$	$90° - \theta_{2r}$	$a_{2l} = 11$	$d_{2l} = 11$	$-30°$ to $50°$
Left knee $3l$	θ_{3l}	$a_{3l} = 11$	0	$-120°$ to $0°$

Move Z_1 along axis Z. The transformation matrix $Trans(0, 0, z_1)$

$$^0A_1 = \begin{bmatrix} 1 & 0 & 0 & 0 \\ 0 & 1 & 0 & 0 \\ 0 & 0 & 1 & z_1 \\ 0 & 0 & 0 & 1 \end{bmatrix}. \tag{4.1}$$

Similarly: $^1A_2 = Trans(0, d_{2r}, 0)Trans(a_{2r}, 0, 0)Rot(y, \pi/2 - \theta_{2r})$:

$$^1A_2 = \begin{bmatrix} s\theta_{2r} & 0 & c\theta_{2r} & a_2 \\ 0 & 1 & 0 & d_{zr} \\ -c\theta_{2r} & 0 & s\theta_{2r} & 0 \\ 0 & 0 & 0 & 1 \end{bmatrix}. \tag{4.2}$$

$^2A_3 = Trans(a, 0, 0)Rot(y, \theta_{3r})$:

$$^2A_3 = \begin{bmatrix} c\theta_{3r} & 0 & s\theta_{3r} & a_3 \\ 0 & 1 & 0 & 0 \\ -s\theta_{3r} & 0 & c\theta_{3r} & 0 \\ 0 & 0 & 0 & 1 \end{bmatrix}. \tag{4.3}$$

Transformation matrix of each coordinate relative to the base coordinate

$$^0T_i = {}^0A_1{}^1A_2 \cdots {}^{i-1}A_i, i = 1,2,3. \tag{4.4}$$

Based on the coordinate transformation matrixes, the forward kinematic functions of the exoskeleton robot can be developed:

$$^0[X,Y,Z,1] = {}^0T_i \cdot {}^i[x,y,z,1], \tag{4.5}$$

in which $^i[x,y,z,1]$ stands for the coordinate vector of a specific position in the ith joint coordinate. $^0[X,Y,Z,1]$ stands for the coordinate vector of the position in the base coordinate.

Based on the coordinate value of one position in one joint, the coordinate value of the position in the base coordinate can be obtained. Using the forward kinematic function (4.5), we can calculate the coordinate values of every center of gravity in the base coordinate:

$$m_1 : \left[l_1, 0, z_1 \right] \tag{4.6}$$

$$m_{2r} : \left[a_{2r}, l_{2r} s\theta_{2r}, d_{2r}, z_1 - l_{2r} c\theta_{2r} \right] \tag{4.7}$$

$$m_{3r} : \left[a_{2r}, a_{3r} s\theta_{2r} + l_{3r} s(\theta_{2r} - \theta_{3r}), d_{2r}, z_1 - a_{3r} c\theta_{2r} - l_{3r} c(\theta_{2l} - \theta_{3l}) \right] \tag{4.8}$$

$$m_{2l} : \left[a_{2l}, l_{2l} s\theta_{2l}, d_{2l}, z_1 - l_{2l} c\theta_{2l} \right] \tag{4.9}$$

$$m_{3l} : \left[a_{2l}, a_{3l} s\theta_{2l} + l_{3l} s(\theta_{2l} - \theta_{3l}), d_{2l}, z_1 - a_{3l} c\theta_{2l} - l_{3l} c(\theta_{2l} - \theta_{3l}) \right]. \tag{4.10}$$

Suppose that the angles of the hip and knee joints on the right and left sides is zero, one can calculate the coordinate value of every center of gravity. It can be found that the results are the same with the initial position, demonstrating the correctness of the kinematic model. After determining the trajectory of every joint, the displacements of every joint screw slider are also needed to perform the position control of exoskeleton joints. The schematic diagram of exoskeleton rehabilitation robot prosthesis joint is illustrated in Figure 4.33. Motor drives the rotation of the ball screw through the coupling so as to move the hip joint slider 2 and knee joint slider 5 fixed on the screw nut. The slider motion drives the hip joint rod 3 and knee joint rod 6 to move so as to make the thigh rod 4 and calf rod 7 swing.

Define the vertical position of thigh skeleton and calf skeleton relative to the horizontal plane as the initial zero position (as illustrated in Figure 4.34). Swing the thigh forward relative to zero position as the positive angle and backward as the negative position. Swing the knee joint backward relative to the zero position as the positive angle. L_1 is the distance between the hip joint slider and the center of hip joint when the hip joint is at the zero position. L_2 is the distance between the knee joint slider and the center of knee joint when the hip joint is at the zero position. ($L_1 = 129.17$ mm, $L_2 = 137.44$ mm)

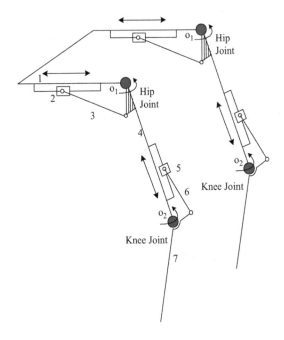

FIGURE 4.33   Schematic diagram of exoskeleton rehabilitation robot prosthesis joint.

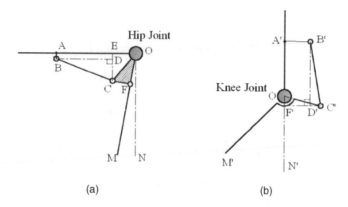

FIGURE 4.34   (a) Geometrical relationship of hip joint rods; (b) geometrical relationship of knee joint rods.

1. **Geometrical relationship between hip joint angle and displacement of hip joint slider**
   As illustrated in Figure 4.34a, $\angle MON = \theta_h$ is the rotation angle of hip joint. $\overline{AB}, \overline{BC}, \overline{OC}$, $\angle COF$ are the design parameters, whose values are fixed. Referring to the figure, we have

$$
\begin{cases}
\overline{AO} = \overline{AE} + \overline{EO} = \sqrt{\overline{BC}^2 - \overline{CD}^2} + \overline{OC} \cdot c(\angle COE) \\
\angle COE = 90° - \angle COF - \theta_h \\
\overline{CD} = \overline{CE} - \overline{ED} = \overline{OC} \cdot s(\angle COE) - \overline{ED}
\end{cases}
\tag{4.11}
$$

Based on the mechanism's design parameters, the relationship between the rotation angle and slider displacement of hip joint can be obtained:

$$
\begin{aligned}
l_h &= L_1 - \overline{AO} \\
&= L_1 - \sqrt{l_{BC}^2 - \left[l_{OC} \cdot s(60° - \theta_h) - l_{AB} \right]^2} - l_{OC} \cdot c(60° - \theta_h)
\end{aligned}
\tag{4.12}
$$

2. **Geometrical relationship between knee joint angle and displacement of knee joint slider**
   As illustrated in Figure 4.34b, $\angle M'ON' = \theta_k$ is the rotation angle of knee joint. $\overline{A'B'}, \overline{B'C'}, \overline{O'C'}, \angle C'OM'$ are the design parameters. Similarly, referring to the figure, we have

$$
\begin{cases}
\overline{A'O} = \overline{A'F'} + \overline{OF'} = \sqrt{\overline{B'C'}^2 - \overline{C'D'}^2} + \overline{OC'} \times c(\angle C'OF') \\
\angle C'OF' = \angle C'OM' - \theta_k = 120° - \theta_k \\
\overline{C'D'} = \overline{C'F'} - \overline{A'B'} = \overline{OC'} \cdot s(\angle C'OF') - \overline{A'B'} \\
\overline{OF'} = \overline{OC'} \cdot c(\angle C'OF')
\end{cases}
\tag{4.13}
$$

The relationship between the rotation angle and slider displacement of knee joint is

$$
\begin{aligned}
l_k &= L_2 - \overline{A'O} \\
&= L_2 - \sqrt{l_{B'C'}^2 - \left[l_{OC'} \cdot s(120° - \theta_k) - l_{A'B'} \right]^2} - l_{OC'} \cdot c(120° - \theta_k)
\end{aligned}
\tag{4.14}
$$

4.1.4.3.4 Dynamic Analysis

Dynamic model analysis of the exoskeleton robot aims to get the required torque and power of joint motion, and to select appropriate motor parameters so as to drive the load, and also provide theoretical foundations for the active control of robot. The forward dynamics is to solve the motion of exoskeleton, including the joint displacement, velocity, and acceleration based on the driving force/torque of every joint. It is mainly used for system simulation. The inverse dynamics aims to solve the required joint force/torque based on the known joint displacement, velocity and acceleration, and system's mass inertia. It can be used for actuator selection and real-time control of the robot [110]. There are two methods to develop the robot's dynamic model: the Newton–Euler method and the Lagrangian mechanics. When we use Newton–Euler function, we have to get the acceleration based on the kinematics and develop models for every component, the computation of which is complex. Lagrangian mechanics is used here to obtain the system's dynamic feature without calculating the internal force between the components. The Lagrangian function is

$$F_i = \frac{d}{dt}\frac{\partial L}{\partial \dot{q}_i} - \frac{\partial L}{\partial q_i}, i = 1, 2, \cdots, n \tag{4.15}$$

in which $L = K - P$ is the Lagrangian function. K is the kinematic energy of the system. P is the potential energy, and q_i is the generalized coordinate of the robot system determined by rectilinear coordinate or angular coordinate. F_i is the generalized force or torque. $n = 5$ is the DOF of the system.

The system includes supporting elements, right hip, left hip, right knee, and left knee, as illustrated in Figure 4.35.

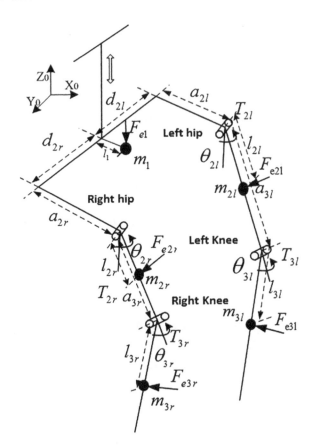

FIGURE 4.35 Simplified model of exoskeleton.

The definitions of mechanical parameters are as follows:

F_{e1}: force exerted from external load to the supporting system (body trunk).
F_{e2r}: force exerted from external load to exoskeleton right thigh (right thigh).
F_{e3r}: force exerted from external load to exoskeleton right calf (right calf).
F_{e2l}: force exerted from external load to exoskeleton left thigh (left thigh).
F_{e3l}: force exerted from external load to exoskeleton left calf (left calf).
F_1: generalized force of the supporting mechanism.
T_{2r}: generalized torque of the right hip joint.
T_{3r}: generalized torque of the right knee joint.
T_{2l}: generalized torque of the left hip joint.
T_{3l}: generalized torque of the left knee joint.

Based on the position coordinates of the center of gravity of every component (4.6–4.10), calculate the potential energy and kinematic energy.

a. The velocity, kinematic energy, and potential energy of the supporting component

$$v_1 = \dot{z}_1,$$

$$\begin{cases} K_1 = \dfrac{1}{2} m_1 \dot{z}_1{}^2 \\ P_1 = m_1 g z_1 \end{cases}. \tag{4.16}$$

b. The velocity, kinematic energy, and potential energy of right thigh

$$\begin{cases} \dot{x}_{2r} = -l_{2r}\dot{\theta}_{2r}c\theta_{2r} \\ \dot{z}_{2r} = \dot{z}_1 + l_{2r}\dot{\theta}_{2r}s\theta_{2r} \end{cases} \tag{4.17}$$

$$\Rightarrow v_{2r}{}^2 = \dot{x}_{2r}{}^2 + \dot{z}_{2r}{}^2$$

$$\begin{cases} K_{2r} = \dfrac{1}{2} m_{2r} v_{2r}{}^2 \\ P_{2r} = m_{2r} g (z_1 - l_{2r}c\theta_{2r}) \end{cases}. \tag{4.18}$$

c. The velocity, kinematic energy, and potential energy of right calf

$$\begin{cases} \dot{x}_{3r} = a_{3r}\dot{\theta}_{2r}c\theta_{2r} + l_{3r}\left(\dot{\theta}_{2r} - \dot{\theta}_{3r}\right)c(\theta_{2r} - \theta_{3r}) \\ \dot{z}_{3r} = \dot{z}_1 + a_{3r}\dot{\theta}_{2r}s\theta_{2r} + l_{3r}\left(\dot{\theta}_{2r} - \dot{\theta}_{3r}\right)s(\theta_{2r} - \theta_{3r}) \end{cases} \tag{4.19}$$

$$\Rightarrow v_{3r}{}^2 = \dot{x}_{3r}{}^2 + \dot{z}_{3r}{}^2$$

$$\begin{cases} K_{3r} = \dfrac{1}{2} m_{3r} v_{3r}{}^2 \\ P_{3r} = m_{3r} g \left(z_1 - a_{3r}c\theta_{2r} - l_{3r}c(\theta_{2r} - \theta_{3r})\right) \end{cases}. \tag{4.20}$$

d. The velocity, kinematic energy, and potential energy of left thigh

$$\begin{cases} \dot{x}_{2l} = -l_{2l}\dot{\theta}_{2l}c\theta_{2l} \\ \dot{z}_{2l} = \dot{z}_1 + l_{2l}\dot{\theta}_{2l}s\theta_{2l} \end{cases} \tag{4.21}$$

$$\Rightarrow v_{2l}^2 = \dot{x}_{2l}^2 + \dot{z}_{2l}^2$$

$$\begin{cases} K_{2l} = \dfrac{1}{2}m_{2l}v_{2l}^2 \\ P_{2l} = m_{2l}g(z_1 - l_{2l}c\theta_{2l}) \end{cases} \tag{4.22}$$

e. The velocity, kinematic energy, and potential energy of left calf

$$\begin{cases} \dot{x}_{3l} = a_{3l}\dot{\theta}_{2l}c\theta_{2l} + l_{3l}(\dot{\theta}_{2l} - \dot{\theta}_{3l})c(\theta_{2l} - \theta_{3l}) \\ \dot{z}_{3l} = \dot{z}_1 + a_{3l}\dot{\theta}_{2l}s\theta_{2l} + l_{3l}(\dot{\theta}_{2l} - \dot{\theta}_{3l})s(\theta_{2l} - \theta_{3l}) \end{cases} \tag{4.23}$$

$$\Rightarrow v_{3l}^2 = \dot{x}_{3l}^2 + \dot{z}_{3l}^2$$

$$\begin{cases} K_{3l} = \dfrac{1}{2}m_{3l}v_{3l}^2 \\ P_{3l} = m_{3l}g(z_1 - a_{3l}c\theta_{2l} - l_{3l}c(\theta_{2l} - \theta_{3l})) \end{cases} \tag{4.24}$$

The robot system has five DOFs. Its total kinematic energy and potential energy are

$$\begin{cases} K = \dfrac{1}{2}m_1v_1^2 + \dfrac{1}{2}m_{2r}v_{2r}^2 + \dfrac{1}{2}m_{3r}v_{3r}^2 + \dfrac{1}{2}m_{2l}v_{2l}^2 + \dfrac{1}{2}m_{3l}v_{3l}^2 \\ P = P_1 + P_{2l} + P_{2r} + P_{3l} + P_{3r} \end{cases} \tag{4.25}$$

Lagrangian function is

$$L = K - P$$
$$= \dfrac{1}{2}m_1v_1^2 + \dfrac{1}{2}m_{2r}v_{2r}^2 + \dfrac{1}{2}m_{3r}v_{3r}^2 + \dfrac{1}{2}m_{2l}v_{2l}^2 + \dfrac{1}{2}m_{3l}v_{3l}^2 - P_1 - P_{2l} - P_{2r} - P_{3l} - P_{3r} \tag{4.26}$$

Get the derivative and partial derivative of L, and substitute it into the dynamic function (4.15) to get the generalized force/torque function of every component. As the computation process is complex, the process will not be listed here. Only the formulas are listed:

$$\begin{cases} F_1 = \dfrac{d}{dt}\dfrac{\partial L}{\partial \dot{z}_1} - \dfrac{\partial L}{\partial z_1} \\ T_{ir} = \dfrac{d}{dt}\dfrac{\partial L}{\partial \dot{\theta}_{ir}} - \dfrac{\partial L}{\partial \theta_{ir}}, \quad i = 2,3. \\ T_{il} = \dfrac{d}{dt}\dfrac{\partial L}{\partial \dot{\theta}_{il}} - \dfrac{\partial L}{\partial \theta_{il}} \end{cases} \tag{4.27}$$

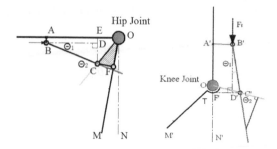

FIGURE 4.36 Force analysis of the crank-slider mechanism of the hip and knee joints.

Considering the impact of external load to the exoskeleton, the required active force and torque for joint motion are

$$
\begin{cases}
F_{a1} = F_1 + F_{e1} \\
T_{air} = T_{ir} + F_{eir} \times r_{eir}, & i = 2,3. \\
T_{ail} = T_{il} + F_{eil} \times r_{eil}
\end{cases}
\tag{4.28}
$$

Based on the requirements of robot motion, the required torque of each joint should be transformed into the driving torque of the motor. We take the knee joint as an example.

First, deduce the relationship between the driving force F_1 of the slider on the calf and the joint torque. Referring to the geometric feature in Figure 4.36, the force on the crank OC' transformed from the driving force of the slider is

$$
F_k = \frac{F_t \sin\theta_2}{\cos\theta_1}.
\tag{4.29}
$$

Now transform it into the torque exerted on the knee joint:

$$
T_k = F_k \cdot L_{OC'}.
\tag{4.30}
$$

$L_{OC'}$ is the force arm, i.e., the distance form C' to the rotation center of knee joint.

If the required rotation torque of knee joint T_k is known, the thrust force of the rod F_t can be obtained. And based on the torque transformation equation of the screw nut, calculate the required torque T_k of the motor:

$$
T_{mk} = \frac{F_t P_h}{2\pi\eta i_c},
\tag{4.31}
$$

where P_h is the pitch, η is the transmission efficiency of the screw nut, and i_c is the transmission ratio.

Motor driving torque of the exoskeleton hip joint is the same as the above, but the supporting component is directly driven by the screw nut. The required motor torque can be calculated through (4.31). Based on the exoskeleton dynamic equations, one can write a MATLAB® program to do the simulation. The relating physical parameters of the robot system are listed as follows:

$$a_{2r} = 0.338\ \text{m},\ a_{3r} = 0.422\ \text{m},\ a_{2l} = 0.338\ \text{m},\ a_{3l} = 0.422\ \text{m},\ d_{2r} = 0.25\ \text{m},\ d_{2l} = 0.25\ \text{m}$$

$$m_1 = 35.16\ \text{kg},\ m_{2r} = 4.3\ \text{kg},\ m_{3r} = 0.56\ \text{kg},\ m_{2l} = 4.3\ \text{kg},\ m_{3l} = 0.56\ \text{kg}$$

$$l_1 = 0.08\ \text{m},\ l_{2r} = 0.26687\ \text{m},\ l_{3r} = 0.055785\ \text{m},\ l_{2l} = 0.26687\ \text{m},\ l_{3l} = 0.055785\ \text{m}$$

Patients follow the motion of exoskeleton robot when doing passive rehabilitation trainings. The required active force/torque of every exoskeleton joint in the gait mode is calculated to provide reference for exoskeleton control. Set the gait cycle as 2 s. The angle of hip and knee joints of both legs is illustrated in Figure 4.37a,b. There is a half time phase between the two legs. The data comes from the gait analysis device. We should calculate the corresponding angular velocity and angular acceleration. The maximum displacement of center-of-gravity shift is 15 mm, the trajectory of which is represented by $z_1 = -0.015 \cos (2\pi t)$. The displacement of center of gravity is illustrated in Figure 4.37c.

There are interactive forces exerted from human body to the exoskeleton joint when human wears on the exoskeleton. If the active contraction of human muscle is not considered, humans will follow the motion of exoskeleton. Thus, the gravity of all the parts of human body exerts forces on exoskeleton joints and the supporting mechanism. One can calculate exoskeleton's carrying capacity according to the gravities of different parts of human. Note that one should leave some design margin, so we can suppose that human weight is 100 kg. Referring to Table 4.2 to get the ratio of total body weight of different parts, the forces exerted on the exoskeleton are $F_{e1} = 613.2$ N, $F_{e2r} = 142$ N, $F_{e3r} = 51.5$ N, $F_{e2l} = 142$ N, $F_{e3l} = 51.5$ N. In one gait cycle, the calculated active force/torque of the drive units is illustrated in Figure 4.38. The required driving force of the supporting mechanism fluctuates with the motion of human body and exoskeleton, the maximum value of which is 1,250 N.

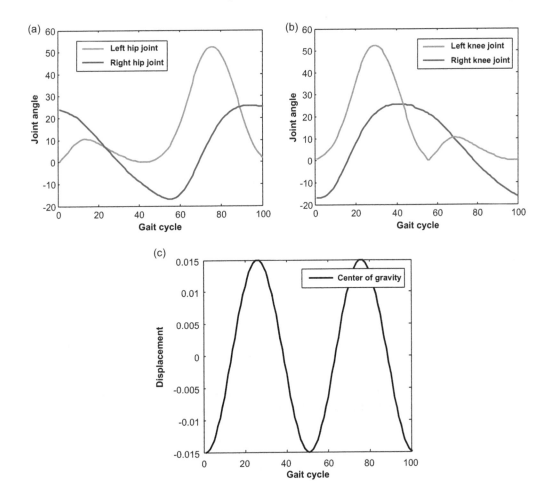

FIGURE 4.37   (a) Hip joint and (b) knee joint angles in one gait cycle; (c) displacement of center of gravity in one gait cycle.

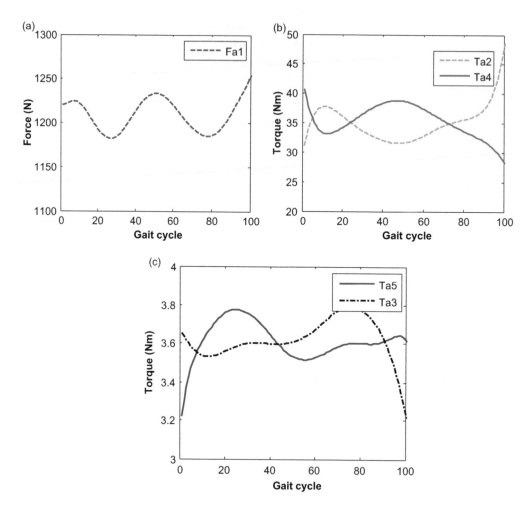

FIGURE 4.38 (a) The required driving force of the supporting platform; (b) the required driving torque of hip joint; (c) the required driving torque of knee joint.

The maximum value of the required driving torque of hip joint is approximately 50 Nm, while that of the knee joint is approximately 4 Nm. As the weight of human calf and exoskeleton calf is relatively smaller, the required driving torque is relatively smaller for the knee joint. The data above can be used for exoskeleton motor selection.

Transform it into the required motor driving moment. In one gait cycle, the calculated moment of the motor is illustrated in Figure 4.39. The maximum value of motor moment of the supporting mechanism is approximately 1.1 Nm, while that of the hip joint is 0.75 Nm and that of the knee joint is 0.031 Nm.

Besides, the force when muscle contracts to make the joint move is larger than that in the passive mode. Based on the joint torque information of human gait cycle in Figure 4.19, the required active torque of hip joint is 85 Nm and that of the knee joint is 80 Nm when we take the person weighing 100 kg as the example. The data can be used as a reference of the required driving torque of exoskeleton joints. To meet the requirements of lower-extremity exercise, we should determine the motor power of the robot system based on the dynamic analysis results. The power values of AC servo motor of the knee and hip joints are 400 W and 200 W, and the power of the supporting mechanism is 750 W. The rated torques of the above motors are 0.64 Nm, 1.3 Nm, and 2.4 Nm, while the maximum torques are 1.9 Nm, 3.8 Nm, and 7.1 Nm, respectively. As the timing pulley is

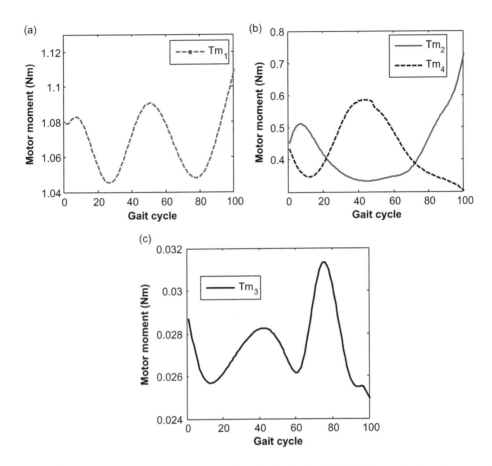

FIGURE 4.39 (a) The required motor moment of supporting mechanism; (b) the required motor moment of hip joint; (c) the required motor moment of knee joint.

applied in the transmission of exoskeleton joints, the transmission ratios of the hip and knee joint are 1:1 and 11:18, respectively. The calculated maximum driving forces on the ball screw are 4,341 N, 5,308 N and 8,022 N. We can now transform them into the maximum torque of exoskeleton joint. The values are 269 Nm and 362 Nm, respectively. Motors need to work in the rated range and meet the requirements of active and passive training of human joints.

4.1.5 HARDWARE SYSTEM FOR LOWER-EXTREMITY EXOSKELETON ROBOT

Based on the preset requirements and functions, the hardware system for lower-extremity exoskeleton robot includes the myosignal amplifier, myosignal data aquisition (DAQ) instrument, and motion controller. The myosignal amplifier is used to amplify the original sEMG signal collected by AgCl patch electrodes. It enhances the output impedance so as to do the data acquisition and recording in the next step. The myosignal DAQ instrument is used to acquire, record, process, transmit, and display the sEMG signal amplified by the amplifier. Motion controller transforms the order from upper computer into motor control pulses, sends the pulses to the motor actuator, and controls the corresponding external numerical I/O.

4.1.5.1 EMG Signal Amplifier

The circuit of EMG signal amplifier includes pre-amplifier (the gain is 10 to enhance the capacity of resisting disturbance and reduce the influence from noises), the circuit schematic of which

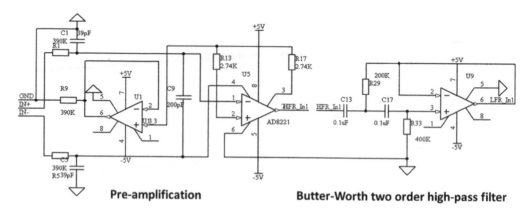

Pre-amplification   **Butter-Worth two order high-pass filter**

FIGURE 4.40   Circuit schematics of the pre-amplifier and second-order Butterworth high-pass filter.

is illustrated in Figure 4.40. Second-order Butterworth high-pass filter (the cutoff frequency is 10 Hz) is used, and the circuit schematic is illustrated as in Figure 4.40. Third-order Butterworth low-pass filter (cutoff frequency of 500 Hz) is used together with the high-pass filter, and it controls the signal frequency spectrum within the range of 10–500 Hz. The circuit schematic of it is illustrated in Figure 4.41. The circuit schematic of the main amplifier (gain of 500) is illustrated in Figure 4.42. Proportional translation (the input of the applied signal acquisition card is 0–3 V, so the proportional translation is needed as required). Low-pass resistance capacitance (RC) filter (filtering the high-frequency noise from operational amplifier (OP) chips, external disturbance, etc.) and a voltage follower (increasing the input impedance and reducing the output impedance) are illustrated in Figure 4.42. The pre-amplifier and the main amplifier are both designed using the AD8221 chips with common-mode rejection ratio, thus being able to restrain broadband interference and linear distortion. At the same time, the working noise of the chip is low. When the working frequency is 1 kHz, the maximum input voltage noise of AD8221 amplifier is $8\,\text{nV}/\sqrt{\text{Hz}}$. When the working frequency is 0.1–10 Hz, there is only point to point noise with 0.25 uV of the AD8221. The range of the gain is 1–1,000, which meets the application requirements. Other OP chips are mainly used in the filter circuit, whose accuracy requirements are lower. Thus, the OP27 chips with lower cost are adopted. A sample of the above myosignal amplifier is illustrated in Figure 4.43.

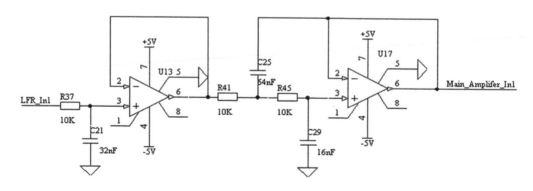

Butter-Worth three order low-pass filter

FIGURE 4.41   Circuit schematics of the third-order Butterworth high-pass filter.

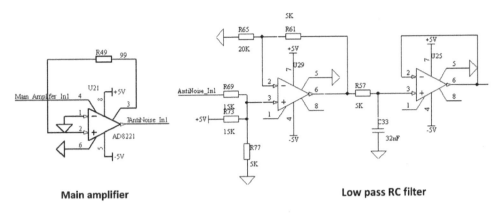

Main amplifier **Low pass RC filter**

FIGURE 4.42 Circuit schematics of the main amplifier and low-pass RC filter.

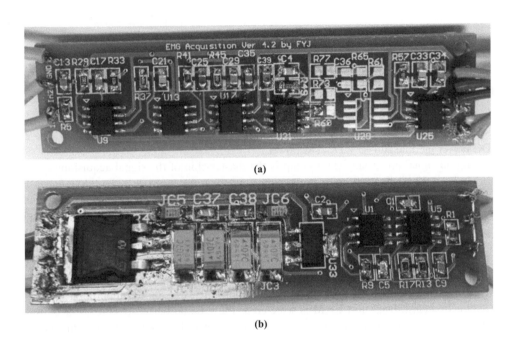

(a)

(b)

FIGURE 4.43 Myosignal amplifier sample. (a) The front; (b) the reverse.

4.1.5.2 EMG Signal DAQ Instrument

The system block diagram of the EMG signal DAQ instrument is illustrated in Figure 4.44. The system is composed of the plaque of the DAQ instrument, signal acquisition card, and embedded computer with PC/104 interface.

The plaque of the DAQ instrument is mainly used for signal transformation between signal amplifier and signal acquisition card, external digital signal input and output, and providing power for the various modules. The resources on the plaque include two integrated drive electronics (IDE) interfaces for x8 signal amplifier (including ±12 V power, ground (GND), signal line, IDE interface connecting the aviation connectors, through which it connects with the signal amplifier), nine pairs of digital I/O (on-off control of the power of external signal amplifier through external I/O), in-line interface of PC 104, two groups of 2 × 17 pin interface (connected with signal acquisition card to transfer external digital signal into the card), 2 × 9 pin interface (connected with signal acquisition

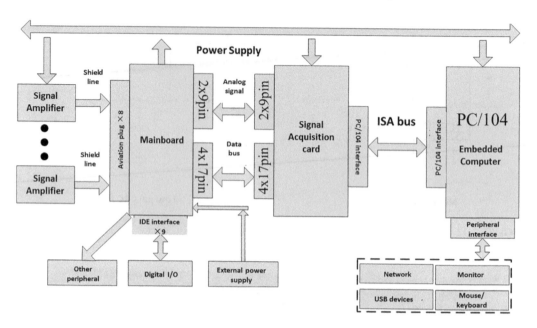

FIGURE 4.44   Block diagram of the EMG signal DAQ instrument.

card to transfer external analog signal into the card, including the analog ground), and the ±12 V DC/DC power module and +5 V DC/DC power.

The digital signal processing (DSP) chip is the master chip of the signal acquisition card. The chip includes a 32-bit floating point processing unit; thus, it can process digital signal faster. It also has a 12-bit analog-to-digital converter (ADC) with 16 channels to meet the requirements of myosignal analog quantity acquisition, a 6-DMA (direct memory access) channel that supports ADC to transform, read, and transfer the analog/digital (A/D) signal faster. Complex programmable logic device (CPLD) is the companion chip. Using the programmability and parallel processing of CPLD, the logic computing and transforming of industry standard architecture (ISA) control bus and chip control bus and the external digital I/O extension are performed. The CPLD has 116 I/O and 1,270 logic blocks, completely satisfying the requirements of logic computing and I/O of the data acquisition card. Dual-port RAM is selected as the rotation buffer to store the acquired data or order that is not read in time to ensure that the operation system on the upper computer without real-time property is able to receive data from the acquisition card fast and with no omission and DSP is able to have enough memory space to store the following orders when the former mission has not been completed. The dual-port RAM chip has an 8K capacity and a 16-bit high-speed dual port. Considering the data transfer rate, life cycle of the system development, and system maturity, ISA control bus is selected in the data acquisition card to do signal transfer with upper computer. Based on the DSP processing capacity, storage capacity of the dual-port RAM, and the frequency distribution of the collected myosignal, the maximum sampling frequency is set as 2 kHz. As the frequency range of sEMG is 20–500 Hz. The acquisition card is able to meet the requirements of real-time acquisition of sEMG signal. The hardware block diagram is illustrated in Figure 4.45.

The PH-450 integrating the Intel Atom N450 chip group is selected as the embedded computer with PC/104 interface. It has low power consumption, high stability, and high performance and is suitable for real-time control, data acquisition, information recording, video displaying, visual manipulation, and networking.

The sample of signal acquisition card is illustrated in Figure 4.46.

The sample of EMG signal DAQ instrument and its inner structure is illustrated in Figures 4.47 and 4.48, respectively.

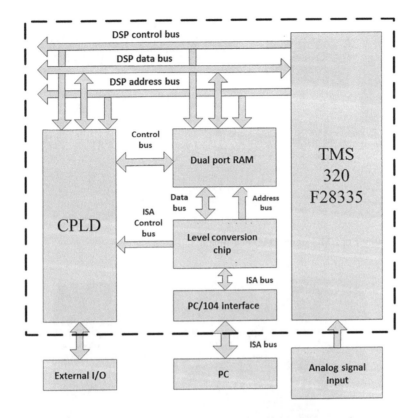

FIGURE 4.45 Block diagram of the ISA control-bus–based signal acquisition card system.

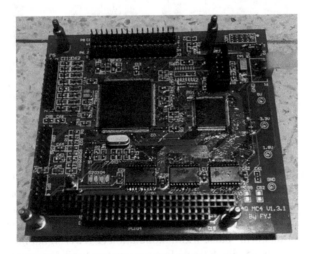

FIGURE 4.46 Sample of the ISA control-bus–based signal acquisition card.

4.1.5.3 Motion Controller

The system block diagram of the motion controller is illustrated in Figure 4.49, including the signal exchanging board, motion control board, and the computer.

The signal exchanging board is mainly used in the signal transformation between motion control board and servo actuator, the signal input of external limit switch, the input and output of external digital signal, and providing power for the various modules. The resource on the board includes

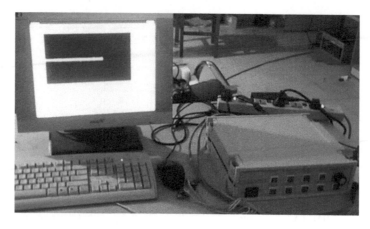

FIGURE 4.47   Sample of EMG signal DAQ instrument.

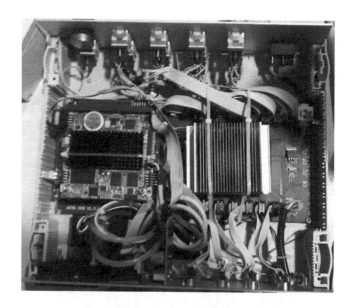

FIGURE 4.48   Inner structure of the sample of EMG signal DAQ instrument.

6 DB15 interfaces (including actuator power, pulse signal line, encoder signal line, servo enabler, servo alertor, analog signal line), among which the pulse signal is transformed into differential signal from signal channel signal through a 26LS31 chip. The encoder signal line transforms the differential signal into signal channel signal and sends it to the control board through a TLP2631 chip. The analog signal transforms pulse width modulation (PWM) signal into voltage signal; every axis is equipped with three-limit switch (including the positive limit, the negative limit, and the zero position, with a sum of 18), and every axis is equipped with a pair of I/O (to meet the requirement of external I/O extension), PC104 in-line interface, two groups of 2×17 pin interfaces (connected with motion control board to achieve data transformation between motion control board and signal exchanging board), an advanced technology eXtended (ATX) power interface, and a power-line terminal (providing different kinds of power input).

The DSP chip is again selected as the master chip of the motion control board. A CPLD is selected to perform logic computing and digital I/O extension. Different from signal acquisition

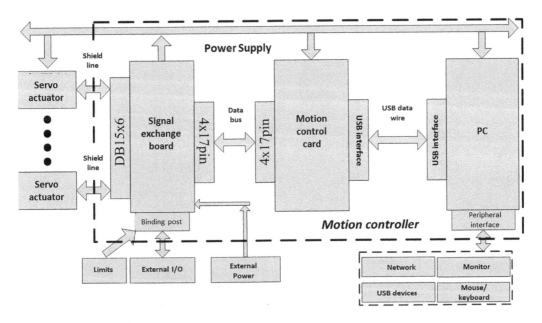

FIGURE 4.49 System block diagram of the motion controller.

board, as the transmission rate of ISA bus is slow, the industrial equipment using this interface has gradually fallen into disuse. Thus, the widely applied USB interface is adopted in the motion control. Its transmission rate is faster, and the error rate is lower. Besides, the transport protocols are mature, and the development is easier. The USB chip of CY7C68013A is selected to perform the data transmission in the motion control board. The chip supports USB 2.0 transmission protocol. The maximum transmission bit rate is 480 Mbps, supporting 8-bit or 16-bit external data interface. It is embedded with 8051 microprocessor and 16K RAM, qualified for the requirements of the data transmission between motion control board and the computer. EEPROM (Electrically Erasable PROM) is also equipped. It is based on I^2C bus with storage capacity of 64 Kbit and starter programs for loading USB chips. Meanwhile, to extend the RAM space of DSP chip, SRAM—IS61LV25616 with the storage capacity of 16*256K is also used. When the motion control board is in service, the trajectory data containing potential, velocity, and control orders is sent to motion control board from computer through the USB interface and is stored in the RAM of USB chips. Meanwhile, the logic computing is performed by the CPLD, and it transforms the data into control signal for USB chips to complete the reading of RAM data in USB chip from DSP chips. DSP generates the feedback data, and then the USB control signal is generated by CPLD. It controls the USB chips to transfer the DSP feedback data to the computer to achieve the data communication between computer and motion control board. DSP performs the interpolation based on the trajectory data generated by the computer and transforms it into command pulse. The command pulse outputs in the form of PWM impulse wave through CPLD. Meanwhile, the servo actuator inputs the A/B phase pulses from motor encoder to CPLD through the exchanging board. After the decoding by phase discrimination and frequency division module, position feedback of the motor axis is achieved. Moreover, when DSP accesses the CPLD, real-time monitoring of the positive and negative limits, the zero position, alarm signal of the motor actuator can be achieved. With the wide application of USB interface, the embedded computer is selected, such as the PH-4501 integrating Intel Atom N450 chip group. Personal computer is of course another choice. The block diagram of USB-interface–based motion control board is illustrated in Figures 4.50 and 4.51.

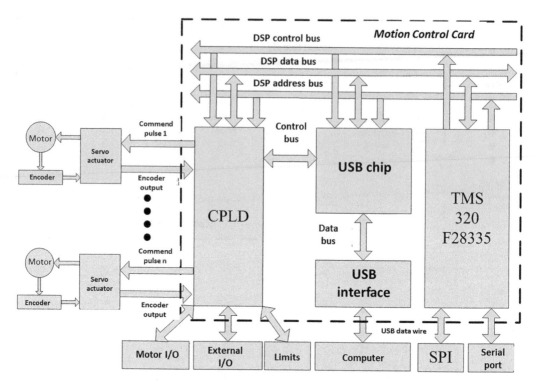

FIGURE 4.50   Block diagram of USB-interface–based motion control board.

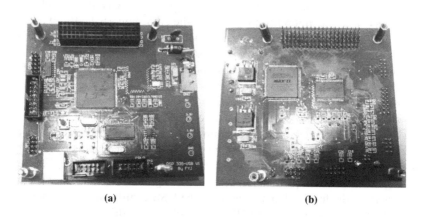

(a)   (b)

FIGURE 4.51   Sample of USB-interface–based motion control board. (a) The front; (b) the reverse.

4.1.6   SOFTWARE SYSTEM FOR LOWER-EXTREMITY EXOSKELETON ROBOT

The research group also developed the exoskeleton robot rehabilitation system software and EMG signal DAQ software and the control interface for human–machine interaction using Microsoft Visual Basic 6.0 to call the application programming interface (API) function library in the computer to provide easy access for doctors to manipulate and control the device (Figure 4.52).

4.1.6.1   Software for EMG Signal Collection

The software for EMG signal detection is illustrated in Figure 4.53, including the compound treatment mode and signal collection mode. The compound treatment mode is responsible for the

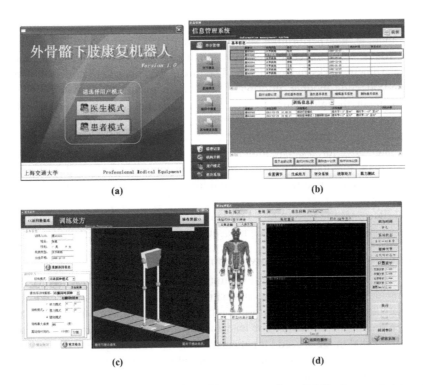

FIGURE 4.52 The application software interface of lower-extremity rehabilitation exoskeleton. (a) Access interface; (b) information management interface; (c) prescription management interface; (d) information display interface.

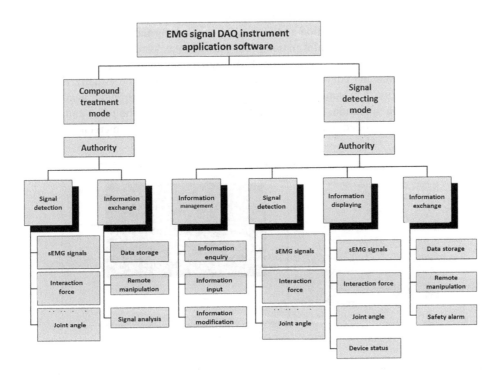

FIGURE 4.53 Structure of the EMG signal DAQ instrument application software.

coordination of EMG signal and exoskeleton, identifying the authorization of the user through the authorization module, and performing signal detection and signal communication based on the requirements from exoskeleton controller. The signal collection mode is the mode when the EMG signal DAQ instrument works independently. The mode is composed of information management module, signal collection module, information display module, and information communication module. Among them, the information management module inputs, inquires, and modifies the basic information and treatment information of the patients. Signal collection module acquires the sEMG signal, interactive force signal, and joint angle signal. Information display module displays the sEMG signal, interactive force signal, joint angle signal, and equipment conditions through visualization methods to the manipulator and user. Information communication module stores the relevant data and provides available interface for remote information operation and sets off the alarm when emergencies occur.

Figure 4.54 illustrates the EMG signal DAQ instrument application software interface, in which (a) is the access interface and (b) is the signal acquisition and display interface.

4.1.6.2   Software for Lower-Extremity Rehabilitation System

The structure of the software for lower-extremity rehabilitation training system is illustrated in Figure 4.55, including the doctor mode and patient mode. The doctor mode is mainly used for doctors to input and inquire the basic information and disease symptoms of the patients and to prescribe based on the diagnosis results. The load and input of prescriptionare performed through the software. The remedial mode is used for patients with lower-extremity diseases (including the joint patients, paraplegia patients, stroke patients, and central nerve injured patients) to do rehabilitation exercises based on prescription. It aims to recover lower extremity's range of motion to normal level and promotes muscle force recovery to prevent muscle atrophy, so that the patient is able to regain active walking ability gradually. There are five functional modules in the remedial mode: (1) Rehabilitation training. It includes the training mode (active/passive F/E mode, active/passive walking training mode) and muscle force detection mode. The training parameters, such as the training time, training intensity, and amplitude, etc., can be modified by the doctors in the training process based on the practical situation and requirements. (2) Information management. With this module, one can inquire the basic information of the patients, the corresponding prescriptions, and relating cases. (3) Data display. It illustrates the sEMG signal, human–machine interaction information, joint angle, and velocity curves to the medical staff and users in the visualization method in real time. (4) Information communication. It stores the related data and provides available interface for remote information operation. (5) Motion control. In this module, the robot and rehabilitation bed can be manually controlled. It also has the emergent operation when emergency happens.

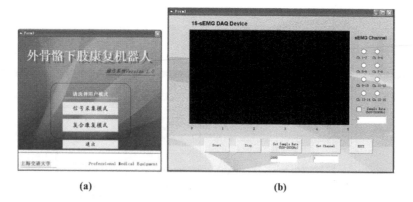

(a)   **(b)**

FIGURE 4.54   EMG signal DAQ instrument application software interface. (a) Access interface; (b) signal acquisition and display interface.

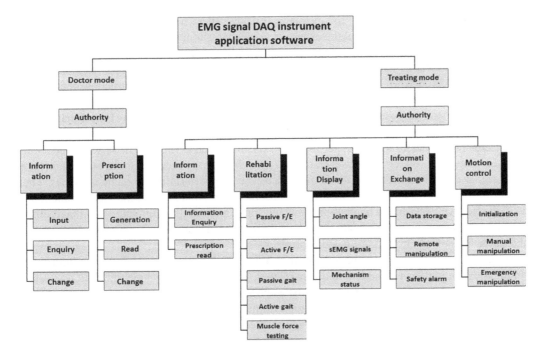

FIGURE 4.55   Structure of the software for lower-extremity rehabilitation training system.

The application software interface for lower-extremity rehabilitation exoskeleton is illustrated in Figure 4.52, where (a) is the login interface. Users log into the system through this interface. (b) is the information management interface. Users input, inquire, modify the information through this interface. (c) is the prescriptionmanagement interface. Users input, inquire, modify, and confirm prescriptionthrough this interface. (d) is the information display interface. The information, such as sEMG signal and joint angles, is displayed to patients and medical staff via this interface.

4.2   MULTI-SOURCE-SIGNAL–BASED BIOELECTROMECHANICAL HUMAN–MACHINE INTERFACE AND ACTIVE COMPLIANCE CONTROL

Active rehabilitation is the rehabilitation method in which patients perform the F/E and walking exercises through the motor ability of themselves with assistance from the rehabilitation devices. It provides muscle with enough exercises so as to accelerate the rehabilitation process and improve rehabilitation efficacy. However, there is a key problem in the active rehabilitation, i.e., the accurate identification of human movement intent. Only when real-time and accurate prediction and identification of human movement intention are achieved, the appropriate assistive force can be exerted to patients by controlling the rehabilitation equipment in the process of rehabilitation exercises. It is a prerequisite for helping patients complete rehabilitation exercises more effectively. Thus, the key points to achieve coordinated control of exoskeleton and human body and provide real-time, stable, and appropriate auxiliary training are to select appropriate signal source and establish effective human–machine interface.

At present, common signal resources of human–machine interface are composed of joint angle/angular velocity meter, force sensor, accelerometer, etc. These signals are able to reflect the current joint angle/angular velocity, the interactive force between human and exoskeleton, contact force and its distribution between human/exoskeleton and the ground, movement acceleration, etc. Yet, all these data are static and hysteretic. Thus, they can't be used to predict and identify human movement. Moreover, considering the mechanical delays, there would be 200 ms delay using the traditional signal sources to control the exoskeleton mechanism in real time, and this will give rise to bad influences on the coordinated control of human–exoskeleton system. Thus, signal sources that are able to reflect human movement intention in advance are needed.

EMG signal is able to reflect human muscle contraction state and contraction condition in advance, together with the functional status of nerve and muscle. Because of this advantage, EMG signal has been studied by more and more research institutions and applied in clinical diagnosis. It has been used in the human–machine interface for exoskeleton, e.g., the HAL series, ORTHOSIS exoskeleton robot, and a series of upper-limb exoskeletons, such as the ones in Saga University and Shanghai Jiao Tong University. However, there is great fuzziness in EMG signal. A totally different EMG signal could be collected even from the same person performing the same activities. Thus, further research has to be done to improve the accuracy of motion identification and prediction, to develop effective EMG-based human–machine interface integrating traditional signal that is able to reflect accurate movement information, such as the joint angle and force, and to achieve real-time and stable human–machine coordinated control.

Human–machine interface is the link between human and exoskeleton robot and the information communication platform of human and exoskeleton. Using human–machine interaction interface, the movement status of human joints could be acquired to provide information source for exoskeleton control. To provide effective rehabilitation training for the patients, exoskeleton robot should possess intelligence. Thus, an efficient interaction interface is the prerequisite for intelligent control of the robot [111].

In fact, there is interactive force between human and exoskeleton. It is closely related to human movement intention. While doing active training, muscle contracts to generate force and move the joint, and the leg bound with exoskeleton will exert force on exoskeleton. When the contraction force is not enough, exoskeleton is able to compensate it to perform the desired activities. While doing passive training, exoskeleton is able to provide the force for joint movement. Once the aim of human movement is determined, the muscle contraction force and the force provided by exoskeleton should be predicted accurately. Thus, it is of great significance to develop human–machine interface. Referring to the mechanism of force generation of skeletal muscle, the activation degree of muscle could be characterized by sEMG signal, which laid a foundation for calculating muscle force by EMG signal. Lloyd predicted the muscle force and joint torque on the basis of Hill-type model by processing EMG signal [112,113], while he did not establish a systematic mathematical model for muscle activation and contraction, resulting in the problem of inaccuracy in prediction. Thus, it is necessary to bring in the contact force in human–machine interaction interface when the interactive force between human and exoskeleton can be measured by corresponding force sensor. The human–machine interaction interface should include hardware, such as EMG DAQ instrument, force sensor, angle transducer, data acquisition card, processor, etc. The actual status of human body and joint torque should be acquired through body dynamics analysis.

To analyze the torque exerted on the exoskeleton when human muscle contracts, dynamic analysis of human lower limbs should be done by considering human–machine interaction interface, and the mechanical model of skeletal muscle should be verified at the same time. Based on the forward dynamics, we can measure the EMG signal to characterize the activation degree of the muscle. One can further calculate the muscle force through the mechanical model of skeletal muscle based on the collective attribution of molecular motor. Next, calculate the active joint torque during muscle contraction based on the joint arm from geometric anatomy. On the other hand, we should solve the joint torque using inverse dynamics by detecting the interactive force between human and exoskeleton. By comparing the torque with the calculated result from forward dynamics, we can verify the effectiveness of the muscle mechanical model and lay the foundation for further control application of human–machine interface in exoskeleton robot.

4.2.1 RESEARCH OBJECT

Now we can develop the dynamic model for the knee joint. The main movement of the joint is extension/flexion [104]. The driving muscles for knee joint movement are the thigh muscle groups. Among them, flexion is achieved by BF, ST, SM, and extension of the muscle is achieved by QF, including the rectus femoris (RF), vastus intermedius (VI), vastus lateralus (VL), vastus medialus (VM). They are antagonistic muscles to each other. When one muscle group contracts actively, the other group is extended passively to achieve coordinated joint movement. There are also other muscles, such as SR, TF, etc., that are responsible for assisting knee joint movement (Figure 4.56).

The geometric dimensions are illustrated in Table 4.4, referring to [114]. The samples are males with the height of 168.4 ± 9.3 cm and weight of 82.7 ± 15.2 kg.

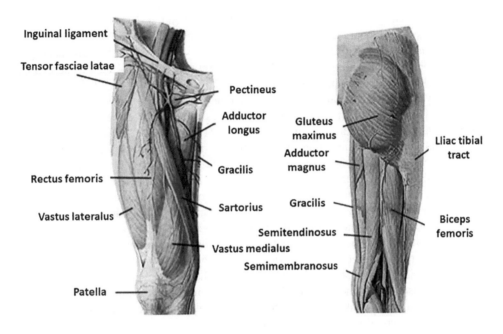

FIGURE 4.56 Muscle distribution of human thigh [104].

TABLE 4.4
Part of the Geometric Dimensions of the Muscles

Muscle	Optimal Length (cm)	Payne Angle (°)	Tendon Resting Length (cm)	PCSA (cm²)
Semimembranosus (SM)	8.0	15	35.9	19.1
Semitendinosus (ST)	20.1	5	26.2	4.9
Biceps femoris(lh) (BFLH)	10.9	0	34.1	11.6
Biceps femoris(sh) (BFSH)	17.3	23	10.0	5.2
Rectus femoris (RF)	8.4	5	34.6	13.9
Vastus lateralus (VL)	8.4	5	15.7	37
Vastus medialus (VM)	8.9	5	12.6	23.7
Vastus intermedius (VI)	8.7	3	13.6	16.8
Sartorius (SR)	57.9	0	4.0	1.9
Tensor fasciae latae (TF)	9.5	3	42.5	2.5

Referring to the skeletal muscle contraction mechanism in Chapter 3, the maximum contraction force is proportional to the physiological cross-sectional area (PCSA) of the muscle. Based on Table 4.4, the cross-sectional area of SR and TF is smaller than that of the QF; the maximum isometric contraction force is also smaller. Thus, the influence on knee joint movement is smaller, and their influence can be neglected. The muscles, including the ST, SM, BF and QF (RF, VI, VL, VM) are main actuators considered here.

4.2.2 Musculoskeletal System of Knee Joint

The musculoskeletal system is the basis for lower-extremity dynamics research. At present, there have been a lot of institutions studying the modeling of musculoskeletal system. In China, the lower-extremity musculoskeletal system consisting of 19 muscles in the hip and thigh was developed by Shang Peng in Shanghai Jiao Tong University [115]. Ji Wenting developed a lower-extremity musculoskeletal system model including 41 muscles and studied the biomechanics related to lower-extremity movement [116]. Xu Meng in Zhejiang University developed a human–machine engineering simulation and an analysis-oriented biomechanical model [117]. Yang Yiyong in Tsinghua University developed a biomechanical model including four rigid bodies and 10 muscle groups for lower-extremity muscle force analysis during squatting [118]. Moreover, Delp in Neuromuscular Biomechanics Laboratory of Stanford University developed a lower-extremity musculoskeletal system including seven DOFs and 43 muscles in 1990 [119]. Recently, the lab provided an open musculoskeletal system software, namely OpenSim 2.2, with which researchers could conduct biomechanical research. Most of the above systems adopted Hill-type model to perform mechanical property analysis. Because of the complexity of the modeling of musculoskeletal system, it is not the focus of this book, which concentrates on the dynamic analysis and experimental verification of knee joint based on the above research results and the existing musculoskeletal systems.

The extension/flexion of knee joint is the relative movement of calf to thigh. It is achieved by the torque generated by the thigh muscle contraction. As illustrated in Figure 4.57, there are mainly eight muscles related to knee extension/flexion. Among them, flexion is achieved by BF, ST, SM, and extension of the muscle is achieved by QF, including the RF, VI, VL, and VM. Every muscle is represented by muscle force linear model. The lower-extremity skeletons include the pelvis, femur, tibia, fibula, scutum, and foot skeletons. We now define local coordinate in each skeleton and regard the pelvis as the base coordinate.

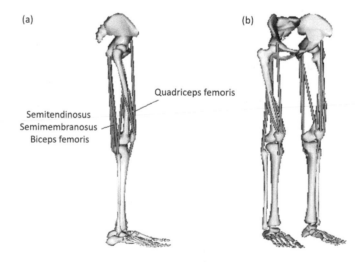

FIGURE 4.57 Musculoskeletal system model for lower extremity (including linear model of eight muscles in knee joint). (a) Side view; (b) front view.

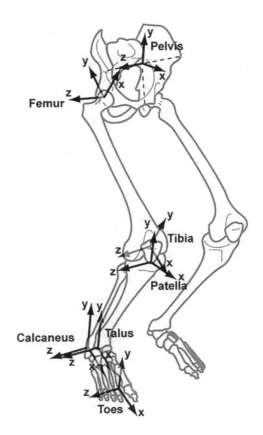

FIGURE 4.58 The coordinate definition of each bone [118].

As illustrated in Figure 4.58, the definitions of coordinates are as follows. Axis Z points to the outer side of human body. Axis Y directs to the near-end from the far-end of each limb. Axis X is orthogonal to axis Y and Z. The origins of each axis are as follows. Coordinate P of pelvis is the midpoint of the left side and right side of iliac crest. Coordinate F of femur is the center of caput femoris. Coordinate T of tibiofibular is the midpoint of the ankles inside and outside femur. The coordinate of patella is on the apex of patella bone [116].

The start point and end point of attachment points of each muscle can be acquired through anatomy. The positions of muscle attachment points in each local coordinate are illustrated in Table 4.5, when the initial hip and knee joint angles are zero. The data comes from the sample data from OpenSim software.

The angles of hip and knee joint change, and the attachment points of each muscle also change in the base coordinate. Among them, the coordinate whose attachment point is on the thigh bone (femur) is mainly affected by hip joint angle. The coordinate whose attachment point is on the calf bone (patella, tibia, and fibula) is affected by both the hip and knee joint angles. Thus, there is a need to transform the position of attachment point in local coordinates to the base coordination. When the angles of hip and knee joints are known, the position of attachment points of each muscle in the base coordinate can be acquired, and the length of muscle in the angle can be calculated together with the length variation and contraction speed of the muscles.

4.2.2.1 Geometric Parameter Computation of Muscles

As illustrated in Figure 4.59, A and B are the start point and end point of one muscle, respectively, and O is the rotation center of the joint.

TABLE 4.5

The Coordinate of the Start and End Points of the Eight Muscles in Right Knee Joint

Knee Joint Motion	Muscle	Attachment Point	Start Point (mm)			Attachment Point	End Point (mm)		
			x	y	z		x	y	z
Flexion	(SM)	Pelvis	−119.2	−101.5	69.5	Tibia	−24.3	−53.6	−19.4
Flexion	(ST)	Pelvis	−123.7	−104.3	60.3	Tibia	−31.4	−54.5	−14.6
Flexion	(BFLH)	Pelvis	−124.4	−100.1	66.6	Tibia	−8.1	−72.9	42.3
Flexion	(BFSH)	Femur	5	−211	23.4	Tibia	−10.1	−72.5	40.6
Extension	(RF)	Pelvis	−29.5	−31.1	96.8	Patella	12.1	43.7	−1
Extension	(VL)	Femur	26.9	−259.1	40.9	Patella	10.3	42.3	14.1
Extension	(VM)	Femur	35.6	−276.9	0.9	Patella	6.3	44.5	−17
Extension	(VI)	Femur	33.5	−208.4	28.5	Patella	5.8	48	−0.6

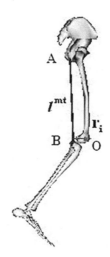

FIGURE 4.59   Definition of muscle moment arm.

Muscle moment arm is the vertical dimension from the joint center to muscle action line, i.e., the distance from point O to line AB in the figure. The computational formula of the moment arm of the ith muscle is as follows:

$$r_i = \frac{\left|\overrightarrow{AO} \times \overrightarrow{AB}\right|}{\left|\overrightarrow{AB}\right|}.$$

(4.32)

The distance between the two attachment points of one muscle includes the length of muscle and tendon. The length changes with the angles of hip and knee joints. The length of the start and end points is

$$l^{mt} = \left|\overrightarrow{AB}\right|.$$

(4.33)

Referring to the literature, the stiffness of the tendon is larger than that of the muscle, and the strain rate of the tendon is only 3.3% when muscle is fully activated. When human is doing normal activities, the stress borne by the tendon is only one-third of the limit with the strain rate being between

2% and 5%. Thus, the change of muscle-tendon length mainly depends on the muscle contraction variation. Neglecting the influence of the tendon length change, the tendon length is regarded as the length in relaxed state:

$$l^{\mathrm{t}} = l^{\mathrm{t}}_{\mathrm{s}}. \tag{4.34}$$

When muscle contracts, the length changes with the angle between muscle and tendon and satisfies the relation

$$l^{\mathrm{m}} \sin \phi = l^{\mathrm{m}}_{\mathrm{o}} \sin \phi_{\mathrm{o}}. \tag{4.35}$$

$l^{\mathrm{m}}_{\mathrm{o}}, \phi_{\mathrm{o}}$ are the optimal length and the Payne angle in the resting state, respectively. The detailed data is shown in Table 4.1.

Thus, the length of the single muscle is

$$l^{\mathrm{m}} = \sqrt{\left(l^{\mathrm{m}}_{\mathrm{o}} \sin \phi_{\mathrm{o}}\right)^2 + \left(l^{\mathrm{mt}} - l^{\mathrm{t}}_{\mathrm{s}}\right)^2}. \tag{4.36}$$

The angle between the muscle and tendon is

$$\phi = \arcsin\left(l^{\mathrm{m}}_{\mathrm{o}} \sin \phi_{\mathrm{o}} / l^{\mathrm{m}}\right). \tag{4.37}$$

Based on the values of $l^{\mathrm{m}}_{\mathrm{o}}, \phi_{\mathrm{o}}$, and $l^{\mathrm{t}}_{\mathrm{s}}$ in the resting state, the angles of hip and knee joints, the length and variation of each muscle, and coordinates of the start and end points of each muscle, the value of the muscle moment arm is illustrated in Figure 4.60.

4.2.2.2 Dynamic Analysis of Knee Joint

4.2.2.2.1 Forward Dynamics of Knee Joint

The F/E of knee joint is controlled by the motor command sent by CNS. It is transferred in the form of action potential (AP) on the surface of muscle fibers. The forward dynamics of knee joint aims to calculate the active joint moment through the activation degree of muscle featured by the

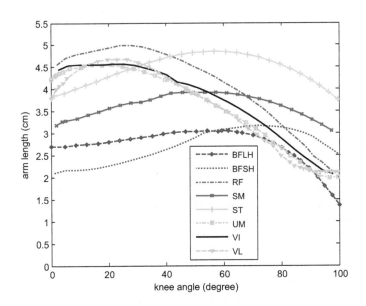

FIGURE 4.60 The muscle moment arm changing with knee joint angle.

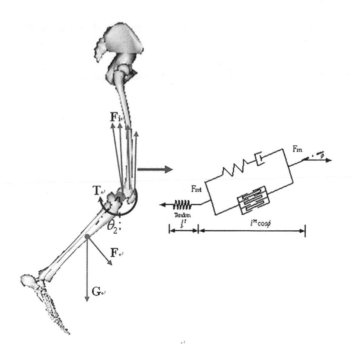

FIGURE 4.61 Dynamics of knee joint.

EMG signal, the active contraction force calculated by the mechanical model of the muscle, and the anatomy information about human joints (Figure 4.61).

Based on Eq. (2.58) of skeletal muscle force, the passive force is mainly determined by the length variation Δl^m and contraction velocity v. The contraction velocity of the muscle equals the ratio value of contraction amount to the contraction time Δt. The active muscle force is related to the factors such as muscle activation degree, muscular physical parameters, etc., where the activation degree β is featured by EMG signal illustrated by Eq. (2.64). When $\beta = 1$, muscle force reaches its maximum value F_{ma}. The force along the direction of tendon is calculated by Eq. (2.58). Thus, the total moment exerted on the joint center is

$$T = \sum_{i=1}^{8} F_i^{mt} r_i, \tag{4.38}$$

where F_i^{mt} is the muscle force of the ith muscle. Based on the data from muscle anatomy, the real-time detected EMG signal, joint angle, and the joint moments can be calculated by the mechanical model of the muscle.

4.2.2.2.2 Inverse Dynamics of Knee Joint

The inverse dynamics aims to calculate the corresponding angular velocity and angular acceleration through measuring the joint angle and develop the calf inverse dynamics equation to calculate the joint moment through the interactive force between calf and exoskeleton measured by airbag force sensor:

$$T' = J_\omega \dot{\omega}_k + G \times r_g + F \times r_f, \tag{4.39}$$

in which J_ω is the moment of inertia around axis Z of the knee joint. $\dot{\omega}_k$ is the angular acceleration. G is the gravity of calf. F is the interactive force between calf and the airbag. r_g and r_f are the force arms of gravity and pressure, respectively.

According to the balancing condition, the active muscle moment should be equal to the inverse joint moment:

$$T - T' = 0. \tag{4.40}$$

4.2.2.2.3 *Computation of the Parameters in Muscle Mechanical Model*

Theoretically, the joint moment calculated through forward dynamics should be equal to the measured moment value from the inverse dynamics. However, due to individual differences, the anatomia data would be different. Thus, there is a need to quantize the parameters in muscle models. As physiological rules should be obeyed when muscle contraction is controlled, optimization should be done and mechanical indices (such as the total energy consumed, mechanical work) should be limited to the minimum level [100]. The objective function is set as the quadratic sum of the moment errors here, and least square method is applied to solve the parameters in the model.

$$\min: \left(\sum_{i=1}^{8} F_i^{\mathrm{mt}} r_i - T' \right)^2. \tag{4.41}$$

$$\sigma_i = \frac{F_i^{\mathrm{mt}}}{A_i}, \tag{4.42}$$

where A_i is the PCSA of the ith muscle, σ_i is the muscle contraction force in unit area (muscle active stress).

4.2.3 MULTI-SOURCE INFORMATION FUSION BASED ON FORCE INTERACTION

The signal needs to be acquired by the human–machine interaction interface including the EMG signal of muscle and the interactive force between human and exoskeleton joints. The human–machine interface is composed of sensors, data acquisition unit, processor, etc. The corresponding hardware includes EMG DAQ instrument, force sensor, angular sensor, data acquisition card, DSP processor, etc. The interaction interface is integrated in the system control platform of exoskeleton robot. Data acquisition card can be used to collect the interacting information between human and exoskeleton in real-time and do the A/D transformation of the analog signal and then send it to the motion controller and computer to be processed. As the EMG signal is actually the electric signal of both the control signal of neural system and the feedback signal of the sensing organs (such as the muscular spindle and tendon organ) in the muscle; it is of great fuzziness and cannot reflect human movement intention directly. On the other hand, the features of EMG signal are highly coupled with the fatigue degree of the muscle. The sEMG signal of the same person doing the same activity is different if the muscle becomes fatigued or body status and surrounding environment are different. Thus, it is impossible to do real-time and accurate prediction of human movement intention and joint movement depending only on the sEMG signal. Thus, multi-source information fusion is needed to identify accurate movement intention.

4.2.3.1 Multi-Source Biosignal Acquisition

Traditional methods detect joint angle and angular velocity through angle encoder and interactive force through force sensor. In this way, real-time and accurate joint information and interactive force information between human and exoskeleton can be acquired, but these pieces of information can be acquired only when the activities are finished. Thus, it only reflects the hysteretic and quasi-static information about human movement and is not able to predict movement accurately in advance. However, the prediction about human movement intention is able to provide effective control information of human movement for exoskeleton robot and is of great significance to the

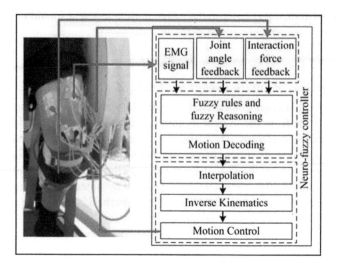

FIGURE 4.62 Neurofuzzy controller of the exoskeleton robot.

coordinated control of the human–exoskeleton robot system. It can further promote the applications of exoskeleton robot in the field of assistive movement and assistive physical treatment.

The sEMG signal is the direct reflection of muscle's control signal and is generated 200 ms ahead of muscle contraction. Thus, it is the appropriate signal source for human movement prediction. Compared with the electroencephalograph, sEMG signal is easier to detect with lower mixing degree. But it still possesses strong fuzziness and is coupled with the environmental factors and body status. Depending only on sEMG signal is not able to accurately predict and identify movement intention. Thus, it should be integrated with traditional angular signal and force signal to perform more accurate prediction of human movement.

As illustrated in Figure 4.62, sEMG signals that are able to reflect human intention in advance, the joint angle, angular velocity, and interactive force information that are able to reflect human movement information are used. sEMG signals are acquired through AgCl patch electrodes and the self-made sEMG signal DAQ instrument. One can acquire the active contraction force through the sEMG-based biomechanical model for active skeletal contraction force, the joint angle information through angle transducer, and human–machine interactive force through the airbag force sensor placed on the calf. Information fusion and movement intention decoding are implemented through neurofuzzy network [120], and kinematics decoding and movement control of exoskeleton robot are conducted through the neurofuzzy network controller.

Note that the detecting device of interactive force is composed of airbag, gas tube, air pump, force sensor, and the controller. The force detecting device is developed based on the manometric mechanism of gas-filled electronic sphygmomanometer. Two pressure airbags are wrapped in the front and back sides of human leg, respectively, as illustrated in Figure 4.63. The method is as follows. First, the impulse signal is sent by the controller to control the air pump. The value of the pressure is detected by the force sensor to acquire the interactive force between human leg and exoskeleton. By calibration, the measurement range of the force detecting device is −200 to 200 N.

4.2.3.2   The Neurofuzzy-Network–Based Multi-Source Information Fusion and Movement Intention Identification

As there are two DOFs in the existing exoskeleton robot, i.e., the hip joint and the knee joint, real-time joint information can be provided by the exoskeleton when the thigh is bound with the exoskeleton and the interactive force between calf and airbag is measured by the airbag force sensor fixed to the calf. The EMG detecting electrodes are stuck to the belly of thigh muscle. We then acquire

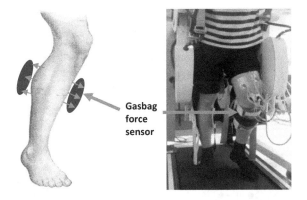

FIGURE 4.63   Force sensor.

the EMG signal of each muscle through the EMG DAQ instrument when the muscle contracts for further signal processing. The experimental devices are illustrated in Figure 4.64, and the detailed introduction can be referred to in Chapter 5. Figure 4.64a illustrates the position of EMG electrodes and airbag after human leg is bound with the exoskeleton. Figure 4.64b illustrates electrode position on the rear side of the thigh. We set the sampling frequency of EMG signal as 2,000 Hz and record the data every 400 sampling intervals. Furthermore, we set the sampling points as 400 and the sampling period as 500 μs. Thus, a group of data is recorded every 0.2 s; i.e., the recording period is $\Delta T = 0.2$ s.

Through the Takagi–Sugeno–Kang FNN [121,122], the multi-source information fusion and movement intention identification can be achieved. However, the structure of the FNN will affect the prediction error. To evaluate the performance of different networks, FNNs with three different levels of complexity, including the simple, medium, and complex, are developed with different fuzzy rules, respectively. There are five layers in each network. The topological structures of networks with simple and medium complexities are illustrated in Figure 4.65.

The first layer is the input layer. The inputs include active contraction force estimated from the sEMG signal and the joint angle and angular velocity sampled by sensors, defined as $O_i^1 = ch_i$ ($i = 1, 2, …, n$).

The second layer is the fuzzification layer. There are four neurons in this layer corresponding to the four fuzzy linguistic variables of each EMG signal input channel, respectively: ZO (zero),

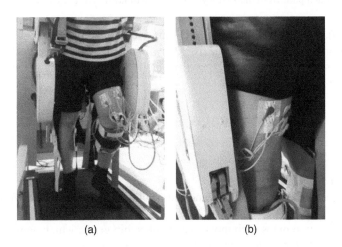

(a)   (b)

FIGURE 4.64   (a) Front view of human–machine interface; (b) rear view of human–machine interface.

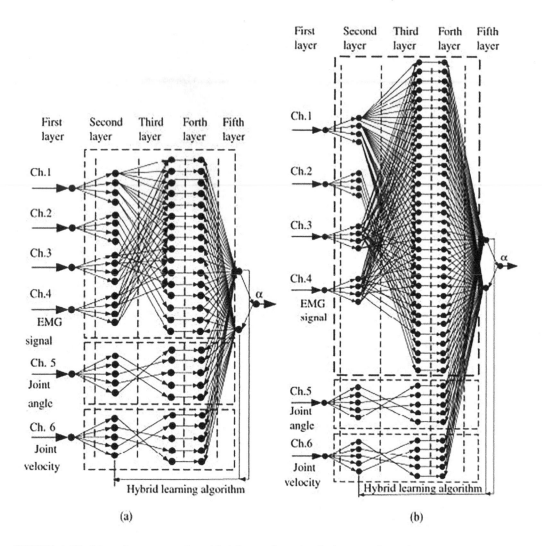

FIGURE 4.65 Neurofuzzy networks with joint angle and velocity proprioception: (a) simple network; (b) normal network. Each path from the first layer to the fourth layer is a fuzzy rule.

PS (positive small), PM (positive medium), PB (positive big). As for the angle and velocity input, there are five neurons corresponding to the five fuzzy linguistic variables, respectively: NB (negative big), NS (negative small), ZO (zero), PS (positive small), PB (positive big). Generalized bell membership function in Eq. (4.43) is used.

$$f(x;\alpha,\beta,\gamma) = \frac{1}{1+\left|(x-\gamma)/\alpha\right|^{2\beta}},$$ (4.43)

where

   x—independent variable,

   α, β, γ—variables that determine the shape and position of the membership function.

The membership function maps each input to a membership grade, which represents the activation level of the corresponding muscle and that of the ankle joint, denoted as $O_i^2 = \mu_{mfi}(ch_k)$.

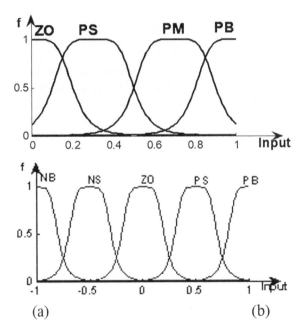

FIGURE 4.66 Fuzzy membership functions: (a) four fuzzy linguistic variables; (b) five fuzzy linguistic variables.

The third layer is the fuzzy reasoning layer. The three networks with different complexity are different mainly in this layer. The complex network includes all the possible combinations of the neurons (Figure 4.66).

The fuzzy rules of the normal and simple networks are simplified based on anatomical knowledge and the results of previously performed experiment. The antecedent with multiple parts is resolved by logic operator (AND) and outputs a membership grade of support for the rule. The fuzzy rules of the simple neural network are illustrated in Table 4.6, in which OUT is the corresponding sEMG signal.

The output of the third layer is denoted as (4.44):

$$O_i^3 = \mu_{A^i}(\xi) = \hat{\Pi}\left(\mu_{A_1^i}(\xi_1), \ldots, \mu_{A_k^i}(\xi_k)\right), \tag{4.44}$$

in which

A_i—the fuzzy set of the antecedent part of the ith rule, $A^i = A_1^i \cap A_2^i \cdots \cap A_k^i$,

K—the number of the sub-antecedent,

ξ_i—the input,

Π—product operator,

$\mu_A(\xi)$—membership degree of the ith rule when the input is ξ.

The fourth layer is the output layer of the fuzzy rules. The weighted output of the ith rule is

$$O_i^4 = \mu_{A^i}(\xi) \cdot f_i, \tag{4.45}$$

where $f_i = a_i \cdot ch_1 + b_i \cdot ch_2 + c_i \cdot ch_3 + d_i \cdot ch_4 + e_i$ and a_i, b_i, c_i, d_i, e_i are the parameters of the output membership functions.

TABLE 4.6

Fuzzy Rules of Simple Network

Rule Number	Fuzzy Rules
1	IF Ch1 is ZO and Ch3 is ZO and Ch4 is ZO, THEN OUT is ZO
2	IF Ch1 is ZO and Ch3 is PS and Ch4 is PS, THEN OUT is ZO
3	IF Ch1 is ZO and Ch3 is PM and Ch4 is PM, THEN OUT is PS
4	IF Ch1 is ZO and Ch3 is PB and Ch4 is PB, THEN OUT is PM
5	IF Ch1 is PS and Ch3 is ZO and Ch4 is ZO, THEN OUT is ZO
6	IF Ch1 is PS and Ch3 is PS and Ch4 is PS, THEN OUT is ZO
7	IF Ch1 is PS and Ch3 is PM and Ch4 is PM, THEN OUT is PS
8	IF Ch1 is PS and Ch3 is PB and Ch4 is PB, THEN OUT is PM
9	IF Ch1 is PM and Ch3 is ZO and Ch4 is ZO, THEN OUT is ZO
10	IF Ch1 is PM and Ch3 is PS and Ch4 is PS, THEN OUT is ZO
11	IF Ch1 is PB and Ch3 is ZO and Ch4 is ZO, THEN OUT is PS
12	IF Ch1 is PB and Ch3 is PS and Ch4 is PS, THEN OUT is PM
13	IF Ch2 is ZO, THEN COM is ZO
14	IF Ch2 is PS, THEN COM is PS
15	IF Ch2 is PM, THEN COM is PM
16	IF Ch2 is PB, THEN COM is PB
17	IF Ch5 is NB, THEN ANG is NB
18	IF Ch5 is NS, THEN ANG is NS
19	IF Ch5 is ZO, THEN ANG is ZO
20	IF Ch5 is PS, THEN ANG is PS
21	IF Ch5 is PB, THEN ANG is PB
22	IF Ch6 is NB, THEN VEL is NB
23	IF Ch6 is NS, THEN VEL is NS
24	IF Ch6 is ZO, THEN VEL is ZO
25	IF Ch6 is PS, THEN VEL is PS
26	IF Ch6 is PB, THEN VEL is PB

The fifth layer is the defuzzification layer. The EMG signal and artificial proprioception are fused in this layer. The final output is the weighted average of all the outputs of fuzzy rules, which represent the predicted angle of dorsiflexion/plantar flexion, computed as

$$O_i^{\,5} = y_l = \frac{\sum_{i=1}^{r} \mu_{A^i}(\xi) \cdot f_i}{\sum_{i=1}^{r} \mu_{A^i}(\xi)}, \qquad (4.46)$$

where r is the number of rules.

The combination of back propagation algorithm and least square method is used to learn and obtain the parameters of the membership function $\{\alpha_i, \beta_i, \gamma_i\}$ and the consequent parameters $\{a_i, b_i, c_i, d_i, e_i\}$. The learning process has two steps: first, fix the parameters $\{\alpha_i, \beta_i, \gamma_i\}$, and the best set $\{a_i, b_i, c_i, d_i, e_i\}$ that makes the error quadratic sum $(y_m - y_{out})^2$ (y_{out} is the actual output, and y_m is the ideal output) minimum is resolved according to the training samples $\{\xi_m, y_m\}$; second, the output error is back-propagated, back propagation algorithm is used to adjust the parameters $\{\alpha_i, \beta_i, \gamma_i\}$.

The output of the neurofuzzy network is the predicted joint torque. Theoretically, joint torque can be directly used as a control signal. However, EMG signal contains a lot of uncertainties, and it is hard to obtain accurate transfer functions of the human–machine integrated system. This will lead to a huge error if the output is directly used as the control signal. Therefore, position control mode is applied here, and the angle of the EMG feeding forward item can be calculated by

$$T = J\alpha + mgl\sin\theta + Fd$$

$$A(\text{sEMG}) = \frac{1}{2}\alpha(\Delta T)^2 \qquad , \tag{4.47}$$

where
  J—the inertia of calf,
  α—angular acceleration of knee,
  m—mass of calf,
  l—distance between gravity center of calf and knee joint,
  F—interactive force,
  d—distance between center of F and knee joint.

Now we can substitute the acquired $\theta(T)$, $\Delta\theta$, and $A(\text{sEMG})$ into Eq. (4.48) to acquire the predicted joint angle. During the experiments, we should modify and smooth the trajectory using the method of real-time linear interpolation.

$$\theta(T + \Delta T) = \theta(T) + k(\Delta\theta + A(\text{EMG})), \tag{4.48}$$

in which
  $\theta(T + \Delta T)$—joint angle in the next moment,
  $\theta(T)$—joint angle at this moment, obtained through angle encoder,
  $\Delta\theta$—angle correction value obtained based on interacting force, which can be obtained through the pressure of airbags,
  $A(\text{sEMG})$—the EMG feeding forward item derived from detected sEMG signal by neurofuzzy network in (3.47),
  k—the proportional coefficient that adjusts the assistance level of the exoskeleton.

$$\Delta V = \left(1 - \frac{P_0}{P_t}\right)V_0 = Sr\Delta\theta$$

$$\Delta\theta = \left(1 - \frac{P_0}{P_t}\right)V_0 \Big/ Sr \qquad , \tag{4.49}$$

in which
  P_0—original pressure of the gasbag,
  P_t—pressure of current time,
  V_0—volume of air in the gasbag,
  S—contact area,
  r—distance between the joint center and the gasbag.

Based on the above algorithm, the real-time prediction of joint angle can be achieved through sEMG, joint angle, and human–machine interactive force.

The experiments include movement intention identification and assistive motion. Among them, the comparison between the ankle joint and knee joint resulting from the movement intention identification is used to evaluate the performance of neural networks with different complexities. The experiment has been carried out with a healthy male subject of age 26 (A) and a healthy male subject of age 24 (B). The experimental setup consists of the exoskeleton robot with artificial proprioceptor, a PC, a self-made DAQ card, a programmable multi-axis controller (PMAC2-Lite of the Delta Tau

Data Systems, Inc., Chatsworth, CA), and a self-made EMG signal processor and a 3D gait analysis system (Vicon MX system of Vicon Company).

The experiment is divided into two stages: the neurofuzzy adaptive learning stage and the human–machine coordinated control stage. During the experiments, subjects sit on the chair and do the flexion and extension of ankle joint. In the first stage, sEMG signals are sampled for every motion, meanwhile the motion angles of the subject's ankle are recorded by the Vicon. Recorded data are used as the training sample to adapt the parameters in the neurofuzzy network mentioned above. In the second stage, the exoskeleton follows the subject's specified motions in real time. The stage lasts about 10 min in one experiment. The Vicon system and angle encoder record the angles of the human ankle and the parallel exoskeleton ankle, while the PC records the outputs of the neurofuzzy controller with proprioception (controller C). To evaluate the effectiveness of the artificial proprioception in the real-time coordinated control of the ankle exoskeleton, neurofuzzy controllers without proprioception (controller A) and with joint angle proprioception (controller B) are also established. These controllers are achieved by setting the corresponding weights of the networks to zero. Neurofuzzy controllers with different styles and complexities are tested, respectively, during the experiment. They are denoted as A–C, A–N, A–S, B–C, B–N, B–S, C–C, C–N, and C–S, where A, B, C represent the controllers A, B, and C, and C, N, S denote complex, normal, and simple complexities, respectively. Eight kinds of movements are used as the test samples: slow small dorsiflexion, slow big dorsiflexion, fast small dorsiflexion, fast big dorsiflexion, slow small plantar flexion, slow big plantar flexion, fast small plantar flexion, and fast big plantar flexion. T_{m} values equal to 100 and 200 ms are chosen, respectively, during the experiments.

In the assistive motion experiments, the real-time performance and the effectiveness of the movement intention identification method proposed here are verified through wearing exoskeleton to do assistive F/E. During the experiment, first we extract the real-time feature of sEMG signal from the experimental results and do the offline prediction and comparison of the joint moment. Then the subject puts on the exoskeleton. The exoskeleton works in the torque mode. The ankle of the robot is connected with a spring, the other end of which is fixed. In this way, the total output moment of the exoskeleton and human is measured. The subjects are required to do F/E with 20% of the maximum contraction force. The characteristic values of the real-time detected EMG signal are acquired through the differential method and traditional method, and then the joint moment is calculated. The control torque of the exoskeleton robot is the difference between the target joint torque and the active joint torque. In the experiments, we set the target torque as twice of the active joint torque and then sample and analyze the human–machine interactive force and the output knee joint torque of the exoskeleton. There are ten groups in the experiments, each lasting for 2 min.

The experimental results of the nine controllers are shown in Figure 4.67, which demonstrates the dynamic angles of dorsiflexion/plantar flexion. The results show that the outputs of controllers with proprioception follow the motion better than the others. Specifically, Figure 4.67 (i) is the result of the controller with joint angle, velocity proprioception, and simple complexity. It is clear that the dashed line without mark follows the solid line with the smallest error compared to the others.

Mean square deviation (MSD) is used to compare the accuracy of these neurofuzzy controllers.

$$\delta = \sqrt{\frac{\sum (y_{\mathrm{out}} - y_{\mathrm{m}})^2}{n}}, \qquad (4.50)$$

y_{out}—output of the neurofuzzy controller,
y_{m}—measured angle of the human ankle,
n—number of sample points.

Tables 4.7 and 4.8 illustrate the mean square difference of controllers with different types and different levels of complexities under different activities. Referring to the tables, the simple controller

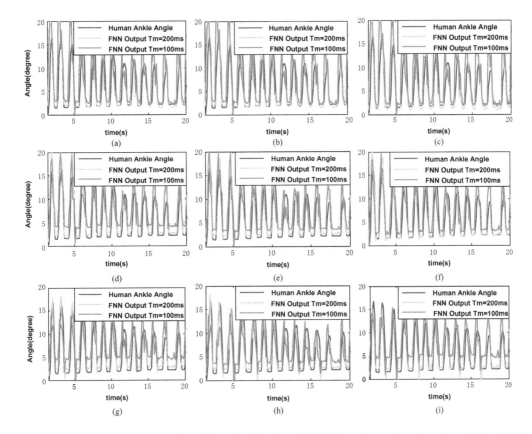

FIGURE 4.67 Experimental results of slow dorsiflexion. (a)–(c) Experimental results of controllers A–C, A–N, and A–S; (d)–(f) experimental results of controllers B–C, B–N, and B–S; (g)–(i) experimental results of controllers C–C, C–N, and C–S. The three curves denote the subject's ankle joint (solid line), the output of the neurofuzzy network when T_m is 51.2 ms (dashed line without mark), and the output of the neurofuzzy network when T_m is 102.4 ms (dashed line with mark), respectively.

with joint angle feedback and angular velocity feedback has smaller MSD value; thus, it can be regarded as owning the best prediction performance. Meanwhile, neural network with complex structure with feedback has a larger MSD value, indicating a degraded prediction performance.

In the assistive motion experiments, the offline prediction results for joint moments are illustrated in Table 4.9 and Figure 4.68. The control torque error obtained from differential method is 6.4% smaller than that obtained from the traditional method. Among them, joint moment of the autoregressve (AR) model has the smallest error. The experimental results of online assistive motion are illustrated in Figure 4.69. The output torque of the exoskeleton is twice the value of the assistive torque and is almost equal to the target torque. Thus, it can be recognized that the proposed controller can predict human motion intention and achieve the assistive motion for the wearer. However, there are still some observable errors in the experiments. It is probably due to the fact that the differential method is not able to extract all the information in sEMG signal. The fuzzy understanding of the generation and transmission of sEMG signal leads to the error in the motion control of exoskeleton robot.

4.2.4 HUMAN–MACHINE COORDINATED CONTROL MECHANISM

Human locomotion system is a closed-loop control system with proprioceptors. Real-time feedback of lower-extremity motion status is the prerequisite for closed-loop control and human–machine

TABLE 4.7
Experimental Results of Subject A

Action		Controller	$T_m = 51.2\,\text{ms}$			$T_m = 102.4\,\text{ms}$		
			Simple	Normal	Complex	Simple	Normal	Complex
Dorsiflexion	Slow and small	Controller A	2.4506	2.2199	2.2223	3.9096	3.7427	3.7226
		Controller B	1.9417	1.9772	2.0824	2.7536	3.0486	3.1265
		Controller C	1.5795	1.4897	1.7288	2.804	2.331	3.3011
	Fast and small	Controller A	4.9704	5.7735	5.7804	8.6585	9.578	9.5729
		Controller B	3.1083	3.2092	3.4167	5.8277	5.9151	6.4066
		Controller C	1.6654	2.1839	1.985	5.0276	3.8207	4.1975
	Slow and big	Controller A	2.933	2.8192	2.8208	4.2705	4.5379	4.5503
		Controller B	2.2812	2.4322	2.2395	3.0529	3.4284	3.152
		Controller C	1.9918	1.8236	1.8561	3.1286	3.0673	3.0884
	Fast and big	Controller A	4.2443	4.8066	4.8233	8.6585	9.578	9.5729
		Controller B	4.5285	4.6775	4.3458	7.9072	8.1023	8.6943
		Controller C	4.0202	3.9347	4.7328	7.2596	7.4109	7.6096
Plantar flexion	Slow and small	Controller A	2.3734	2.6257	2.8213	2.9837	3.3272	3.5139
		Controller B	1.5804	1.7243	2.0783	2.4425	2.6293	3.3362
		Controller C	1.2904	1.5608	1.8357	2.1838	2.3842	2.5896
	Fast and small	Controller A	1.6697	1.9499	2.0016	2.3008	2.482	2.5652
		Controller B	1.0844	1.1805	1.1527	2.2697	2.0237	2.1428
		Controller C	1.1048	1.1927	1.2917	2.4112	2.4063	2.4985
	Slow and big	Controller A	2.1003	2.1834	2.2345	2.1429	2.4554	2.4879
		Controller B	1.1909	1.5999	1.519	1.6822	2.2296	2.4499
		Controller C	1.0983	1.3922	1.0249	2.0975	2.4286	1.9235
	Fast and big	Controller A	3.3378	3.6894	3.9293	4.3277	5.1042	5.8845
		Controller B	2.2307	2.5199	2.2765	3.3413	3.5112	3.3598
		Controller C	1.602	1.8578	1.9881	3.3547	3.271	3.2421
	Average		2.3491	2.5343	2.5911	3.9498	4.1172	4.2912

coordinated control [123]. However, for the lower-extremity–paralyzed patients, body neural system of most patients is broken, and most of the proprioceptors of lower extremity are not able to work. Patients have to perceive with other sensory organs through the assistance from external devices so as to achieve the closed-loop control. The development of artificial sensory feedback makes it possible, and it has been successfully applied in surgical robots, industrial robots, virtual reality, and video games. Its feedback methods include visual feedback, auditory feedback, electric stimulation, and haptic simulation [78,85]. Referring to the experimental results, electric stimulation and haptic simulation achieve the best performance among all the methods [79]. Considering the safety and comfort, airbag force sensor is adopted in the mechanism to detect the joint angle information. We can adjust the pressure of airbag placed on lower extremity or arm to feed back the joint angle and moment information, thus developing the extended proprioceptor feedback. Hence, we can connect the exoskeleton robot system and body motor system, which are initially two independent control systems, through the bioelectromechanical human–machine interaction interface, so as to rebuild the body closed-loop control system and achieve active compliance control of the human–exoskeleton system through this interface.

This section will start with the closed-loop control mechanism of human motor control system, then simulate human closed-loop control system, propose the FNN controller integrating sEMG sensor and proprioceptor, and develop the motor control pathway from human to exoskeleton robot. The FNN controller fuses the sEMG signals which are able to reflect human motion intention in

TABLE 4.8
Experimental Results of Subject B

Action		Controller	$T_m = 51.2\,\text{ms}$			$T_m = 102.4\,\text{ms}$		
			Simple	Normal	Complex	Simple	Normal	Complex
Dorsiflexion	Slow and small	Controller A	3.1779	4.3147	4.0548	2.6637	2.8494	2.4684
		Controller B	2.4699	3.2951	3.2082	2.7243	3.0886	2.9584
		Controller C	1.3589	1.7046	1.5763	1.9204	2.5709	2.1626
	Fast and small	Controller A	3.853	3.6112	3.6398	6.2643	6.8353	6.4819
		Controller B	2.9088	2.9576	3.7428	5.0516	5.654	5.2104
		Controller C	2.7444	2.3227	2.7671	4.5111	4.2585	4.8397
	Slow and big	Controller A	2.5274	2.411	2.3799	3.3592	4.481	3.9747
		Controller B	2.3846	2.0357	2.9687	3.1777	3.3486	3.271
		Controller C	1.7818	2.6082	1.6818	2.6307	3.0356	3.5356
	Fast and big	Controller A	4.1662	3.8897	3.8517	7.6615	8.7196	8.2162
		Controller B	3.5115	3.4421	4.1843	7.8482	7.9023	8.5224
		Controller C	3.973	4.8323	3.747	6.802	7.8415	8.3238
Plantar flexion	Slow and small	Controller A	2.3972	2.6129	2.6091	3.5249	3.2972	2.9924
		Controller B	1.9783	1.5105	1.5804	2.3306	2.5896	2.3755
		Controller C	1.2891	2.0357	1.7608	2.2208	2.6293	3.3362
	Fast and small	Controller A	3.4878	4.1753	4.0207	4.6711	7.0797	10.4967
		Controller B	2.1989	2.1805	2.5966	3.8132	4.0671	4.482
		Controller C	1.6293	2.8466	2.8411	3.7962	3.7949	3.8301
	Slow and big	Controller A	3.5191	4.2203	4.039	3.1993	3.8134	5.0357
		Controller B	2.495	2.181	2.6062	2.3807	2.6709	2.8002
		Controller C	1.6352	2.9054	2.8483	1.8217	2.8757	3.1714
	Fast and big	Controller A	2.2834	4.7368	4.3422	3.1502	4.6579	5.8348
		Controller B	2.1353	2.3827	3.164	3.6367	3.9271	4.2353
		Controller C	1.997	2.282	2.9142	3.1286	3.8451	4.6894
	Average		2.5793	2.9789	3.0469	3.8454	4.4097	4.7185

TABLE 4.9
RMS Values of the Estimated Torque Errors with Different Methods

	Differentiated Power Spectrum Estimation (Nm)	Normal Power Spectrum Estimation (Nm)
AR Model	0.4780	0.5257
Welch	0.5039	0.5894
Short-time Fourier transform (STFT)	0.7623	0.7502

advance and human–machine interactive force and joint angle which accurately reflect lower-extremity motion information. Meanwhile, through the extended physiological proprioception (EPP) feedback, we can achieve information feedback (such as joint angle and moment), complete the information feedback pathway from exoskeleton robot to human, and develop the real-time bidirectional human–machine information interaction interface and rebuild human closed-loop motor control system. Based on this human–machine interaction interface, the kinematic and dynamic models of exoskeleton robot can be developed; we can further determine the control strategy for exoskeleton robot control system, thus achieving the coordinated control of human–exoskeleton robot system. At last, one needs to analyze, compare, and verify the effectiveness of the developed

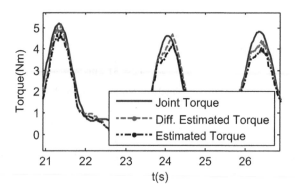

FIGURE 4.68 Time–torque curve.

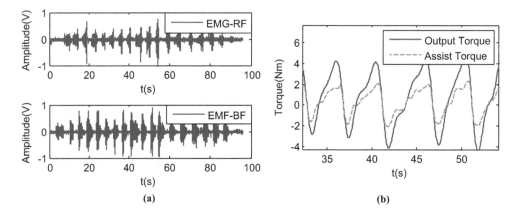

FIGURE 4.69 (a) Raw sEMG signal; (b) output torque and assistive torque.

human–machine interaction interface and the coordinated control strategy through experiments. The details are as follows.

4.2.4.1 Local Closed-Loop Control Mechanism in Motorium

Human somatic motorium is a perfect control system full of effective information exchanges. For a healthy person, the active voluntary exercise is generated by human brain. More specifically, it is controlled by somatic nervous system (SNS). As illustrated in Figure 4.70, neural signals send the information, such as motion intentions, from upper motor neurons to the ones through corticospinal tract to control the contraction of muscle fibers and finally drive the musculoskeletal system to complete target activities. Meanwhile, human detects motion status, such as muscle contraction velocity, contraction force, and joint angle, through proprioceptors and feedback to CNS to do active or reflective feedback adjustment for human motion [124]. Thus, human somatic motion control system is a typical closed-loop control system with feedback pathway for proprioceptors, which can be seen as the biological foundation of human stable motion [125].

However, for most patients with paralysis of lower extremity and some patients with lower-extremity diseases, the neural pathway is damaged, leading to the fact that motor neural signal cannot be sent to muscle fibers and cannot control the movement effectively. On the other hand, patients are unable to apperceive the motion status of lower extremity when the feedback neural pathway is damaged. It leads to the breakdown of the closed loop of human motion control, resulting in the disability to control human motion accurately and stably.

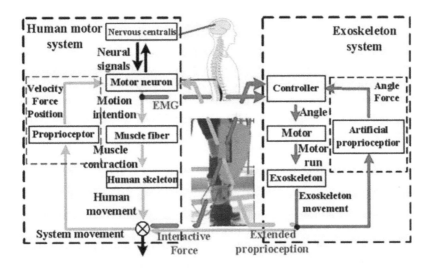

FIGURE 4.70 Control system of exoskeleton and its information interaction with human body. Nerve signal of motor neurons are transmitted forward to control skeletal muscles. The joint torque, velocity, etc., are fed back to the human body via EPP.

4.2.4.2 Closed-Loop Control Mechanism for Exoskeleton Robot

For the exoskeleton robot alone, its closed-loop motion control system is similar to that of the regular electromechanical system, including the forward channel and feedback channel. As illustrated in Figure 4.70, human is the host, releasing the control signal with the joint angle of the exoskeleton robot as the feedback signal. It calculates the target joint angle and moment through the motion controller and controls the motor to drive the exoskeleton to complete corresponding joint rotation. The joint angle and moment feedback is able to increase system accuracy in the exoskeleton robot closed-loop control system. Note that due to the influence of response time of motors, mechanical inertia, mechanism clearance, and external disturbance, there are delay of response time and position errors between control signal and mechanical output.

4.2.4.3 Requirement Analysis of Bioelectromechanical Integration

For healthy people, the somatic motor control system is an independent motion control system that is able to control human body to perform various activities independently and efficiently. Similarly, exoskeleton robot system is also a complete control system which is able to control exoskeleton mechanism to perform various activities. However, for the human–exoskeleton integrated system, there should be effective information exchange channels between the two systems which are originally independent to achieve active compliance control or coordinated control. For a patient whose lower-extremity motor nerve is damaged, the function of brain and upper motor neuron is still intact, but the channel from lower motor neurons to muscle fiber is unable to work, or the sensory organ neural channel is broken, leading to motor function injury. For exoskeleton robot, it has complete motion function and is the ideal device to replace the motor function of lower extremity. Yet, without effective human–machine integration strategy, it would be hard for the users to control the exoskeleton to do voluntary motion by self-consciousness or detect the motion status of the exoskeleton robot, resulting in the incoordination between human body and exoskeleton. Thus, effective integration and fusion of human and exoskeleton robot is needed to put exoskeleton robot into clinical rehabilitation. We should then develop efficient bioelectromechanical integration interface to enable the exoskeleton to detect human motion intention in real time and eliminate the error generated by the response time of the system. Meanwhile, we need to also detect the motion status of exoskeleton and human body in real time just as the user is controlling his body so as to control the exoskeleton to do voluntary motion, assistive motion, and physical rehabilitation treatment. As illustrated in Figure 4.70, to integrate human and exoskeleton as a bioelectromechanical integrated system, the motion control channel from human to exoskeleton robot is developed here to deliver human motion control information to exoskeleton system. Meanwhile, one can develop information feedback channel from exoskeleton robot to human to deliver exoskeleton motion information to wearer so as to detect mechanism motion status in real time and realize the coordinated control of human–exoskeleton robot system.

4.2.5 BIOELECTROMECHANICAL INTEGRATED COORDINATION CONTROL STRATEGY

4.2.5.1 Bidirectional Interaction Interface Based on EPP and sEMG

As illustrated in Figure 4.71, to realize human–machine integrated coordinated control, there are two channels in the established human–machine interaction interface: motion control channel and information feedback channel. Through sampling of the sEMG signal of human skeletal muscle, human–machine interactive force, and joint angle, the motion control channel fuses the multi-source information and predicts human motion using the FNN. It also generates motion control signal to control the motors and the rotation of exoskeleton joints based on the dynamic and kinematic models of exoskeleton robots. Referring to the above discussion, as sEMG signals are able to reflect human motion intention in advance, it is able to alleviate or eliminate the exoskeleton motion delay generated by system response time when using sEMG signal as the control signal. Thus, sEMG signal is the ideal information source for human–machine interface.

The information feedback channel acquires the pressure of the gasbag used for information feedback through detection of the joint angle and angular torque in real time and controls the pressure in the gasbag by the pressure-controlling device composed of baroreceptor, air pump, and air valve. It feeds back the information to human in the form of air pressure, enabling the information perception through haptic method. Conventional visual feedback is able to feed back human motion information to the user in real time. However, patients have to acquire other information through visual sense. Thus, long-time visual feedback is not a good choice. Meanwhile, visual sense is unable to feed back mechanical information, such as joint torque, but dynamics is of great significance to rehabilitation treatment. As the human is able to perceive haptic simulation information in real time safely and sensitively, haptic feedback is a better way to feed back information compared to visual feedback.

As shown in Figure 4.71, the EPP system features an air pressure sensor, a gasbag, and a pneumatic control system. The air pressure sensor detects the pressure of the gasbag that is mounted on

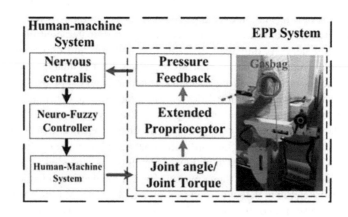

FIGURE 4.71 EPP system based on pressure feedback.

the arm. Information including the joint angle and joint torque is transmitted to human body by the air pressure of the gasbag, which is controlled by the pneumatic control system. The feedback pressure can be determined as follows:

$$P_1 = P_0 + k_1 \cdot \theta$$
$$P_2 = P_0 + k_2 \cdot T_{\text{knee}}, \tag{4.51}$$

in which

P_1, P_2—the pressures that feed back joint angle and torque information,

P_0—original pressure,

k_1, k_2—proportional coefficients,

θ—joint angle,

T_{knee}—joint torque.

4.2.5.2   Human–Machine Coordinated Control Strategy

The motion pattern of the human–exoskeleton robot system includes two kinds, the passive training mode and active training mode. In the passive training mode, exoskeleton drives human to do exercises. In this process, exoskeleton is able to conduct periodic motion according to the trajectory and speed defined in the computer. Human is bound with the exoskeleton so that human lower extremity is able to move in the same pace with the exoskeleton. In this mode, exoskeleton is the master, and human user can be regarded as the external load or disturbance of the exoskeleton. The human–exoskeleton robot system is simplified into a single system. Thus, closed-loop PID controller of the exoskeleton itself is selected to develop the dynamic and kinematic models for the exoskeleton mechanism to realize the accurate movement in the passive training mode.

Active training mode is the mode where human drives the exoskeleton to move. In this process, human performs active voluntary motion. The exoskeleton tries to generate the same movement as human does by signal acquisition, analysis, and processing. In this mode, human lower extremity is the master, and the exoskeleton is the slave. As the joint torque of exoskeleton is far greater than that of human, mechanism movement will also act on human lower extremity. Different from passive training mode, exoskeleton cannot be simplified as the external load or disturbance of human, and human and exoskeleton should be considered as a whole. As with the control strategy for the human–machine system, the fusion of human and exoskeleton control systems is needed to realize the coordinated control of human–machine integrated system.

Taking the active training mode of signal DOF (knee joint of exoskeleton) as an example, the control strategy of human–exoskeleton system is illustrated in Figure 4.72. The process is as follows. When human does the voluntary motion, signal acquisition module detects the sEMG signal of the skeletal muscles, human–machine interactive force, and joint angle in real time. The motor control signal is then generated to drive the joint movement through multi-source signal fusion, motion intention decoding, solving inverse kinematics, and motion control. As human is bound with the exoskeleton, relative displacement will give rise to interactive force, and it will be the auxiliary force or resistant force from exoskeleton to human. By controlling the interactive force, this auxiliary force can be reduced. Meanwhile, for patients whose lower-extremity perception function is damaged, the controller turns joint motion information into gasbag pressure, making it possible for the patients to perceive lower-extremity motion status so as to modify and control the movement.

4.2.5.3   Human–Machine Integrated System Modeling

Referring to the above discussion, one can see that coordinated control of human–machine integrated system can only be achieved by effective fusion of the control systems of human and exoskeleton. For practical application, effective intervention and control of somatic nerve center cannot be achieved based on current technologies. A better method is the external stimulation to human sensory organ to develop reflex arc in the nerve system so as to achieve fast response. This effect

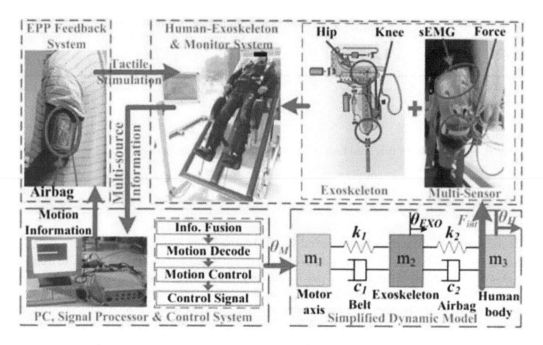

FIGURE 4.72 Human–machine integrated coordinated control strategy.

is expected to be applied in the gasbag haptic feedback module in the system so that external perception units are effectively used in the motion control system. On the other hand, in the human–exoskeleton system, what is under effective control is only the motion control system of exoskeleton robot system. Thus, to realize the coordinated control of the human–machine integrated system, the control model of the system should be further studied and designed.

In the passive training mode, exoskeleton robot controls the movement through the PID controller. The input is the target joint angle, and the output is the exoskeleton joint angle.

Figure 4.73 shows the control block diagram of the active mode, where F_{req} is the required assistive force; F_{int} is the interactive force; F_a is the actual assistive force; k_p, k_i, and k_d are coefficients of the PID controller; and s is the complex variable for the Laplace transformation. The transfer function H maps the pulses onto the angular increment of exoskeleton joint. T is the transfer function from features of sEMG signal to active joint torque τ_{sEMG}; $d\theta_{act}$ is applied as the feedforward item and is the product of k_s and τ_{sEMG}. G_1, G_2, G_3, and G_4 represent interaction dynamics between the pilot and the exoskeleton and the kinematics of the pilot limb and exoskeleton leg (e.g., velocity, position, or a combination thereof). T_m and T_s are delays of motor and sensor.

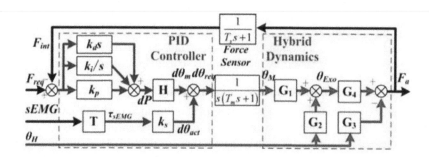

FIGURE 4.73 Control block diagram of active mode.

The exoskeleton knee is powered by a single actuator that generates an angular displacement θ_M. There is a belt-driven motor axis and ball screw, which can be interpreted as a spring-damper connection. The interactive force, F_{int}, between human leg and exoskeleton leg is detected by two airbags mounted on the front and back of human shank respectively. It is also interpreted as a spring-damper connection in this example. k_1, k_2, c_1, and c_2 represent the stiffness and damping of the belt and airbag.

4.2.6 EXPERIMENTAL RESULTS OF ACTIVE COMPLIANCE CONTROL

4.2.6.1 Experiment 1

4.2.6.1.1 Experimental Process

During the experiment, the subject's left leg is bound with the exoskeleton. The hip joint is fixed, and the thigh cannot move. As human knee joint corresponds to exoskeleton knee joint, knee angle is acquired through the sensor on the exoskeleton. The gasbag connected with gas tube is bound with the calf to detect the interactive force between the exoskeleton and human calf. The human calf is fixed to the gasbag with bandage. EMG electrodes are placed on the muscle belly of each muscle to observe and record the activation condition. The location of the EMG signal electrodes is illustrated in Figure 4.74.

First, the gasbag is charged, and then the subject moves his/her calf. The contraction intensity is recorded by the EMG signal, and the joint angle is acquired by the exoskeleton. In this process, the pressure in the gasbag changes with the pressure from the calf. The pressure is used to feature the interactive force between calf and the exoskeleton (Figure 4.75).

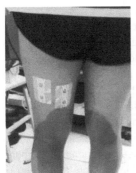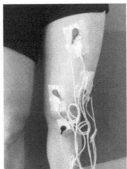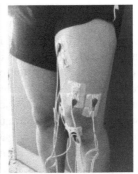

FIGURE 4.74 The location of the electrodes of the eight muscles.

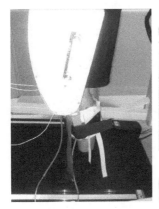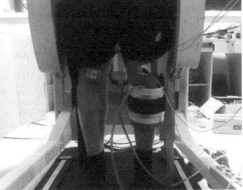

FIGURE 4.75 Acquisition of interactive force and EMG signal.

4.2.6.1.2 Measurement of EMG Signal's Characteristic Value

EMG characteristic value: Measure the EMG signal of the eight muscles at the same time. EMG signal on the BF belly is used to represent the signal of the long head and short head of the BF. EMG signal of VI is featured by that of RF. SM and ST are located at the middle point of the line between ischial tuberosity and medial tibial, and their signals are detected by one electrode. As EMG signal is weak, it is amplified by 6,826.7 times by the amplifier. In the experiment, subjects are required to use full strength, and we record the EMG for 5–10 s. After each maximum voluntary contraction (MVC) test, subjects rest for 5 min. MVC test for each muscle is repeated three times to ensure that the data acquired by the force sensor is the maximum muscle force. We process the EMG signal to obtain the characteristic value at the maximum muscle force. The data is illustrated in Table 4.10. When the calf buckles backward, the maximum muscle force of BF, SM, and ST exerted on the gasbag reaches 218.5 N, and the MVC of BF is the largest. When the calf buckles forward, the maximum muscle force of QF is about 154.44 N. The MVC of RF located in the middle of the thigh is the largest.

4.2.6.1.3 Relation between Characteristic Frequency and Contraction Force

To verify the steady-state relation between the isometric contraction force and AP frequency, RF is selected for the experiments. The characteristic frequency of the EMG signal is used to determine the activation degree, and the EMG electrodes are placed on the belly of RF. First, the gasbag is charged, and then the subject moves his calf. In this process, RF contracts, and the contraction intensity is recorded by the EMG signal. As the calf's position is fixed, there won't be any displacement of the calf. Therefore, the pressure in the gasbag changes with the force exerted by the calf. The pressure is used to represent the interactive force between calf and the exoskeleton. In this way, the EMG signal under a different contraction status is acquired.

One group of comparisons between the characteristic frequency of the EMG signal and the pressure of the gasbag is illustrated in Figure 4.76a. EMG signal has been filtered (divided by the enlargement factor) to calculate the corresponding root mean square (RMS) value and characteristic frequency (FRE) value. Referring to the figure, RMS value and characteristic frequency change with the pressure of the gasbag, indicating that the characteristic frequency of EMG signal can also reflect accurately the muscle contraction force. Besides, in the low-frequency stage when muscle starts to contract, characteristic frequency follows the changing trend of pressure better.

One group of real-time data of gasbag pressure and EMG characteristic frequency is illustrated in Figure 4.76b. Referring to the figure, when EMG characteristic frequency is higher, the pressure exerted on the gasbag is higher; i.e., the contraction force is larger. Note that when EMG characteristic frequency rises to its maximum and does not change with time any more (the dotted line in the figure), the force still increases for a period of time. This is because under the same activation

TABLE 4.10

MVC and Maximum Characteristic Frequency (MFR) of Each Muscle

Muscle	MVC (mV)	MFR (Hz)	Maximum Muscle Force (N)
Semimembranosus (SM)	157.99	65.3	218.5
Semitendinosus (ST)			
Biceps femoris(lh) (BFLH)	517.74	132.6	218.5
Biceps femoris(sh) (BFSH)			
Rectus femoris (RF)	612.63	118.1	154.44
Vastus intermedius (VI)			
Vastus lateralus (VL)	378.14	141.6	154.44
Vastus medialus (VM)	376.85	82	154.44

degree, the recruitment number of muscle fibers increases. When EMG characteristic frequency reaches its maximum, RMS is still increasing to its maximum (MVC value). At this time, all the muscle fibers are activated, and muscle force reaches its maximum.

The experimental results and the theoretical relation between frequency and muscle force are illustrated in Figure 4.76c. It can be noted from the figure that the experimental results agree well

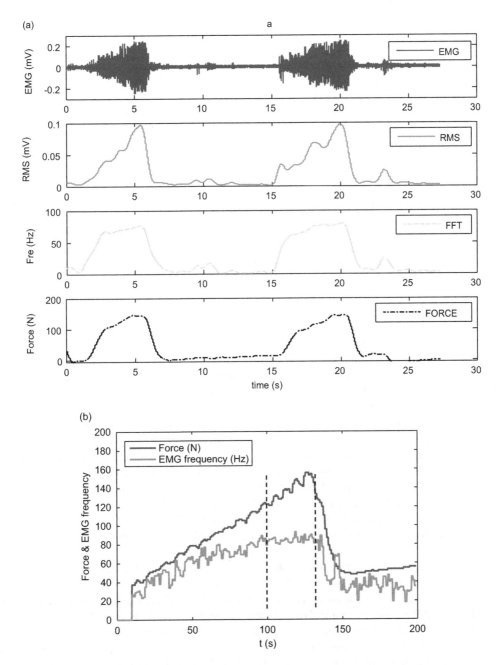

FIGURE 4.76   (a) Raw EMG signal, RMS and characteristic frequency and the comparison with interactive force. (b) Interactive force and EMG frequency.

(*Continued*)

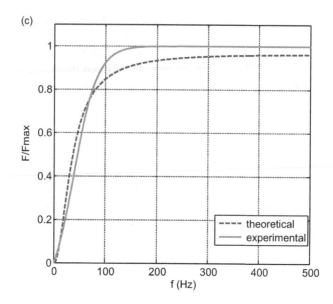

(c)

FIGURE 4.76 (CONTINUED)   (c) Comparison between experimental curve and theoretical curve.

with the theoretical results, and the slope of the curves is almost the same when muscle force increases with AP frequency. However, there is an obvious delay between the experimental and theoretical curves in the stage close to saturation, and the experimental results are larger than the theoretical results all the time after saturation. It is because it is a slow asymptotic process when the force reaches its maximum from the perspective of theoretical deduction.

4.2.6.1.4   Knee Joint Extension Experiment

The former experiment reveals preliminarily the relation between EMG's frequency-domain features and muscle active contraction force. In fact, there are multiple muscles taking part in the extension of calf, including QF (RF, VI, VL, and VM). Active moment is generated by each muscle to drive the knee joint to extend. Thus, the total moment of these muscles should be analyzed and compared with the calculated results with inverse dynamics. As the subjects have had enough rest, there is no muscle fatigue here. In the experiment, the calf exerts pressure on the gasbag, and the pressure increases gradually. Then, the force decreases after a period, and the muscles stop contracting. Myoelectric apparatus is used to record the EMG signal generated by each muscle and do the preprocessing to calculate the RMS and FRE of the four muscles (in which the values for RF and VI are the same). As illustrated in Figure 4.77, RMS rises faster than FRE, and RMS stays longer at the maximum range than FRE. As muscle force decreases, RMS and FRE both decrease quickly. The FRE and RMS of RF are larger than that of VL and VM, indicating that in the process of knee joint extension, RF is activated and reaches its maximum earliest.

As the experiments are carried out when subjects are fully at rest, the adenosine triphosphate (ATP) in sarcoplasm can be regarded to be in saturation. Referring to the muscle force model, the main factors affecting muscle force are the cross-sectional area and the activation degree (including the AP frequency and the recruitment number of muscle fibers). Based on the RMS and FRE values of the EMG signal, we can calculate the activation degree of each muscle and the muscle force. The active moments of each muscle are illustrated in Figure 4.78. Among the three muscles, the active moments generated by RF and VI are the largest with the highest activation degree.

When the calf and the exoskeleton are first bound together, muscles do not contract to generate force, and the calf is in static equilibrium; i.e., the passive forces of each muscle, gravity of the

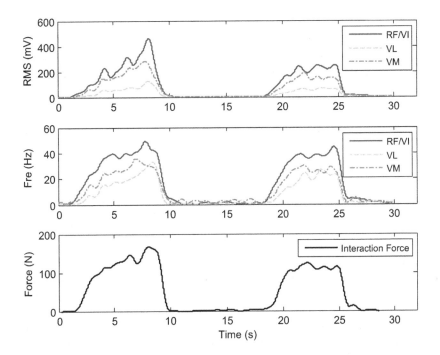

FIGURE 4.77 Comparison of RMS, characteristic frequency, and interactive force of the muscles in knee joint extension.

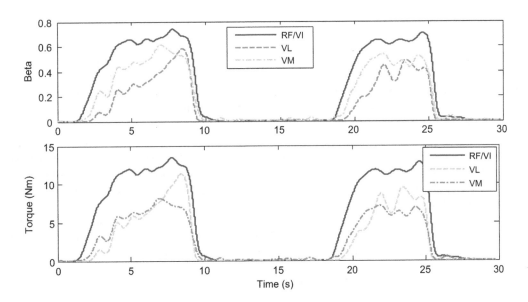

FIGURE 4.78 The activation degree and active torque of each muscle in knee joint extension.

calf, and the initial value of gasbag pressure are in equilibrium. When the calf extends forward, the interactive force between calf and exoskeleton is recorded with the force sensor. The value is the counterforce to resist muscle contraction. As the gasbag is located in the middle of the calf, the interactive force arm is half of calf length. The value for the subject is about 369 mm; thus, the interactive force arm is 185 mm. In the experiment, knee joint is fixed, and the inertial force of the calf is also ignored. We can calculate the inverse torque (T-inverse) of knee joint based on the

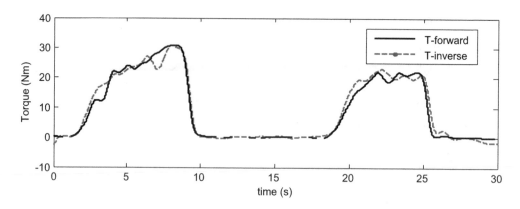

FIGURE 4.79 Comparison between active torque and inverse torque in knee extension.

inverse dynamics equation (4.39) and compare with muscle active torque (T-forward). The results are illustrated in Figure 4.79. It can be inferred that the active torque calculated from the mechanical model follows well the inverse torque. In the initial stage of muscle contraction, the torque increases quickly and reaches its maximum. It stays for a period of time and decreases quickly when the muscle starts to relax. The maximum torque generated is about 30 Nm. It indicates the effectiveness of muscle force prediction with biomechanical models, thus verifying the biomechanical model based on the collective feature of molecular motors from experiment. It lays a foundation for further human–machine interface application studies.

4.2.6.1.5   Knee Joint Flexion Experiment

In the experiment, the knee joint flexes and exerts pressure on the gasbag. The muscles taking part in the flexion include BF (both long head and short head), ST and SM. Myoelectric apparatus is used to record the raw EMG signal generated by each muscle and do the preprocessing to calculate the RMS and FRE of the four muscles, as illustrated in Figure 4.80b. Compared with SM/ST, the raw EMG signal of BF is stronger, indicating that the activation degrees of the two muscles are higher, which can also be noted from the RMS and FRE values. As muscle activation level increases, the contraction force becomes larger, together with the counterforce on the gasbag.

If we calculate the activation degree of each muscle based on the RMS and characteristic frequency, the muscle force and the active torque predicted by the biomechanical model can be illustrated as shown in Figure 4.81. In the flexion process, the active torque of BF is the largest and that of ST is the smallest. Biceps femoris(long head, lh) (BFLH) generates force faster and is the first to contract, with the maximum torque of about 15 Nm.

The total torque of the four muscles is illustrated in Figure 4.82. We can calculate the inverse torque of the knee joint based on the inverse dynamics via recording the pressure of gasbag and the joint angle and then compare it with muscle's active torque. It can be inferred that the active torque calculated from biomechanical model follows well the inverse torque. The maximum muscle torque is about 27 Nm in the flexion process.

4.2.6.2   Experiment 2

4.2.6.2.1   Experimental Process Description

To verify the feasibility of the pneumatic haptic feedback device and evaluate the effectiveness of the human-machine coordinated control strategy, the gasbag pressure feedback experiment, the following exercise, auxiliary exercise and resistance exercise in the active mode are implemented, together with human–machine coordination experiments with gasbag pressure feedback. The experiment devices include the lower-extremity exoskeleton robot, PC, self-made EMG DAQ instrument,

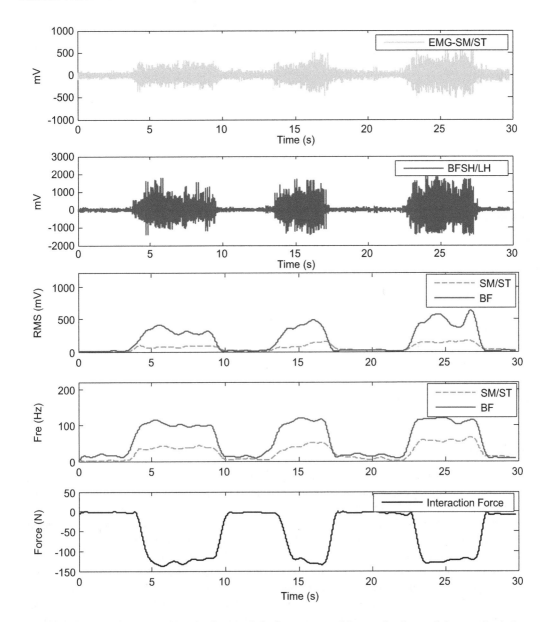

FIGURE 4.80 Comparison of RMS, characteristic frequency, and interactive force of the muscles in knee joint flexion.

feedback pneumatic system, self-made signal processing card and the main control card. Three healthy subjects with the age of 27, 25, and 24 participated in the experiment. The target object is the knee joint. Two channels of sEMG signal are selected as the control signal source for knee joint F/E, including channel 1 (BF) and channel 2 (QF). Meanwhile, human-machine interactive force and joint angle are also selected as the control signal, together with the sEMG signal.

In the gasbag pressure feedback experiment, the joint angle of the exoskeleton robot is selected randomly. We can turn the joint angle into gasbag pressure with Eq. (4.1) and control the gasbag pressure that changes with the set joint angle using the pressure control units. Then, one should further record the gasbag pressure in real-time and observe the relation between joint angle and real pressure of the gasbag.

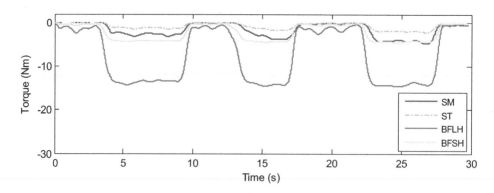

FIGURE 4.81   Active torque of each muscle in knee joint flexion.

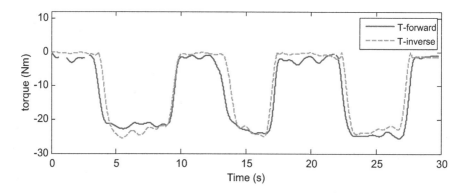

FIGURE 4.82   Comparison between active torque and inverse torque in knee flexion.

In the active training experiments, subjects are required to do voluntary movements. In this process, the assistive forces are set as 0, 20, 40, 60, −20, −40, and −60 N, in which 0 N represents the pure following motion, while positive force is for auxiliary motion and negative force is for resistant motion. Two groups of experiments are conducted for each force value. Subjects are required to do 20 times active F/E depending on his own condition. The experiment stops when the subject feels tired to avoid the influence of fatigue. In this process, the subject's lower extremity is bound with the exoskeleton limb. Two motion controllers with and without sEMG feedforward item are selected. They are applied to control the exoskeleton robot to do following motion, auxiliary motion or resistant motion according to the preset force. The interactive forces are detected and recorded in real time to find out the relation between human–machine interactive force and the preset force, joint angle, etc. They are used to compare the performance of different motion controllers to verify the effect of sEMG feedforward item on human motor intent prediction, and the promoting effect on increasing the compliance of the human–machine system.

The experiment was divided into two stages: the neurofuzzy adaptive learning stage and the human–machine coordinated control stage. In the first stage, sEMG signal and the interactive force were sampled under different joint angles. Meanwhile, the subject adapted his/her movement to the pressure feedback and learned to control the machine by the EPP feedback. The recorded data was used as the training sample to adapt the parameters in the neurofuzzy network. In the second stage, the controller with and without EMG feedforward items were used to control both legs of the exoskeleton to follow the subject's specific motions in real time. The duration of each experiment was about 5 min. The performance of different controllers was discussed after the experiments. Subjects also controlled the knee joint of exoskeleton to 0°, 30°, and 60°, according to the pressure feedback that indicated the joint information in the second stage. Since the SNS of the subjects were healthy, in order to avoid the effect of the proprioception of the subjects, further experiments converted the pressure feedback according to (4.52), and also let the subjects control the knee joint of exoskeleton to 0°, 30°, and 60°, according to the pressure feedback.

$$\theta = \lambda\theta_t + d\theta \qquad (4.52)$$

in which
θ—feedback angle,
λ—proportional coefficient and was set to 0.9 in experiment,
θ_t—real angle,
$d\theta$—angle offset and was set to $-10°$ in experiment.

Due to the conversion, the real angles were 11.11°, 44.44°, and 77.77°, respectively

4.2.6.2.2 Experimental Results

The experimental results of EPP feedback are shown in Figure 4.83. The solid line is the joint angle of the exoskeleton knee, and the dashed line is the pressure of the feedback gasbag. The pressure is amplified by a factor of 0.01 to make it convenient to compare the two values. The angle changed rapidly on purpose to test the performance of the feedback system. The result shows that the pressure of the gasbag can change with the joint angle and can feed back the joint angle precisely; besides, there exists a time delay of about 100 ms.

The experimental results of motion following are shown in Figure 4.84. The interactive force of the controller without the EMG feedforward item is larger. The average value is 22.6567 N ± 35.7659 N after 100 tests, while the average value of the controller with EMG feedforward item is 12.4673 N ± 25.4695 N, which is 44.97% smaller than the previous one.

The experimental results of active compliance control are shown in Figure 4.85. During the motion following F/E experiments, the interactive force remains in the range of −10 to 10 N, and the RMS value is 4.35 N. It indicates that the exoskeleton joint can follow the movement of human knee. The RMS value of the errors between the required assistive force and interactive force is shown in Table 4.11. The average RMS value of force error during active F/E, when the assistive or resistive force is 20, 40, and 60 N, respectively, is shown in Figure 4.86. The average RMS value of angle error during coordinated control is shown in Figure 4.86.

Figure 4.87 illustrates the experimental results of human–machine integrated coordinated control. Among them, (a) is the real joint angle feedback coordinated control, and (b) is the transferred

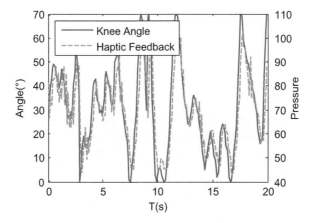

FIGURE 4.83 Knee angle and haptic feedback.

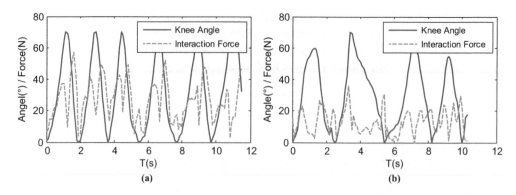

FIGURE 4.84   Experimental results of (a) controller without EMG feedforward item and (b) controller with EMG feedforward item.

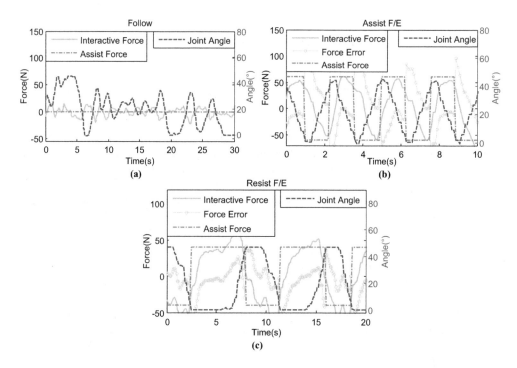

FIGURE 4.85   Active compliance control experiments. (a) Follow F/E; (b) assist F/E; and (c) resist F/E.

TABLE 4.11
RMS Values of Errors between the Required
Assistive Force and Interactive Force

	Assist F/E (N)	Resist F/E (N)
0 N	4.35	
20 N	7.62	6.26
40 N	13.37	11.15
60 N	18.45	16.42

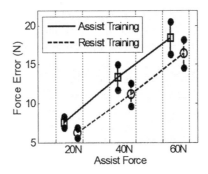

FIGURE 4.86 Errors between the required assistive force and interactive force during active F/E, when assistive force is 20, 40, and 60 N.

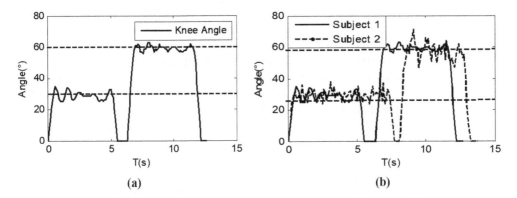

FIGURE 4.87 Human–machine integrated coordinated control experiment results. (a) Real joint angle feedback coordinated control; (b) transferred joint angle feedback coordinated control.

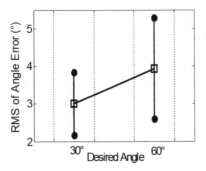

FIGURE 4.88 RMS values of errors between desired angle and real angle, when desired angle is 30° and 60°.

joint angle feedback coordinated control. When the required angles are 0°, 30° and 60°, the RMS are 6.9780°, 7.7946° and 9.6750°, respectively.

As illustrated in Figure 4.88, when the desired joint angle are 30° and 60° in the coordinated control experiments, the RMS values of errors are 2.9956° and 3.9385°, respectively.

4.2.6.2.3 Experimental Results Analysis

The results of gasbag pressure feedback experiment illustrate that the gasbag pressure is able to change with joint angle accurately in real time. Thus, the pneumatic control system works well, but there are still some delay between the gasbag pressure and joint angle. This is caused by the delay of the mechanical units, such as force sensors and air pumps. The average delay is about 100 ms, which is relatively short compared to human response time. Thus, force information feedback through haptic method of gasbag is feasible.

In the motion following experiment, the interactive force error of the controller without the EMG feedforward item is larger than that with EMG feedforward item, indicating that sEMG signal are able to be applied for predicting human motion intention in advance. The sEMG, joint and force integrated multi-source information fusion method for motion control is promising to realize the real-time decoding of human motion intention and motion control, while there are still some interactive forces between human and the exoskeleton, i.e., there are some prediction errors. Thus, further studies should be conducted on the improvement of sEMG processing and prediction algorithm.

The results of active compliance control experiment show that human–machine interactive force is maintained near the preset value, indicating that exoskeleton is able to follow the voluntary motion of the wearer and provides certain assistive force or resistive force according to the preset value in the process. Thus, it is able to meet the basic active rehabilitation training requirements for the patients with lower-extremity dyskinesia. However, during the extension and flexion process, there would be some fluctuation of the human–machine interactive force, as illustrated in Figure 4.85. Through the sEMG feeding forward item and differential feature extraction method, the real-time prediction of human motion intention is relatively more accurate. The error is more obvious in the assistive motion process, in which the RMS of assistive force error is also higher, as illustrated in Figure 4.85b. This is because that the assistive force is in the same direction as that of lower-extremity movement. During F/E, the direction of auxiliary force needs to change quickly, which poses higher requirements for the accuracy and lead time of motion intention prediction. On one hand, there are still some improvement to be made in the motion intention prediction method based on sEMG signal and multi-source biosignal. A better understanding of the closed-loop control mechanism of human body will help to better model the artificial neural network or other nonlinear controllers to improve the accuracy of motion prediction. On the other hand, the accuracy of the hybrid dynamic model for human–exoskeleton integrated system is to be improved. The dynamic model in the book has been simplified, with the parameter set based on the statistical results of normal people. For special users, there must be some error. Thus, the further optimization of the hybrid dynamic model for human–exoskeleton system will help to increase the accuracy of motion intention prediction and exoskeleton motion control.

In the information feedback experiment, subjects are able to perceive lower-extremity motion status and control the motion based on corresponding feedback. It indicates that the gasbag haptic feedback module can be used to extend physiological proprioceptor, feed back joint motion status, establish the information channel from robot to human, and achieve the closed-loop control of human–machine system and its coordinated control. The reason for the error may be that although gasbag pressure is able to reflect joint motion information accurately, there is still fuzziness in the process when the human uses haptic sense to perceive. As there is a lack of long-time training, the pressure and its changes cannot be perceived accurately, leading to the control error, so long-time training may be useful to reduce the error. On the other hand, as the original closed-loop control system is broken and a human–machine integrated closed-loop system is rebuilt, the original motor reflex arcs are in a mess, and a certain amount of training time is needed for human body to adapt to the new system. Human has to learn the original motion control mode in the later stage of rehabilitation, which has a considerable effect on the whole rehabilitation process. Thus, it is necessary to conduct further research on the feedback method for practical applications.

The rehabilitation requirements posed by patients with lower-extremity motion impairments have been analyzed first in this chapter to determine the basic structure of the exoskeleton robot followed by corresponding design, optimization, and prototype development. According to the patients with different diseases, degrees, ages, bed-type, seat-type, and standing-type auxiliary mechanisms have been developed. Through the static and kinematic analyses for the mechanism, we proved that the structures meet the application requirements and further developed the dynamic model for lower-extremity exoskeleton. Lower-extremity motion features have been studied in terms of the joint motion range, gait feature, center of gravity motion feature, and the design indices for the lower-extremity exoskeleton robot system have been determined. Further, the design requirements have been discussed: (1) joint range of motion. It should meet the requirements of real motion. The ranges of motion of the hip and knee joints should be able to achieve human gait and joint F/E motion. (2) stability of the robot system. It should be ensured that the mechanism will not fall down when moving forward. (3) dynamic features. Sufficient motor power should be guaranteed, which is of great significance in exoskeleton design.

The multi-functional exoskeleton robot designed based on bionics has some leading features. The structure is compact, and the range of motion of every joint is large. The knee joint is 0–110°, and the hip joint is −26° to 56°, which meets the requirements for human gait and normal joint swing. As servo motors are adopted, the control accuracy is high and the output torque is large. Straight-line motion mechanism on the mobile platform is used to adjust the height of hanger so that it can be used for people with the height of 158–190 cm. The robot can also adjust the center of gravity when doing rehabilitation exercises, in accordance with the gait feature. The safety belt on the hanger is used to support the human body to prevent patient from falling down and ensure the stability of the exoskeleton robot system. We introduced the parallel mechanism into the optimization design of exoskeleton robot. A three-RPS mechanism is selected to form the bionic design of the ankle joint. The structure is compact with two rotational DOFs and has a high stiffness, meeting the requirements of ankle joint.

Based on the preset requirements and functions of lower-extremity rehabilitation exoskeleton robot system, the myosignal amplifier, EMG DAQ instrument, and motion controller are designed and developed. At last, based on the hardware, the software for exoskeleton robot rehabilitation training system and EMG DAQ is developed. Based on an artificial FNN, motion identification algorithm based on the multi-source signals, including joint angle, human–machine interactive force, and sEMG signal, has been proposed. Through motion identification experiment, compare the performance of neurofuzzy networks with different topologies. The best network structure is selected based on experimental results. Compared with traditional algorithm, the proposed method reduces the prediction error by 6.4%, thus laying a solid foundation for human–machine coordinated control. The human–machine interaction interface is developed for exoskeleton robot, including EMG DAQ instrument, force sensor, angular sensor, data acquisition card, and DSP processor. The interface is integrated in the control system platform of the exoskeleton robot.

To achieve active compliance control of human–exoskeleton robot, we developed a bidirectional human–machine integrated information interface. Based on the interface, the dynamic and kinematic model is developed for exoskeleton robot, and the coordinated control strategy and control model are also established for the human–machine integrated system. Through the controller which fuses sEMG signal, joint angle, and interactive force, real-time motion decoding and the active motion control of human–exoskeleton robot system have been achieved. The gasbag that extends physiological proprioceptor to feed back joint angle is used to help patients with lower-extremity impairments achieve closed-loop motion control. With the object of knee joint, the experiment proves that the FNN is able to do real-time decoding of human motion intention. The gasbag-type physiological proprioceptor is able to feed back joint motion information in real time, replacing part of the functions of proprioceptors. Bidirectional human–machine integrated information interface helps to develop the closed-loop system for the human–machine system, achieving human–machine coordinated control.

The force interaction mechanism is analyzed to develop the relationship between the EMG signal and muscle force, laying a foundation for human–machine interface application in exoskeleton robot control. So far, the mechanism of the lower-extremity exoskeleton rehabilitation system and control strategies have been determined. The corresponding rehabilitation strategy will be composed on this basis in the next chapter, and the performance of the developed lower-extremity exoskeleton rehabilitation system on clinical application will also be evaluated.

4.3   IMPROVING THE TRANSPARENCY OF THE EXOSKELETON KNEE JOINT BASED ON ENERGY KERNEL METHOD OF EMG

It is recognized that when using robotic exoskeletons during the later phase of the whole training schedule, e.g., Stage V or Stage VI according to Brunnstrom's six-stage classification [126], the voluntary effort or active participation of the patient plays a key role in shortening training period and improving training quality [127]. This demands the ability of the robotic exoskeleton to provide compliant motion or to be possibly "transparent" to the patient during physical training. Combining the early-phase needs, a robotic exoskeleton is then expected to be capable of running in both "robot-in-charge" and "patient-in-charge" modes. The former mode indicates that the exoskeleton (both structure and actuator) ought to be as stiff as possible in order to implement precise position control (especially for lower-limb devices). However, the tough structure and drive form impose a large impedance on the device and dramatically increase the difficulty for achieving a good transparency. The researchers in this domain have long been puzzled by this contradiction, aimed at which, many pioneering and insightful studies have been conducted.

With respect to hardware-level improvements, several lightweight devices with structural compliance (e.g., the LOPES exoskeleton [128] using SEAs and the powered KNee EXOskeleton (KNEXO) exoskeleton [129] using pleated pneumatic artificial muscles (PPAMs), etc.) have been developed in order to facilitate transparent control. Moreover, LOPES can even achieve variable impedance actuation by installing SEAs with different stiffnesses. For such kinds of strategies, despite better intrinsic compliance, compromises on positioning accuracy and load capacity are often inevitable. In principle, the dynamic positioning error and the lower load capacity of intrinsically compliant devices are hard to compensate, but fortunately, the large-impedance defect of stiff devices which are qualified for precise position control and heavy load, can be relieved by cybernetic (software) level techniques. A representative example is inertia compensation [130], which is promising to provide a better transparency for low-frequency limb swinging motions, while it must be stabilized with the help of passive dynamics of human limbs, and in theory, there always remains a minimum residue inertia. The method of generalized elasticity [131,132] improves the transparency of the device using a conservative force field, and it can effectively reduce the interactive torques, with the limitation that human movements need to be roughly known in advance. The method of using adaptive oscillators [133,134] provides another way of improvement, which does not need strictly prescribed trajectory or user-specific calibration, while the application is limited to periodic motion, and it is not suitable for devices with high actuation stiffness as the machine is supposed to adapt to the frequency of human motion. Considering comprehensively the advantages and limitations of existent studies and the key problems in this domain, one would expect that the following features can be guaranteed simultaneously for an improved exoskeleton: (1) a stiff actuation structure; (2) transparency can be achieved for any irregular, unspecified movements; (3) theoretically, the perceptible device inertia can be reduced to an arbitrarily small level; (4) the device is able to adapt to any user rapidly without calibration or parameter identification. Aimed at these goals, this section proposed an iterative prediction–compensation control scheme based on the understanding of human motor intent, and the core idea is to turn the device into a virtual "copy" of the user's joint in terms of the dynamics and cybernetic features.

Despite the primary task of transparent control to decrease or minimize the interactive force/torque, human–machine interactive mechanism (HMIM) is still unclear up to date. In fact, all the issues discussed previously lead us to a common solution, i.e., building a clearly structured cybernetic model for muscular contraction based on a deep understanding of biomechanics, which thus serves as the theoretical basis for introducing EMG-based estimates to the control system and explaining HMIM. For this purpose, the semiphenomenological biomechanical/cybernetic model of skeletal muscle introduced earlier [135] can be applied. Moreover, this section adopts and improves the highly robust energy kernel method based on the oscillator model of EMG that we proposed earlier [136]. To realize transparency by synchronized movements, in the iterative prediction–compensation controller, an online adaptive predictor is designed using focused time-delay neural network (FTDNN), which is responsible for motor intent understanding and user movement prediction, while the compensator is designed using the normal force–position control paradigm based on the conventional understanding of HMIM. Finally, taking knee joint as the object, initial experiments are conducted to validate the effectiveness of the proposed control strategy.

4.3.1 REAL-TIME EXTRACTION ALGORITHM OF ENERGY KERNEL OF EMG

Extracting the characteristic energy of the energy kernel is equivalent to identifying the elliptic boundary for area calculation. In Chapter 3, this is conducted via a "linear fencing" method, which, however, is not fast enough to meet real-time demands. Here, a "discrete box counting" method is proposed. For a signal segment containing N data points, first identify the outmost boundary of the rectangle enveloping the elliptic shape; then divide the x- and y-direction legs into n_1 and n_2 segments, respectively. This results in a mesh consisting of $n_1 \times n_2$ boxes. Next, count the number of state points falling into each box, and denote it as p_{ij} ($i = 1, 2, \ldots n_1; j = 1, 2, \ldots n_2$). The plot of p_{ij} vs. the center coordinates of the boxes looks like a mountain-shaped surface, with its peak corresponding to the central region of the ellipse. A predefined threshold thr is supposed to "cut" the mountain and produce a flat top surface for area computation, as shown in Figure 4.89a. A 2D moving average method is then applied in order to prevent the case that p_{ij} in the central region is smaller than thr, which would affect the effectiveness of area computation:

$$\bar{p}_{i,j} = \frac{1}{9} \sum_{i=1,j=1}^{n_1,n_2} \left(\begin{matrix} p_{i-1,j-1}, p_{i-1,j}, p_{i-1,j+1}, p_{i,j-1}, p_{i,j}, \\ p_{i,j+1}, p_{i+1,j-1}, p_{i+1,j}, p_{i+1,j+1} \end{matrix} \right), \tag{4.53}$$

where $p_{i,j}$ is the averaged value of p_{ij}. Finally, sum up the area of all the boxes whose $\bar{p}_{ij}$'s are bigger than thr:

$$S = \sum s_{ij} \mid \bar{p}_{ij} > thr, i = 1,2,\ldots,n_1; \ j = 1,2,\ldots,n_2, \tag{4.54}$$

where s_{ij} denotes the area of each box and S is the elliptic area of energy kernel that is used to calculate the characteristic energy, as shown in Figure 4.89b. Here, we use a window width of $N = 600$ (with 1/30 increment, sampling rate, 2,000 Hz), a thr of 3, and $n_1 = n_2 = 10$.

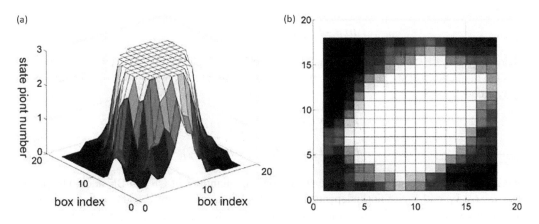

FIGURE 4.89 (a) 3D plot of the state point numbers of the boxes distributing on the phase plane; (b) top view of the plot. Note that the white boxes compose the total area of the energy kernel. In this demonstration, $N = 1,000$, $n_1 = n_2 = 20$, and $thr = 3$.

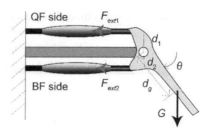

FIGURE 4.90   Mechanical approximation of human knee joint.

4.3.2   HMIM AND ADAPTIVE PREDICTION SCHEME

4.3.2.1   HMIM

Understanding HMIM relies largely on the radical explanation of the generation mechanism of human–machine interactive force/torque, which is the principal target to be eliminated in transparent control. In the domain of impedance control, HMIM is described (but hardly explained) by the general relation between force and stiffness and/or damping. This paradigm is only valid in the vicinity of the system's equilibrium point, unless the interactive force is directly transformed into elastic deformation (position control), while due to the highly nonlinear characteristics of the neuromuscular system and voluntary motion, it is not suitable to handle the fast state transitions in such a global nonlinear state space. Actually, the observable deformation of the interface is the consequence rather than the cause of interactive force, as can be illustrated by a simple thought experiment, assuming that human leg and robotic leg are both rigid and the force transducer is ideal, i.e., no deformation will occur during force sensing. Despite that, impedance control cannot be applied to this condition; obviously the interactive force can still be detected if robotic leg motion is inconsistent with human leg. Therefore, normative impedance control is not a predicting tool but only a compensating tool.

The following discussion of HMIM is based on this ideal situation, since we are attempting to analyze the prime cause of interactive force and heading for motion prediction. An abstract mechanical representation of human knee joint's free motion is shown in Figure 4.90, in which the flexion and extension of the shank are considered to be actuated by two virtual muscles on the QF side and the BF side, and the muscle forces are denoted by F_{ext1} and F_{ext2}, respectively. Note that flexion is prescribed as the positive direction of the joint angle θ. The dynamical equation of the system can be easily written as

$$I\ddot{\theta} = -F_{ext1}d_1 + F_{ext2}d_2 + Gd_g\cos\theta, \qquad (4.55)$$

where d_1 and d_2 are the momentum arms of F_{ext1} and F_{ext2}, G denotes the gravity force of the shank with the momentum arm of dg, and I is the inertia of the shank. According to the semiphenomenological model,

$$F_{ext1} = F_a\left(E_{ch1}, L_1, V_1\right) + F_p\left(L_1, V_1\right)$$
$$F_{ext2} = F_a\left(E_{ch2}, L_2, V_2\right) + F_p\left(L_2, V_2\right), \qquad (4.56)$$

where the subscripts 1 and 2 feature the corresponding quantities of QF and BF sides. The parameters L_1, L_2, V_1, and V_2 are not independent variables but are all coupled and can be expressed by the functions of θ and $d\theta/dt$. Thus, the first two terms on the right side of (12) can be denoted as a nonlinear function T_a; then (12) is modified into

$$I\ddot{\theta} = T_a\left(E_{ch1}, E_{ch2}, \theta, \dot{\theta}\right) + Gd_g\cos\theta. \qquad (4.57)$$

For practical control, the angular position is read in a temporally discrete manner with a servo period of Δt; hence, the angular velocity and acceleration can be expressed using forward difference quotient:

$$\dot{\theta} = \left(\theta^{k+1} - \theta^k\right)/\Delta t$$
$$\ddot{\theta} = \left(\theta^{k+1} - 2\theta^k + \theta^{k-1}\right)/\Delta t^2 \tag{4.58}$$

where θ^k, θ^{k-1}, and θ^{k+1} denote the position at the current, previous, and next time, respectively. Then, (14) can be rewritten into the discrete form as

$$I \frac{\theta^{k+1} - 2\theta^k + \theta^{k-1}}{\Delta t^2} = T_a\left(E_{ch1}, E_{ch2}, \theta^k, \frac{\theta^{k+1} - \theta^k}{\Delta t}\right) + Gd_g\cos\theta^k. \tag{4.59}$$

The position θ^{k+1} is supposed to be used as the controlling input of the exoskeleton knee joint. Here, θ^{k+1} is actually the true position of human knee joint because we have been discussing free motion (without exoskeleton). However, error must exist for the predicted position $\tilde{\theta}^{k+1}$, which would result in the interactive torque when putting on the exoskeleton, while according to the ideal-case assumption that human leg is rigidly attached to the robotic leg, θ^k and θ^{k-1} can be considered as the same for both human and robotic legs, since a stiff-type exoskeleton is expected. Consequently, the actual situation with the interactive torque can be described as

$$I \frac{\tilde{\theta}^{k+1} - 2\theta^k + \theta^{k-1}}{\Delta t^2} = T_a\left(E_{ch1}, E_{ch2}, \theta^k, \frac{\tilde{\theta}^{k+1} - \theta^k}{\Delta t}\right) + Gd_g\cos\theta^k + T_{\text{int}}. \tag{4.60}$$

Subtracting (16) from (17), we get

$$I \frac{\tilde{\theta}^{k+1} - \theta^{k+1}}{\Delta t^2} = T_a\left(E_{ch1}, E_{ch2}, \theta^k, \frac{\tilde{\theta}^{k+1} - \theta^k}{\Delta t}\right) - T_a\left(E_{ch1}, E_{ch2}, \theta^k, \frac{\theta^{k+1} - \theta^k}{\Delta t}\right) + T_{\text{int}}. \tag{4.61}$$

The first two items on the right side of (4.61) characterize the torque difference produced by the muscles with and without the exoskeleton. Thus, (4.61) unveils the fact that interactive force/torque is generated by the velocity difference under the two conditions. This can also be explained by the above cybernetic scheme of skeletal muscle, while here the muscles operate in the velocity-control mode. No matter whether the exoskeleton is put on or not, the motor intent of human body is unchanged; i.e., the activation level and the initial length of muscle remain the same, but the contractile velocity diverging from that under unloaded condition gives rise to the "excessive" force—the interactive force. An extreme example is when a muscle goes from isokinetic to isometric contraction, a sudden jump or fall in tension happens [137], and vice versa.

4.3.2.2 Adaptive Prediction Scheme Using FTDNN

The engineering application would be much easier if the exoskeleton can adapt to human knee joint online with only the source signals of EMG, position, and force. For this purpose, predictive neural network with tapped delay line (FTDNN) might be the best choice. As shown in Figure 4.91, the network architecture used in this work has three inputs: the characteristic energies of QF and BF sides and the angular position of the knee joint fed back by the encoder of motor. A third-order tapped delay line is applied to each input, which thus becomes a vector consisting of the quantities at time $k - 2$, $k - 1$, and k (current time), with the output of the predicted position at time $k + 1$. The arrangement of the layers must be able to achieve acceptable training accuracy and meanwhile be concise enough to facilitate real-time training. After many trials, a 16-neuron structure

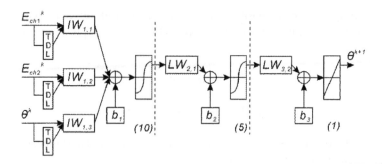

FIGURE 4.91   The architecture of the FTDNN used for active prediction.

(three layers, 10–5–1) is adopted here. The key problem to be solved is that the true/unloaded position of human knee joint is not known, so the position error supposed to train the network cannot be obtained explicitly. However, HMIM enlightens us to deploy the relationship between interactive force and position error $\Delta\theta$. For (4.61), the predicted position can be expressed as

$$\tilde{\theta}^{k+1} = \theta^{k+1} + \Delta\theta. \tag{4.62}$$

Then, (4.61) turns into

$$\frac{I\Delta\theta}{\Delta t^2} \cong \left.\frac{\partial T_a}{\partial\theta}\right|_{\theta^{k+1}} \cdot \Delta\theta + T_{\text{int}}. \tag{4.63}$$

Thus, the position error can be expressed as

$$\Delta\theta = \frac{T_{\text{int}}}{\dfrac{I}{\Delta t^2} - \left.\dfrac{\partial T_a}{\partial\theta}\right|_{\theta^{k+1}}} \cong \frac{\Delta t^2}{I} T_{\text{int}} = \gamma_s T_{\text{int}}. \tag{4.64}$$

It is noteworthy that Δt is a very small quantity compared to I, and the partial differential term in (4.64) is small compared to its left-side term, because the active torque produced by muscle would not change radically with respect to the position; therefore, this term can be neglected. Equation (4.64) indicates that the position error is proportional to the interactive torque by a constant γ_s determined by servo interval and the inertia of human leg. In effect, γ_s does not even need to be absolutely accurate; i.e., it is unnecessary (also impossible) to measure I very precisely only if the network training converges, because it can be merged into the learning rate parameter. Besides, in a practical sense, γ_s would be much larger than the value indicated by Eq. (4.64), which represents the aforementioned ideal rigid contact condition, but human limb is actually flexible with skin and muscle tissue. Variable learning rate training with momentum item [138] is used for the online training. With this scheme, a patient wearing the exoskeleton only needs to make voluntary movements, and soon the device will adapt to his knee joint (in our case, within 1 min). The whole process is very convenient without any parameter identification, so the scheme is not user-specific.

4.3.2.3   Iterative Prediction–Compensation Control Loop

Combining the semiphenomenological model, the prediction scheme provides a rational framework for introducing EMG signal into the predictive control system using the energy kernel method. Yet, this scheme alone is inadequate to perform high quality real-time transparent control, because prediction error always exists under the limitation of network complexity and the incremental training condition. As a result, small oscillations may occur at the static position at which the subject wants to stay. Hence, normal PID-based force–position control used previously in [139] is also applied here between the prediction periods, forming an iterative prediction–compensation control loop. The control strategy is implemented in two steps as follows.

First, let the user (experimental subject) wear the exoskeleton; then let the controller operate under the network training mode during the user's voluntary motion, as shown in Figure 4.92a. Here, three channels of signal, i.e., E_{ch1}, E_{ch2} (collected from the user, displayed together as a bold line), and θ_{exo}^k (fed back by the exoskeleton), are used as the inputs of the FTDNN. Note that these inputs are all treated by the tapped delay line structure (Figure 4.91), and the network is supposed to output the predicted position (θ^{k+1}) of the next servo interval, during which this output then serves as the reference signal that controls the knee joint motor of the exoskeleton. After the nonlinear transformation from angle to pulse number by the transfer function H, the motor driver (G_{drv}) works under the closed-loop position control mode, and the measured position (θ_{exo}^{k+1}) of the exoskeleton limb (G_{exo}) is fed back to FTDNN in real time for next iteration of prediction. Meanwhile, the inter-active torque (T_{int}^{k+1}) calculated from force sensor reading is used to compute the error ($\Delta\theta$) between the predicted position and the real position of the user's knee joint (θ^{k+1}) by the factor γ_s in Eq. (4.64). The computed error is thus used to train the network online. It is clear that in this scheme, training and prediction are conducted simultaneously, and initial transparency is attained during this on-machine process for any user. Then, the resulting network can be regarded as a virtual "copy" of the user's knee joint and is ready for the iterative prediction–compensation control in the next step, while it should be noted that one needs to be cautious when applying the same network/predictor to long term purposes, because long term effects such as potentiation or fatigue may emerge to weaken the prediction performance. Nevertheless, since it is very fast and convenient to retrain the network, such adaptions can be conducted upon the decrease of transparent level.

Next, the iterative prediction–compensation control system is built with the trained network that acts as a predictor, and a compensator is designed using the normal force–position control paradigm with a PID controller, as shown in Figure 4.92b. Here, the predictor and compensator are enabled

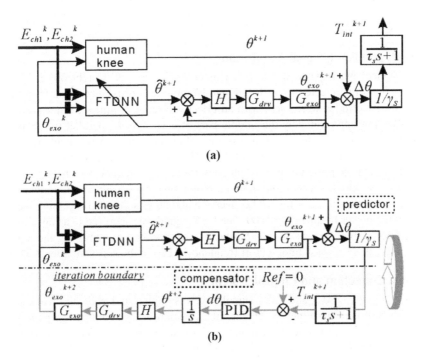

(a)

(b)

FIGURE 4.92 (a) Online training scheme for the predictor, where τ_s is the time constant of force transducer; (b) iterative prediction–compensation control loop comprised of the predictor and the compensator.

iteratively across the iteration boundary to take over the control of knee joint motor, i.e., one prediction period between two compensation periods and vice versa. Specifically, first the exoskeleton reaches the predicted position. Meanwhile, the prediction error ($\Delta\theta$) in the current servo period results in an interactive torque that forms the input of the PID controller in the next servo period. Then, the compensated position (θ_{exo}^{k+2}) again serves as an input of the predictor for another round of prediction. It can be seen from Figure 4.92b that the whole strategy is quite easy to be generalized because the training of the predictor is highly adaptive, and only a normative force-position control method is needed for compensation.

4.3.3 INITIAL EXPERIMENT AND RESULTS

4.3.3.1 Lower-Limb Robotic Exoskeleton

Our standing bed-type exoskeleton adapted from [139] in this section has a very stiff actuation structure as all the powered joints are driven by motor-screw-nut mechanisms, similar to those used in Lokomat [140], ALEX [141], and MINDWALKER [142]. The mechanical structure of the horizontal-type robotic exoskeleton used in this work is shown in Figure 4.93a (3D model) and Figure 4.93b (prototype). For each side of lower extremity, there are totally six DOFs, as shown in Table 4.12. Note that in Figure 4.93a, only DOF 1 and DOF 2 are presented. As shown in Figure 4.93b, the shank part of the machine is composed of two parts, a shank base and a sliding sleeve (position fixed by two pins) connecting with the transducer base, on which the S-type strain gauge force transducer is mounted. The transducer stays in between the transducer base and the shank base, which is fixed to human's leg through a gasbag (to assure the degree of comfort) and a Velcro binding tape. Each time an experimental trial begins, the airbag is charged to a tight but acceptable pressure (controlled by the subject) so that the contact stiffness between human and machine is high enough and meanwhile comfortable. Actually, in our scheme, the gasbag is treated as a virtual part (e.g., like an adipose layer) of human leg. Thus, in the dynamical sense, although the gasbag would not affect force transducing, it will further increase γ_s compared to the situation without the gasbag. Therefore, in this study, γ_s is adjusted to be 0.01 after many trials of network training.

4.3.3.2 EMG and Force Signal Acquisition

One healthy subject participated in the experiment (male, age 29, weight 60 kg, height 174 cm). The EMG signals were collected from the QF and BF muscles of his right thigh. Disposable bipolar Ag–AgCl sEMG electrodes were used, with an effective area of 5 mm × 5 mm for each electrode, which was placed at approximately the middle part of each muscle, parallel to the assumed muscle fiber orientation with an inter-electrode distance of about 20 mm. A self-made EMG acquisition instrument was used, with a sampling rate of 2,000 Hz. The signal successively went through hardware modules of a tenfold pre-amplifier, a high-pass filter (cutoff frequency of 10 Hz), a low-pass filter (cutoff frequency of 500 Hz), a 500-fold main amplifier, and a noise suppressing module. The EMG signal is then sent to the collector for A/D conversion and other software processing including notch rectification at the power frequency (50 Hz). The force signal was acquired in a way almost the same as acquiring EMG signal, except that the hardware was modified by removing the high-pass filter, and was treated with a low-pass filter (cutoff frequency, 5 Hz) in the software after A/D conversion.

4.3.3.3 Data Collection and Control System

All the analog signals (EMG and force signals) were sampled and collected using an NI device (NI USB-6221, National Instruments). The angular position of the robotic knee joint was collected directly via the encoder of the knee joint motor, with the forward and backward interpolations of the nonlinear relationship between pulse number and knee angle (Figure 4.93a). The control system was built in Labview 2010 (National Instruments) on a desktop computer, which receives all the sensor signals and sends control commands to the motion control card.

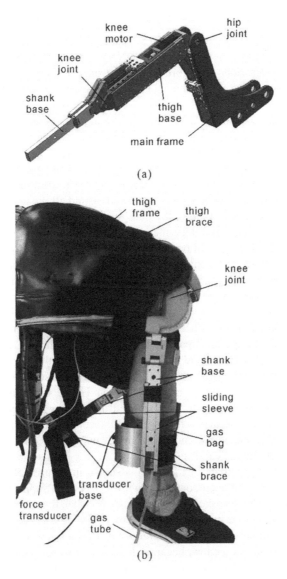

FIGURE 4.93   (a) 3D model of the lower-extremity robotic exoskeleton; (b) the prototype of the exoskeleton worn by the experimental subject.

TABLE 4.12
Configuration of DOFs of the Exoskeleton

DOF Number	Description	Powered or Not
1	Hip flexion and extension	Yes
2	Knee flexion and extension	Yes
3	Thigh length adjustment	No
4	Shank length adjustment	No
5	Hip height adjustment	Yes
6	Hip width adjustment	Yes

4.3.3.4 Results

For each trial, the robotic exoskeleton worked in the patient-in-charge mode (zero-torque mode) for transparency evaluation. Firstly, the predictor (FTDNN) in the control system was trained by the subject using the scheme described in Figure 4.92a. The subject made voluntary and random knee flexion and extension to drive the robotic knee joint. The interactive force decreased gradually with the training process, which thus stopped when the force converged (small oscillations were present before force–position compensation). It is noteworthy that at the beginning, the moving speed of the knee joint was limited for the sake of safety and stability, because the initial output of the network would be random after the initialization of weight matrices in the FTDNN. The adaptability of this training scheme has been validated via several training tests at different times of the day, indicating different physiological statuses of the subject. During each test, the weights of the network were adapted from their random initial values (between 0 and 1), and all the tests converged in less than 1 min. Secondly, the exoskeleton worked in the pure force–position control mode. The subject still made voluntary and random knee motions; meanwhile the dynamic response of the robotic knee joint was observed, and the PID control parameters were adjusted, until the dynamic performance was optimal. Finally, the exoskeleton operated in two modes: (1) iterative prediction–compensation control mode (Figure 4.92b) with the predictor and (2) pure force–position control mode without prediction (Figure 4.92b, lower part). The speed was always limited to approximately 1 rad/s for the purpose of safety.

Here, it should be made clear that since the robotic exoskeleton used in this work is only a prototype, it is not qualified yet to perform patient experiments as in the clinical application scenario. Besides, due to the limits of resource and experimental condition, the mechanical performance as well as the hardware (e.g., force transducer) of the system are still suboptimum, leading to a relatively narrow range of permitted velocity and acceleration. Hence, the primary goal of the current preliminary experiments is to investigate whether the transparency has been improved effectively (i.e., a remarkable decrease in interactive force or impedance) for unspecified or random voluntary movements under mode (1) compared to mode (2), thus evaluating the effectiveness of the proposed control strategy at the methodological level.

A typical set of experimental data of mode (1) is shown in Figure 4.94a, from which one can tell that the interactive force had been controlled within 10 N. The Supplemental Video shows the dynamic response of the robotic exoskeleton under mode (1) when the subject tried to follow the finger pose (pointing angle) of the instructor. The trajectory of θ indicates that the knee joint angle of exoskeleton is irregular without any prescribed frequency. Besides, it is worth noting that the excitement level of the BF muscle is very low, because during such voluntary movements, the subject's knee joint can flex under the effect of gravity without considerably activating the BF muscle. For comparison, a corresponding set of experimental data of mode (2) is shown in Figure 4.94b, in which no EMG related data is presented since pure force–position control is used. It is evident that under this condition, the interactive force increases remarkably, indicating a degraded transparency.

The improvement of transparency can also be investigated by assessing whether the user effort can be decreased in mode (1) or in mode (2). For this purpose, another set of experimental data under mode (2) is shown in Figure 4.95a that includes the EMG signal of QF and BF muscles. For simplicity, here the user effort is estimated via computing the moving average of EMG (EMG_{mv}) with a window width of 100 ms (no overlap). Figure 4.95b shows the user effort during the corresponding motion in mode (1) (top, computed from the data set in Figure 4.94a) and in mode (2) (middle, computed from the data set in Figure 4.95a), respectively. It should be noted that since BF muscle is not activated notably due to the gravity of leg under both modes, only the EMG_{mv} of QF muscle is presented. One can easily tell that the peak value of EMG_{mv} in mode (2) is generally higher than that in mode (1). To be more specific, the trends of EMG_{mv} vs. angular velocity of knee joint are plotted for both modes (bottom of Figure 4.95b), because the movement of the subject is voluntary and random and the user effort cannot be compared directly. The plots show that at high

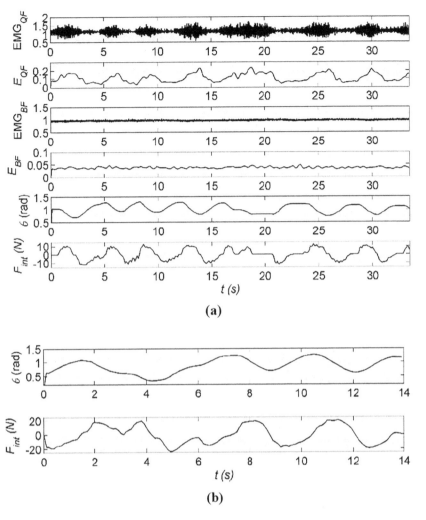

FIGURE 4.94 (a) A typical set of experimental data generated under mode (1); (b) a set of experimental data generated under mode (2). Y-coordinate names: EMG—raw EMG signal; E—characteristic energy of EMG; θ—knee joint angle of exoskeleton; F_{int}—interactive force.

speed (whether positive or negative), the user effort in mode (2) (blue circle) is indeed stronger, while at low speed, the difference is not that remarkable. Besides, for mode (1) there are some data points (red cross) gathering at zero velocity since Figure 4.94a indicates that the subject stopped moving from time to time. Although the user effort is on the whole reduced with the prediction scheme under mode (1), it has to be mentioned that the characterization of user effort using EMG is sometimes not very stable in the experiments, possibly due to the effect of potentiation or fatigue during repetitive trials. Thereby, in order to reliably assess the improvement of transparency, we turned to the direct measurement of impedance with the data of interactive force and velocity.

Figure 4.96a shows three random groups of data produced from three sets of comparing experiments. The data records the relationship between the moving speed of robotic knee joint and interactive force during voluntary random movements. On the whole, the magnitude of interactive force is positively correlated to the speed in an approximately linear manner. This is partly due to the electromechanical delay of the whole system during both network training and compensation control, e.g., the delay of force transducer's response. However, it can be recognized that the

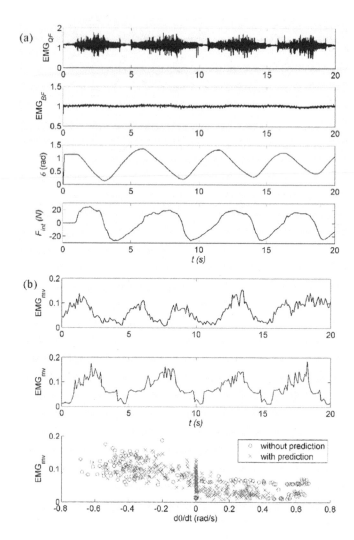

FIGURE 4.95 (a) Another set of experimental data including EMG signal generated under mode (2); (b) comparison between the user effort measured by the moving average of EMG in (a) and that in Figure 4.94a under mode (1); top: mode (1); middle: mode (2); bottom: plots of user effort vs. velocity under the two modes.

impedance under mode (1) (cross) is smaller than that under mode (2) (circle), as indicated by the different slopes of the fitted trends (line). Correspondingly, Figure 4.96b shows the comparisons of the relationships between interactive force and the acceleration of robotic knee joint motion. Distinct from the interactive force–velocity relationship, no explicit trend can be recognized between interactive force and acceleration. However, again, it is easy to tell that the compliance under mode (1) is higher than that under mode (2), as the areas formed by the crosses can be regarded as the "shrunken" versions of those formed by circles. Moreover, the distribution of the data points in mode (1) is denser (i.e., less scattered) than that in mode (2), indicating a higher stability of performance when using the predictor.

According to the results presented in Figure 4.96, the distributions of algebraic impedance (velocity impedance) and inertia (acceleration impedance) can be computed respectively for each data set being compared. Figure 4.97a shows the error bar plot (mean with standard deviation) of the impedance under mode (1) (line with cross) and mode (2) (black line with circle) for the three sets of experiments. The lower mean values for mode (2) make it more evident that the impedance

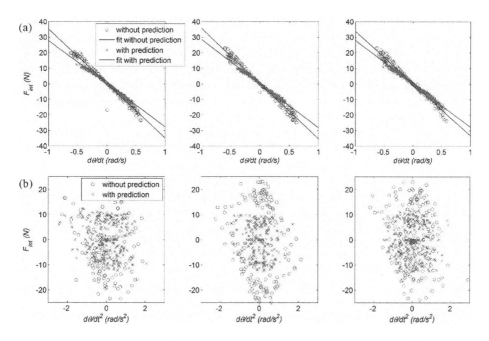

FIGURE 4.96 Comparison of three groups of data from experiments under mode (1) and mode (2) that investigate the relationships between (a) speed and interactive force and (b) acceleration and interactive force.

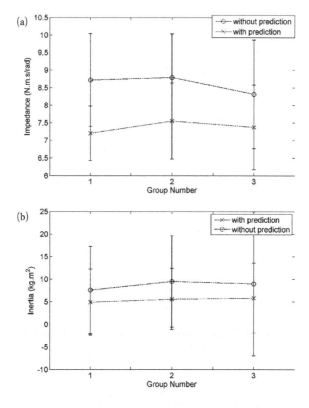

FIGURE 4.97 (a) Error bar plot of the impedance computed from the three groups of data under mode (1) and mode (2); (b) error bar plot of the inertia computed from the three groups of data under mode (1) and mode (2).

is reduced effectively by using the predictor. In the same manner, the error bars for inertia can be plotted, as shown in Figure 4.97b, which indicates that using the predictor can also effectively reduce the inertia of human–machine interaction. Additionally, indeed, the standard deviation of the inertia under mode (1) is apparently smaller than that under mode (2). According to the error bar plots presented in Figure 4.97, it can be concluded initially that the proposed iterative prediction–compensation control strategy brings notable improvement in transparency. Particularly, the performance in impedance reduction is more prominent.

Based on the analysis of the generation mechanism of human–machine interactive force (or HMIM), this section aims at improving the transparency of an exoskeleton knee joint via an iterative prediction–compensation control scheme. The online adaptive predictor is designed based on an FTDNN, where only three inputs of EMG, interactive force, and position are involved, and the activation level of muscle is extracted from EMG using a novel energy kernel method. The compensator is designed with a normative force–position control paradigm. The experiments on the human–machine integrated knee system have validated initially the effectiveness of the proposed control strategy.

REFERENCES

1. Dollar A M, Herr H. Lower extremity exoskeletons and active orthoses: Challenges and state-of-the-art. *IEEE Trans. Robot.*, 2008, 24(1): 144–158.
2. Yagn N. Apparatus for facilitating walking. Google Patents, 1890.
3. Zaroodny S J. Bumpusher-A Powered Aid To Locomotion. No. BRL-TN-1524. Ballistic Research Labs Aberdeen Proving Ground MD, 1963.
4. Gilbert K. *Exoskeleton Prototype Project: Final Report on Phase I.* Schenectady, NY: General Electric Company. GE Tech Rep S-67-1011, 1967.
5. Mosher R S. *Handyman to Hardiman.* Warrendale, PA: Society of Automotive Engineers, 1967.
6. Rosheim M E. Man-amplifying exoskeleton. *Proceedings of the* 1989 *Advances in Intelligent Robotics Systems Conference.* International Society for Optics and Photonics, Philadelphia, PA, 1990.
7. Garcia E, Sater J M, Main J. Exoskeletons for human performance augmentation (EHPA): A program summary. *J. Robot. Soc. Japan*, 2002, 20(8): 822–826.
8. Kazerooni H, Steger R. The Berkeley lower extremity exoskeleton. *J. Dyn. Syst. Meas. Contr.*, 2006, 128(1): 14–25.
9. Zoss A B, Kazerooni H, Chu A. Biomechanical design of the Berkeley lower extremity exoskeleton (BLEEX). *IEEE ASME Trans. Mechatron.*, 2006, 11(2): 128–138.
10. Chu A, Kazerooni H, Zoss A. On the biomimetic design of the Berkeley lower extremity exoskeleton (BLEEX). *Proceedings of the Robotics and Automation, 2005 ICRA 2005 Proceedings of the 2005 IEEE International Conference.* IEEE, Barcelona, Spain, 2005.
11. Guizzo E, Goldstein H. The rise of the body bots [robotic exoskeletons]. *IEEE Spectrum*, 2005, 42(10): 50–56.
12. Huang G T. Wearable robots. *Tech. Rev.*, 2004, 4: 70–73.
13. Walsh C J, Paluska D, Pasch K, et al. Development of a lightweight, underactuated exoskeleton for load-carrying augmentation. *Proceedings of the Robotics and Automation, 2006 ICRA 2006 Proceedings 2006 IEEE International Conference.* IEEE, Orlando, FL, 2006.
14. Walsh C J. *Biomimetic Design of an Under-Actuated Leg Exoskeleton for Load-Carrying Augmentation.* Cambridge, MA: Massachusetts Institute of Technology, 2006.
15. Walsh C J, Endo K, Herr H. A quasi-passive leg exoskeleton for load-carrying augmentation. *Int. J. Hum. Robot.*, 2007, 4(03): 487–506.
16. Gregorczyk K N, Obusek J P, Hasselquist L, et al. Effects of carried weight on random motion and traditional measures of postural sway. *Appl. Ergon.*, 2006, 37: 607–614. doi:10.1016/j.apergo.2005.10.002.
17. Jansen J. ORNL, 2004.
18. Marks P. Power dressing. *New Sci.*, 2001, 172(2316): 32–35.
19. Gogola M, Barth E J, Goldfarb M. Monopropellant powered actuators for use in autonomous human-scaled robotics. *Proceedings of the Robotics and Automation, 2002 Proceedings ICRA'02 IEEE International Conference.* IEEE, Washington, DC, 2002.

20. Kawamoto H, Sankai Y. Power assist system HAL-3 for gait disorder person. In *Computers Helping People with Special Needs*, Miesenberger K., Klaus J., Zagler W., eds. Berlin, Heidelberg: Springer, 2002. 196–203.

21. Yamamoto K, Hyodo K, Ishii M, et al. Development of power assisting suit for assisting nurse labor. *JSME Int. J., Ser. C*, 2002, 45: 703–711.

22. Yamamoto K, Ishii M, Hyodo K, et al. Development of power assisting suit (miniaturization of supply system to realize wearable suit). *JSME Int. J. Ser. C*, 2003, 46(3): 923–930.

23. Low K, Yin Y. An integrated lower exoskeleton system towards design of a portable active orthotic device. *Int. J. Robot. Autom.*, 2007, 22(1): 32–43.

24. Low K, Liu X, Yu H. Development of NTU wearable exoskeleton system for assistive technologies. *Proceedings of the Mechatronics and Automation, 2005 IEEE International Conference*. IEEE, Niagara Falls, ON, 2005.

25. Riener R, Lunenburger L, Jezernik S, et al. Patient-cooperative strategies for robot-aided treadmill training: First experimental results. *IEEE Trans. Neural. Syst. Rehabil. Eng.*, 2005, 13(3): 380–394.

26. Bernhardt M, Frey M, Colombo G, et al. Hybrid force-position control yields cooperative behaviour of the rehabilitation robot LOKOMAT. *Proceedings of the Rehabilitation Robotics, 2005 ICORR 2005 9th International Conference*. IEEE, Chicago, IL, 2005.

27. Von Zitzewitz J, Bernhardt M, Riener R. A novel method for automatic treadmill speed adaptation. *IEEE Trans. Neural. Syst. Rehabil. Eng.*, 2007, 15(3): 401–409.

28. Trailler P, Blanchard V, Perrin I, et al. Improvement of rehabilitation possibilities with the MotionMaker TM. *Proceedings of the Biomedical Robotics and Biomechatronics, 2006 BioRob 2006 The First IEEE/RAS-EMBS International Conference*. IEEE, Pisa, Italy, 2006.

29. HOCOMA. Erigo®: Accelerate early rehabilitation. www.hocoma.com/products/erigo/.

30. Yang C, Zhang J, Chen Y, et al. A review of exoskeleton-type systems and their key technologies. *Proc. IME C J. Mech. Eng. Sci.*, 2008, 222(8): 1599–1612.

31. Dong Y, Yang C. *Study and Preliminary Implementation of the Exercise Control System of Lower Limb Rehabilitation Exoskeleton Robot*. Hangzhou: Zhejiang University, 2008 (in Chinese).

32. Zhang J, Yang C. *The Compliant Exoskeleton Robot Intelligent System Based Fundamental Theory and Application Study*. Hangzhou: Zhejiang University, 2009 (in Chinese).

33. Feng Z. *Walking Rehabilitation Exercise Robot System*. Shanghai: Shanghai University, 2009 (in Chinese).

34. Anam K, Al-Jumaily A A. *Active Exoskeleton Control Systems: State of the Art. Procedia Eng.*, 2012, 41: 988–994.

35. Lo H S, Xie S Q. Exoskeleton robots for upper-limb rehabilitation: State of the art and future prospects. *Med. Eng. Phys.*, 2012, 34(3): 261–268.

36. Kazerooni H, Racine J-L, Huang L, et al. On the control of the Berkeley lower extremity exoskeleton (BLEEX). *Proceedings of the Robotics and Automation, 2005 ICRA 2005 Proceedings of the 2005 IEEE International Conference*. IEEE, Barcelona, Spain, 2005.

37. Kazerooni H, Steger R, Huang L. Hybrid control of the Berkeley lower extremity exoskeleton (BLEEX). *Int. J. Robot. Res.*, 2006, 25(5–6): 561–573.

38. Ghan J, Steger R, Kazerooni H. Control and system identification for the Berkeley lower extremity exoskeleton (BLEEX). *Adv. Robot.*, 2006, 20(9): 989–1014.

39. Aguirre-Ollinger G, Colgate J E, Peshkin M A, et al. Active-impedance control of a lower-limb assistive exoskeleton. *Proceedings of the Rehabilitation Robotics, 2007 ICORR 2007 IEEE 10th International Conference*. IEEE, Noordwijk, Netherlands, 2007.

40. Yang X, Lihua G, Yang Z, et al. Lower extreme carrying exoskeleton robot adative control using wavelet neural networks. *Proceedings of the Natural Computation, 2008 ICNC'08 Fourth International Conference*. IEEE, Noordwijk, Netherlands, 2008.

41. Rosen J, Fuchs M B, Arcan M. Performances of Hill-type and neural network muscle models: Toward a myosignal-based exoskeleton. *Comput. Biomed. Res.*, 1999, 32(5): 415–439.

42. Rosen J, Brand M, Fuchs M B, et al. A myosignal-based powered exoskeleton system. *IEEE Trans. Syst. Man Cybern. Syst. Hum.*, 2001, 31(3): 210–222.

43. Cavallaro E E, Rosen J, Perry J C, et al. Real-time myoprocessors for a neural controlled powered exoskeleton arm. *IEEE Trans. Biomed. Eng.*, 2006, 53(11): 2387–2396.

44. Hashemi J, Morin E, Mousavi P, et al. EMG–force modeling using parallel cascade identification. *J. Electromyogr. Kinesiol.*, 2012, 22(3): 469–477.

45. Kiguchi K, Hayashi Y. An EMG-based control for an upper-limb power-assist exoskeleton robot. *IEEE Trans. Syst. Man Cybern. B Cybern.*, 2012, 42(4): 1064–1071.

46. Suzuki K, Mito G, Kawamoto H, et al. Intention-based walking support for paraplegia patients with Robot Suit HAL. *Adv. Robot.*, 2007, 21(12): 1441–1469.
47. Frisoli A, Sotgiu E, Procopio C, et al. Design and implementation of a training strategy in chronic stroke with an arm robotic exoskeleton. *Proceedings of the Rehabilitation Robotics (ICORR), 2011 IEEE International Conference.* IEEE, Zurich, Switzerland, 2011.
48. Tsai B-C, Wang W-W, Hsu L-C, et al. An articulated rehabilitation robot for upper limb physiotherapy and training. *Proceedings of the Intelligent Robots and Systems (IROS), 2010 IEEE/RSJ International Conference.* IEEE, Taipei, Taiwan, 2010.
49. Gomes M A, Silveira G L M, Siqueira A A. Gait pattern adaptation for an active lower-limb orthosis based on neural networks. *Adv. Robot.*, 2011, 25(15): 1903–1925.
50. Wolbrecht E T, Reinkensmeyer D J, Bobrow J E. Pneumatic control of robots for rehabilitation. *Int. J. Robot. Res.*, 2010, 29(1): 23–38.
51. Rocon E, Belda-Lois J, Ruiz A, et al. Design and validation of a rehabilitation robotic exoskeleton for tremor assessment and suppression. *IEEE Trans. Neural. Syst. Rehabil. Eng.*, 2007, 15(3): 367–378.
52. Jezernik S, Colombo G, Keller T, et al. Robotic orthosis Lokomat: A rehabilitation and research tool. *Neuromodulation: Technol. Neural Interface*, 2003, 6(2): 108–115.
53. Tsukahara A, Hasegawa Y, Sankai Y. Gait support for complete spinal cord injury patient by synchronized leg-swing with HAL. *Proceedings of the Intelligent Robots and Systems (IROS), 2011 IEEE/RSJ International Conference.* IEEE, San Francisco, CA, 2011.
54. Unluhisarcikli O, Pietrusinski M, Weinberg B, et al. Design and control of a robotic lower extremity exoskeleton for gait rehabilitation. *Proceedings of the Intelligent Robots and Systems (IROS), 2011 IEEE/RSJ International Conference.* IEEE, San Francisco, CA, 2011.
55. Hogan N. Impedance control: An approach to manipulation. *Proceedings of the American Control Conference.* IEEE, San Francisco, CA, 1984.
56. Kiguchi K, Tanaka T, Fukuda T. Neuro-fuzzy control of a robotic exoskeleton with EMG signal. *IEEE Trans. Fuzzy Syst.*, 2004, 12(4): 481–490.
57. Miller L M, Rosen J. Comparison of multi-sensor admittance control in joint space and task space for a seven degree of freedom upper limb exoskeleton. *Proceedings of the Biomedical Robotics and Biomechatronics (BioRob), 2010 3rd IEEE RAS and EMBS International Conference.* IEEE, San Francisco, CA, 2010.
58. Yu W, Rosen J, Li X. PID admittance control for an upper limb exoskeleton. *Proceedings of the American Control Conference (ACC).* IEEE, San Francisco, CA, 2011.
59. Culmer P R, Jackson A E, Makower S, et al. A control strategy for upper limb robotic rehabilitation with a dual robot system. *IEEE ASME Trans. Mechatron.*, 2010, 15(4): 575–585.
60. Carignan C, Tang J, Roderick S. Development of an exoskeleton haptic interface for virtual task training. *Proceedings of the Intelligent Robots and Systems, 2009 IROS 2009 IEEE/RSJ International Conference.* IEEE, St. Louis, MO, 2009.
61. Aguirre-Ollinger G, Colgate J E, Peshkin M A, et al. Design of an active one-degree-of-freedom lower-limb exoskeleton with inertia compensation. *Int. J. Robot. Res.*, 2011, 30(4): 486–499.
62. Sugar T G, He J, Koeneman E J, et al. Design and control of RUPERT: A device for robotic upper extremity repetitive therapy. *IEEE Trans. Neural. Syst. Rehabil. Eng.*, 2007, 15(3): 336–346.
63. Nef T, Guidali M, Riener R. ARMin III–arm therapy exoskeleton with an ergonomic shoulder actuation. *Appl. Bionics Biomech.*, 2009, 6(2): 127–142.
64. Nef T, Mihelj M, Riener R. ARMin: A robot for patient-cooperative arm therapy. *Med. biol. Eng. Comput.*, 2007, 45(9): 887–900.
65. Frisoli A, Borelli L, Montagner A, et al. Arm rehabilitation with a robotic exoskeleleton in virtual reality. *Proceedings of the Rehabilitation Robotics, 2007 ICORR 2007 IEEE 10th International Conference.* IEEE, Noordwijk, Netherlands, 2007.
66. Letier P, Motard E, Verschueren J-P. Exostation: Haptic exoskeleton based control station. *Proceedings of the Robotics and Automation (ICRA), 2010 IEEE International Conference.* IEEE, Anchorage, AK, 2010.
67. Schiele A, Visentin G. The ESA human arm exoskeleton for space robotics telepresence. *Proceedings of the 7th International Symposium on Artificial Intelligence, Robotics and Automation in Space*, At Nara, Japan, 2003.
68. Farris R J, Quintero H A, Goldfarb M. Preliminary evaluation of a powered lower limb orthosis to aid walking in paraplegic individuals. *IEEE Trans. Neural. Syst. Rehabil. Eng.*, 2011, 19(6): 652–659.
69. Yang C, Lu Y. Study on the humachine intelligent system and its application. *Chin. J. Mech. Eng.*, 2000, 36(6): 42–47 (in Chinese).

70. Sun J, Yu Y, Ge Y, et al. Research on multi-sensors perceptual system of wearable power assist leg based on interaction force signal and joint angle signal. *J. China Univ. Sci. Tech.*, 2009, 38(12): 1432–1438 (in Chinese).

71. Fleischer C, Hommel G. Calibration of an EMG-based body model with six muscles to control a leg exoskeleton. Proceedings of the ICRA, Roma, Italy, 2007.

72. Kawamoto H, Lee S, Kanbe S, et al. Power assist method for HAL-3 using EMG-based feedback controller. *Proceedings of the Systems, Man and Cybernetics, 2003 IEEE International Conference*. IEEE, Washington, DC, 2003.

73. Burgess E M, Rappoport A. *Physical Fitness: A Guide for Individuals with Lower Limb Loss*. Darby, PA: DIANE Publishing, 1993.

74. Gailey R. Rehabilitation of a traumatic lower limb amputee. *Physiother. Res. Int.*, 1998, 3(4): 239–243.

75. Cavusoglu M C, Williams W, Tendick F, et al. Robotics for telesurgery: Second generation Berkeley/UCSF laparoscopic telesurgical workstation and looking towards the future applications. *Ind. Robot Int. J.*, 2003, 30(1): 22–29.

76. King C, Higa A T, Culjat M O, et al. A pneumatic haptic feedback actuator array for robotic surgery or simulation. *Stud. Health Tech. Inform.*, 2006, 125: 217.

77. Petzold B, Zaeh M F, Faerber B, et al. A study on visual, auditory, and haptic feedback for assembly tasks. *Presence*, 2004, 13(1): 16–21.

78. Shing C-Y, Fung C-P, Chuang T-Y, et al. The study of auditory and haptic signal in a virtual reality-based hand rehabilitation system. *Robotica*, 2003, 21(02): 211–218.

79. Kaczmarek K A, Webster J G, Bach-Y-Rita P, et al. Electrotactile and vibrotactile displays for sensory substitution systems. *IEEE Trans. Biomed. Eng.*, 1991, 38(1): 1–16.

80. Dilorenzo D J, Edell D J, Koris M J, et al. Chronic intraneural electrical stimulation for prosthetic sensory feedback. *Proceedings of the Neural Engineering, 2003 Conference Proceedings First International IEEE EMBS Conference*. IEEE, Capri Island, Italy, 2003.

81. Arieta A H, Yokoi H, Arai T, et al. Study on the effects of electrical stimulation on the pattern recognition for an EMG prosthetic application. *Proceedings of the Engineering in Medicine and Biology Society, 2005 IEEE-EMBS 2005 27th Annual International Conference*. IEEE, Shanghai, China, 2006.

82. Gasson M, Hutt B, Goodhew I, et al. Invasive neural prosthesis for neural signal detection and nerve stimulation. *Int. J. Adapt. Control Signal Process.*, 2005, 19(5): 365–375.

83. Grill W M, Mortimer J T. Electrical properties of implant encapsulation tissue. *Ann. Biomed. Eng.*, 1994, 22(1): 23–33.

84. Navarro X, Krueger T B, Lago N, et al. A critical review of interfaces with the peripheral nervous system for the control of neuroprostheses and hybrid bionic systems. *J. Peripher. Nerv. Syst.*, 2005, 10(3): 229–258.

85. Fan R E, Culjat M O, King C-H, et al. A haptic feedback system for lower-limb prostheses. *IEEE Trans. Neural. Syst. Rehabil. Eng.*, 2008, 16(3): 270–277.

86. Shinohara M, Shimizu Y, Mochizuki A. Three-dimensional tactile display for the blind. *IEEE Trans. Rehabil. Eng.*, 1998, 6(3): 249–256.

87. Summers I R, Chanter C M. A broadband tactile array on the fingertip. *J. Acoust. Soc. Am.*, 2002, 112(5): 2118–2126.

88. Haga Y, Mizushima M, Matsunaga T, et al. Medical and welfare applications of shape memory alloy microcoil actuators. *Smart Mater. Struct.*, 2005, 14(5): S266.

89. Taylor P M, Hosseini-Sianaki A, Varley C J. An electrorheological fluid-based tactile array for virtual environments. *Proceedings of the Robotics and Automation. 1996 IEEE International Conference*. IEEE, Minneapolis, MN, 1996.

90. Bicchi A, Scilingo E P, Sgambelluri N, et al. Haptic interfaces based on magnetorheological fluids. *Proceedings 2th International Conference Eurohaptics*, Edinburgh, Scotland, 2002.

91. Sabolich J A, Ortega G M, Schwabe IV G B. System and method for providing a sense of feel in a prosthetic or sensory impaired limb. Google Patents, 2002.

92. King C-H, Culjat M O, Franco M L, et al. Optimization of a pneumatic balloon tactile display for robot-assisted surgery based on human perception. *IEEE Trans. Biomed. Eng.*, 2008, 55(11): 2593–2600.

93. Ashton K. That 'internet of things' thing. *RFiD J.*, 2009, 22: 97–114.

94. Brock D L. The electronic product code (epc). Auto-ID Center White Paper MIT-AUTOID-WH-002, 2001.

95. Dirks S, Keeling M. *A Vision of Smarter Cities: How Cities Can Lead the Way into a Prosperous and Sustainable Future*. Cambridge, MA: IBM Institute for Business Value, 2009.

96. Feki M A, Kawsar F, Boussard M, et al. The internet of things: The next technological revolution. *Computer*, 2013, 46(2): 24–25.

97. Sauter T, Lobashov M. How to access factory floor information using internet technologies and gateways. *IEEE Trans. Ind. Inf.*, 2011, 7(4): 699–712.

98. Eberle S. Adaptive internet integration of field bus systems. *IEEE Trans. Ind. Inf.*, 2007, 3(1): 12–20.

99. Li X, Lu R, Liang X, et al. Smart community: an internet of things application. *IEEE Commun. Mag.*, 2011, 49(11): 68–75.

100. Tarouco L M R, Bertholdo L M, Granville L Z, et al. Internet of Things in healthcare: Interoperatibility and security issues. *Proceedings of the Communications (ICC), 2012 IEEE International Conference.* IEEE, Ottawa, ON, 2012.

101. Teller A, Stivoric J I. The BodyMedia platform: continuous body intelligence. *Proceedings of the 1st ACM Workshop on Continuous Archival and Retrieval of Personal Experiences.* ACM, Ottawa, ON, 2004.

102. Sunyaev A, Chornyi D, Mauro C, et al. Evaluation framework for personal health records: Microsoft HealthVault vs. Google Health. *Proceedings of the System Sciences (HICSS), 2010 43rd Hawaii International Conference.* IEEE, Ottawa, ON, 2010.

103. Negus K J, Stephens A P, Lansford J. HomeRF: Wireless networking for the connected home. *IEEE Pers. Commun.*, 2000, 7(1): 20–27.

104. Shilian Gao. *Practical Anatomical Atlas. Lower Extremity Fascicle.* Shanghai: Shanghai Science and Technology Publishing House, 2004 (in Chinese).

105. Xueyan Hu, Xiaopin Yun, Zhongwu Huo. Basic gait characteristics of healthy adults. *Chin. J. Rehabil. Theory Pract.*, 2006, 12: 855–857 (in Chinese).

106. Yuehong Bai, Jun Zhou, Juan Liang. Application of gait analysis in orthopaedic and rehabilitation medicine. *Orthepedic J. China.*, 2006, 14(10): 787–789 (in Chinese).

107. GB/T 10000-1988. Human dimensions of Chinese adults (in Chinese).

108. GB/T 17245-1998. Adults body mass centre (in Chinese).

109. Zhen Huang, Lingfu Kong. *Mechanism Theory and Control of Parallel Robot.* Beijing: Machinery Industry Press, 1997 (in Chinese).

110. Zixing Cai, *Robotics.* Beijing: Tsinghua University Press, 2000 (in Chinese).

111. Hoc JK. From human-machine interface to human-machine cooperation. *Ergonomics*, 2000, 43(7): 833–843.

112. Lloyd D, Besier T. An EMG-driven musculoskeletal model to estimate muscle forces and knee joint moments in vivo. *J. Biomech.*, 2003, 36(6): 765–776.

113. Buchanan T S, Lloyd D G, Manal K, et al. Neuromusculoskeletal modeling: Estimation of muscle forces and joint moments and movements from measurements of neural command. *J. Appl. Biomech.*, 2004, 20: 367–395.

114. Arnold E M,Ward S R, Lieber R L, et al. A model of the lower limb for analysis of human movement. *Ann. Biomed. Eng.*, 2010, 38(2): 269–279.

115. Peng Shang. *Study on the Mechanics Characteristics of Intact Femur and Artificial Hip Joint in Gait Cycle.* Shanghai: Shanghai Jiao Tong University, 2003 (in Chinese).

116. Wenting Ji. *Biomechanical Modelling and Application Study of Human Lower Limb Skeletal Muscle System.* Shanghai: Shanghai Jiao Tong University, 2009 (in Chinese).

117. Meng Xu. *Ergononia Simulation Analysis Objected Human Biomechanical Model.* Zhejiang: Zhejiang University, 2006 (in Chinese).

118. Yiyong Yang, Chao Hua, Rencheng Wang. Redundant muscular force analysis of lower limbs during squat lifting. *J. Tsinghua Univ. (Sci & Tech)*, 2004, 44(11): 1493–1497 (in Chinese).

119. Delp S L, Loan J P, Hoy MG, et al. An interactive graphics-based model of the lower extremity to study orthopaedic surgical procedures. *IEEE Trans. Biomed. Eng.*, 1990, 37(8):757–767.

120. Zhou S M, Xu L D. A new type of recurrent fuzzy neural network for modeling dynamic systems. *Knowl. Syst.*, 2001, 14(5): 243–251.

121. Lee W-J, Ouyang C-S, Lee S-J. Constructing neuro-fuzzy systems with TSK fuzzy rules and hybrid SVD-based learning. *Proceedings of the Fuzzy Systems, 2002 FUZZ-IEEE'02 International Conference.* IEEE, Honolulu, HI, 2002.

122. Kukolj D, Levi E. Identification of complex systems based on neural and Takagi-Sugeno fuzzy model. *IEEE Trans. Syst. Man Cybern. B Cybern.*, 2004, 34(1): 272–282.

123. Kandel E R, Schwartz J H, Jessell T M. *Principles of Neural Science.* McGraw-Hill, New York, 2000.

124. Sherrington C S. On the proprioceptive system, especially in its reflex aspect. *Brain*, 1907, 29(4): 467–482.

125. Todorov E, Jordan M I. Optimal feedback control as a theory of motor coordination. *Nat. Neurosci.*, 2002, 5(11): 1226–1235.

126. Brunnstrom S. Motor testing procedures in hemiplegia: based on sequential recovery stages. *Phys. Ther.*, 1966, 46(4): 357–375.

127. Edgerton V R, Roy R R. Activity-dependent plasticity of spinal locomotion: Implications for sensory processing. *Exerc. Sport Sci. Rev.*, 2009, 37: 171–178.

128. Veneman J F, Kruidhof R, Hekman E E G, et al. Design and evaluation of the LOPES exoskeleton robot for interactive gait rehabilitation. *IEEE Trans. Neural. Syst. Rehabil. Eng.*, 2007, 15(3): 379–386.

129. Knaepen K, Beyl P, Duerinck S., et al. Human-robot interaction: kinematics and muscle activity inside a powered compliant knee exoskeleton. *IEEE Trans. Neural. Syst. Rehabil. Eng.*, 2014, 22(6): 1128–1137.

130. Aguirre-Ollinger G., Colgate J E, Peshkin M A, et al. Inertia compensation control of a one-degree-of-freedom exoskeleton for lower-limb assistance: initial experiments. *IEEE Trans. Neural. Syst. Rehabil. Eng.*, 2012, 20(1): 68–77.

131. Vallery H, Duschau-Wicke A, Riener R. Optimized passive dynamics improve transparency of haptic devices. *Proceedings of the IEEE International Conference on Robotics and Automation*, Kobe, 2009, pp. 301–306.

132. Vallery H, Guidali M, Duschau-Wicke A, et al. Patient cooperative control: Providing safe support without restricting movement. *Proceedings of the IFMBE*, Munich, Germany, 2009, pp. 166–169.

133. Ronsse R, Vitiello N, Lenzi T, et al. Human-robot synchrony: Flexible assistance using adaptive oscillators. *IEEE Trans. Biomed. Eng.*, 2011, 58(4): 1001–1012.

134. Ronsse R, Vitiello N, Lenzi T, et al. Adaptive oscillators with human-in-the-loop: Proof of concept for assistance and rehabilitation. *Proceedings of the 3rd IEEE RAS & EMBS International Conference on Biomedical Robotics and Biomechatronics*, Tokyo, 2010, pp. 668–674.

135. Chen X, Yin Y H. A highly efficient semiphenomenological model of a half-sarcomere for real-time prediction of mechanical behavior. *J. Biomech. Eng.*, 2014, 136: 121001-1–121001-9.

136. Chen X, Yin Y H, Fan Y J. EMG oscillator model-based energy kernel method for characterizing muscle intrinsic property under isometric contraction. *Chin. Sci. Bull.*, 2014, 59(14): 1556–1567.

137. Huxley A F. Muscular contraction. *J. Physiol.*, 1974, 243(1): 1–43.

138. Yu C C, Liu B D. A backpropagation algorithm with adaptive learning rate and momentum coefficient. *IEEE Proceedings of the 2002 International Joint Conference on Neural Networks, IJCNN'02*, Honolulu, HI, 2002, pp. 1218–1223.

139. Fan Y, Yin Y. Active and progressive exoskeleton rehabilitation using multisource information fusion from EMG and force-position EPP. *IEEE Trans. Biomed. Eng.*, 2013, 60(12): 3314–3321.

140. Riener R, Lunenburger L, Jezernik S, et al. Patient-cooperative strategies for robot-aided treadmill training: First experimental results. *IEEE Trans. Neural. Syst. Rehabil. Eng.*, 2005, 13(3): 380–394.

141. Banala S K, Kim S H, Agrawal S K, et al. Robot assisted gait training with active leg exoskeleton (ALEX). *IEEE Trans. Neural. Syst. Rehabil. Eng.*, 2009, 17(1): 2–8.

142. Wang S, Wang L, Meijneke C, et al., Design and control of the MINDWALKER exoskeleton. *IEEE Trans. Neural. Syst. Rehabil. Eng.*, 2015, 23(2): 277–286.

5 Clinical Rehabilitation Technologies for Force-Control–Based Exoskeleton Robot

Based on the developed rehabilitation system and control strategy illustrated in former chapters, the detailed condition and requirements for patients with lower-extremity motor injuries such as stroke have been illustrated. Moreover, based on the different requirements in the rehabilitation process, effective passive and active rehabilitation strategies are generated, and the progressive rehabilitation strategy is also proposed to increase the treatment performance, safety, and comfort during the process. Meanwhile, the intelligent management method has also been proposed for the medical resources including the rehabilitation robot to increase the utilization ratio of medical resources to provide better treatment for more patients in time. At last, the safety, usability, and effectiveness of the developed rehabilitation system have been proven through preliminary clinical experiments.

5.1 SYSTEM INTEGRATION FOR LOWER-EXTREMITY EXOSKELETON REHABILITATION ROBOT

The exoskeleton rehabilitation robot system is composed of two main parts: the mechanical structure and control system. The key points in designing exoskeleton robot and its mechanical structure have been discussed in Chapter 4, together with the motor requirements for human lower extremity. The implementation of the exoskeleton robot system will be discussed in this chapter. There should also be a complete control strategy for the robot system and an appropriate rehabilitation strategy for clinical patients. Referring to the existing exoskeleton robot systems, some successful cases include the HAL [1,2], Lokomat [3], lower-extremity powered exoskeleton (LOPES) [4], etc. All these robot systems provide corresponding rehabilitation strategy for training that matches human motion. Enlightened by the above robot systems, our research group developed the hardware system for exoskeleton robot and proposed two rehabilitation modes for different rehabilitation strategies and training methods aiming at different objectives. One is the passive rehabilitation training mode. In this mode, exoskeleton robot drives human to do passive training, during which the robot is the actuator and human is the load. The other mode is the active rehabilitation training mode that puts human in the central role. Human does the exercises based on his/her own intention, which is also the main challenge for exoskeleton robot control. Based on the current research progress, there is a need for effective human–machine interaction interface to control the system based on electromyography (EMG) signal or force tactile signal. For instance, HAL exoskeleton robot adopts artificial neural network to do pattern recognition and prediction control using EMG signal [1]. Kong made use of the contact force information to predict joint angle and control the exoskeleton robot to assist the aged to walk [5]. As EMG signal reflects human muscle force, referring to the process of human–machine interactive force experiment, measuring the EMG signal of muscle is able to predict human muscle contraction force and joint torque, and it can be integrated with the interactive force information between human and exoskeleton measured by force sensor, and it acts as the information source for exoskeleton active training to understand human motion intention, thus controlling the exoskeleton actively and helping the patients to do active rehabilitation.

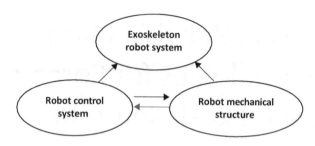

FIGURE 5.1   Exoskeleton robot system components.

As illustrated in Figure 5.1, the exoskeleton robot system is composed of mechanical structure and control system. The mechanical structure is able to meet the requirements of force assistance, gait training, width adjustment, height adjustment, and body support. Hardware and software systems are applied to control the exoskeleton robot to move as required. In the practical clinical application, the robot system generates various rehabilitation strategies for different patients and performs different modes of rehabilitation training to meet the rehabilitation requirements and enhance training effect.

5.1.1 MECHANICAL STRUCTURE OF REHABILITATION ROBOT

Based on the design scheme of lower-extremity exoskeleton robot proposed in Chapter 1, the robot system is developed as illustrated in Figure 5.2. The mechanical structure includes the exoskeleton legs, suspension supporting system, mobile platform, and width adjustment structure. Among them, the suspension supporting system is located on a slider of a linear motion unit (electric cylinder) to adjust the height of the whole exoskeleton system and meet the requirements of people with different heights. The linear motion unit is fixed on the front of control cabinet of mobile platform. The mechanical leg is connected with the width adjustment structure. The joint appliance is fixed inside the mechanical leg to protect human. There are safety belts on the suspension supporting structure. When patients wear the belt, a part of the body weight will be supported by the supporting mechanism to decrease the load on exoskeleton joints.

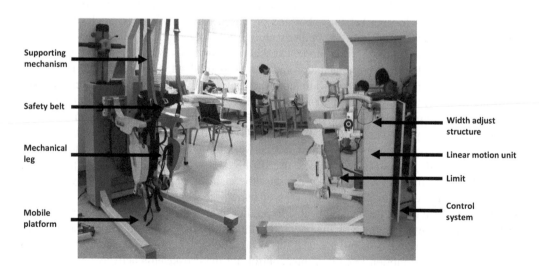

FIGURE 5.2   The developed exoskeleton robot system.

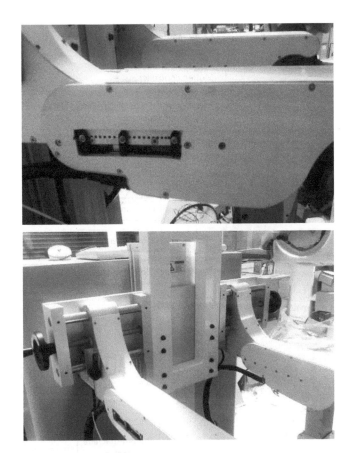

FIGURE 5.3 Safety limits and width adjustment mechanism.

The safety limits and width adjustment mechanism are illustrated in Figure 5.3. The electric position limit switches are adopted as the soft limits, while there are also hard limits in the mechanical structure. There are also safety bottom under the exoskeleton thigh so that patients can receive comprehensive protection when using the exoskeleton. Ball screw transmission is adopted in the width adjustment mechanism. One can rotate the hand shank to adjust the width between two mechanical legs to adapt to people of different sizes.

5.1.2 Rehabilitation Robot Control System

The hardware of exoskeleton robot control system includes the controller, servo motor, actuator, human–machine interface, and peripheral circuit. The controller includes the central processer and the motion controller. The control flow of the system is illustrated in Figure 5.4. First, the doctor generates corresponding rehabilitation strategy based on patients' rehabilitation training requirements. The motion generation and inverse kinematic solution are treated in the central processing unit (CPU) of the computer. The action command is sent to the motion controller, generating pulse signal to the motor actuator to control the servo motor and drive the exoskeleton robot to move. The joint angle, EMG signal, and interactive force are detected by the human–machine interface, and the information is sent to the controller to compose the closed loop.

The components of hardware and software of the control system are introduced as follows.

Controller: Integrated machine produced by Googol Tech Company is selected (model number: GUC-800-TPV/TPG-M0X-L2, Figure 5.5). It is a product integrating CPU (embedded PC) and

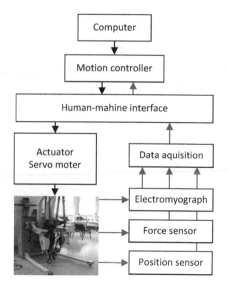

FIGURE 5.4 System control flow.

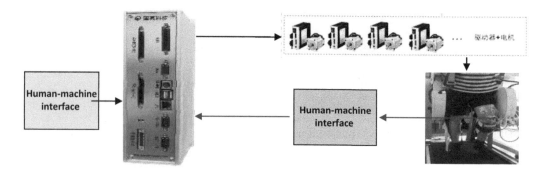

FIGURE 5.5 Hardware for control system.

motion controller. Comparing with the control system composed of industrial computer and motion controller, it has higher reliability, stability, disturbance resistance, and a smaller volume [6], making it suitable for acting as the control kernel. The motion controller is based on the servo motor controller based on digital signal processing (DSP), and it also provides extended interface for fast I/O filed bus, satisfying the requirements of multiple I/O control. Then, the signal from the position limit switch can also be acquired to protect patients' safety.

CPU: It analyzes the signal and generates motion based on the doctor's order. Signal processing refers to digital filtering and conditioning of the signal acquired by data acquisition card. Motion generation unit does the inverse kinematics solution and generates the motion orders based on the processed signal, robot training mode, and the physical dimensions of the robot. The control command is then sent to the motion controller. The computer also has the function of training, monitoring, real-time display, and data recording. They are all realized by the developed rehabilitation software.

Drive unit: Panasonic AC servo motor and actuator are selected (model number: MSMD, Figure 5.6). The servo motor has three control modes: the position, velocity, and torque modes. Based on the analysis in Chapter 1, the motor power values of hip and knee joints are 400 and 200 W, respectively. The motor for supporting mechanism is 750 W with the rated speed of 3,000 rpm. When the motion control card receives the action command from CPU, it programs the motion and sends it to the servo actuator and drives the motor to work.

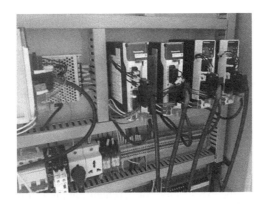

FIGURE 5.6 Servo actuator and peripheral circuit.

5.1.3 Rehabilitation Strategy Generation

Referring to the statistical results of lower-extremity diseases, the patients mainly have lower-extremity joint diseases, hemiplegia, paraplegia, stroke, or nerve injuries. All these patients could be the rehabilitation objects of the exoskeleton robot.

Based on the requirements from the doctor, the evaluation should be done to determine the disease grade before the rehabilitation training is carried out. There are various evaluation methods for different kinds of patients. Some international general evaluation methods are adopted [7]. Evaluation methods for joint disease include Hospital for Special Surgery (HSS) for knee joint and Harris hip score. Evaluation method for hemiplegia is Brunnstrom method. The muscle contraction force can also be evaluated. These evaluation methods are all directed by the software in the computer. Doctors are able to do the evaluation and compare the rehabilitation results with the condition before the training.

The evaluation indices include the parameters, such as joint range of motion (ROM), EMG signal intensity, and muscle force. The data can all be acquired through the human–machine interaction interface of the exoskeleton system and is integrated with the observation of the patients to determine the disease grade.

After the motor ability of the patients are determined by the doctors, corresponding rehabilitation strategy is generated. Then, command is given to control the exoskeleton robot to do the rehabilitation exercise so that the muscle contraction ability of the patients could be increased gradually. In the early stage of rehabilitation training, exoskeleton robot drives the lower extremity of patients to move according to the preset gait or angle. The training is passive. As the rehabilitation process goes forward, patients' lower-limb strength increases, and the walking ability recovers. Patients are expected to take active part in the rehabilitation training process and walk based on their own intention. Exoskeleton robot must be able to recognize patient motion intention quickly to assist patients to walk. Thus, different rehabilitation strategies should be selected in different training stages. The training strategy summarized in this book is listed in Table 5.1, which covers the whole

TABLE 5.1
Rehabilitation Strategy

Early Stage Passive Rehabilitation	Midterm Semi-Active Rehabilitation	Later Stage Active Rehabilitation
1. Patient is flaccid paralyzed and cannot move.	1. Patient's muscle is partly recovered.	1. Patients are able to do some activities.
2. Robot is used to replace human lower limb to move.	2. Passive training and active training are combined.	2. Active control.
3. Joint training and gait training.	3. EMG signal enforcement training.	3. Function training and muscle force training.

rehabilitation process. In the early stage of training, patient follows the motion of robot to recover the motor ability gradually so that muscle could contract to certain extent. EMG signal could be measured to calculate the muscle force representing the recovery degree. During the middle stage of the rehabilitation training, active training could be done integrating the patient's motion intention. Exoskeleton provides assistive force for patients to compensate for the lack of muscle force. The passive training should be combined with active training to help the patients. In the later stage of rehabilitation training, the active control of exoskeleton is implemented to realize human motion and decrease the patient's dependence on the robot.

5.1.4 Rehabilitation Robot System Software

Based on the above analyses, the exoskeleton robot rehabilitation training system software is developed using Microsoft Visual Basic 6.0. An efficient human–machine interaction control interface is also developed to provide convenience for doctors to manipulate and control the system. The software is mainly used to do rehabilitation training for patients with lower-extremity diseases (including patients with lower-extremity joint diseases, hemiplegia, paraplegia, stroke, nerve injuries) so that they can recover muscle force and walking ability.

Main functions: The lower-extremity exoskeleton robot is controlled to move according to scientific data to help patients with lower-limb disease to undergo rehabilitation training.

1. There are four rehabilitation training modes for a patient's lower extremity: passive flexion/extension (F/E), passive gait, active F/E, and active gait. The training parameters, such as stride, frequency of stride, and training times, are able to change according to the practical training requirements. The joint angle, velocity, position could all be displayed in the four modes. There are also functional buttons such as start and stop.
2. Patient information management: There is database storing patient training information, basic information, and evaluation information.
3. Rehabilitation evaluation: Patients' current lower-extremity rehabilitation condition can be evaluated to assess the rehabilitation effectiveness
4. 3D gait simulation: It is used to simulate the 3D dynamic model for the gait training of patients.
5. Training data display: It is used to display the joint angle and velocity curves in the training process in real time.

Main characteristics:

1. Safe: The software is able to do self-check to avoid the abnormal working conditions and protect patients' safety.
2. Scientific: The manipulation flow of the software is developed based on standard rehabilitation processes. The training mode and gait data are recognized by doctors.
3. Rich in functions: Doctors could select different training modes and parameters based on the disease conditions of patients.
4. Friendly in human–machine interface: The software is able to simulate human gait in 3D. The joint angle, velocity, position could all be displayed in real time. The software includes one startup interface (Figure 5.7) and 11 main operation interfaces to provide user convenience.

The prescription interface is illustrated in Figure 5.8. The training mode and training parameters can be selected in this panel, and 3D motion simulation can also be displayed. The resulting output interface is illustrated in Figure 5.9. It is used to monitor the joint training conditions in real time, display the acquired muscle EMG signal, joint angle, and interactive force and is responsible for the start and stop controls of the system.

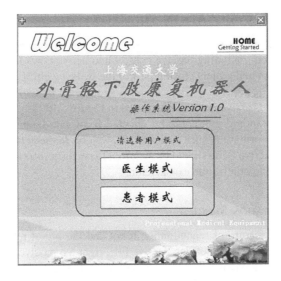

FIGURE 5.7 Startup interface.

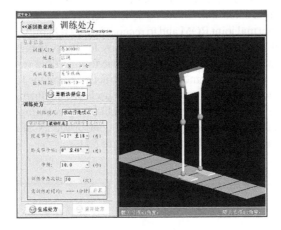

FIGURE 5.8 Prescription generation.

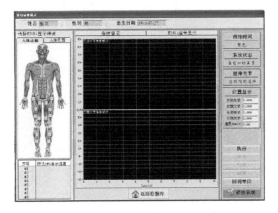

FIGURE 5.9 Training result display.

5.2 COMPOUND REHABILITATION STRATEGY

Based on the above rehabilitation training modes, the control strategies of the exoskeleton robot system should be generated, including passive control and active control. Passive control mode is suitable for critical patients and patients losing part of the walking ability. It uses the standard data (gait, joint angle) to train the patients. Active control is suitable for patients with motor abilities. The control flow of exoskeleton robot system is illustrated in Figure 5.10.

In the passive mode, standard gait could be selected from gait database to do passive training based on patients' basic information, such as height and weight. In the active mode, EMG signal and human–exoskeleton interactive force should be acquired to perform information fusion to recognize human motion intention and control the exoskeleton.

5.2.1 PASSIVE REHABILITATION STRATEGY

Based on the mechanical feature of rehabilitation robot and the preset rehabilitation requirements, passive rehabilitation mode includes left leg passive F/E, right leg passive F/E, two-leg passive F/E, left leg passive gait, right leg passive gait, two-leg passive gait. This mode is mainly for the patients with lower-extremity injuries who did not have physiotherapy after the operation. There is always joint adhesion for these patients because of lack of exercise for a long time. This would lead to the limited joint ROM, which is smaller than that of normal people. Some physical therapy means, such as external assistive flexion and extension, should be done to relieve joint adhesion. These would help the patients to recover to the normal joint ROM and to receive further rehabilitation treatment. Meanwhile, this mode is also helpful in doing assistive physiotherapy for the patients who have lost their motor function, protecting the patients from muscle atrophy due to long-time rest. It can also stimulate the inverted motor nerve channels and promote the reconstruction of motor functions. Human–machine interactive forces are detected in real time, preventing muscle spasm during the motion process.

There are two rehabilitation methods in passive rehabilitation training: one is joint passive training, and the other is gait passive training. They both control the exoskeleton angle to follow the preset value based on kinematics, as illustrated in Figure 5.11.

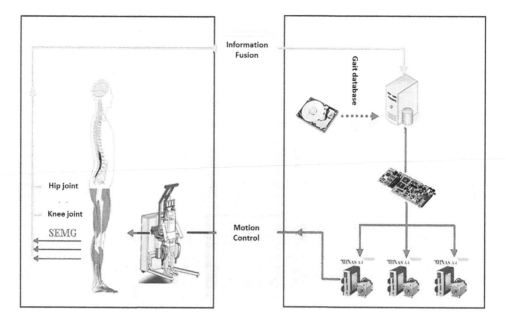

FIGURE 5.10 Control flow of exoskeleton robot system.

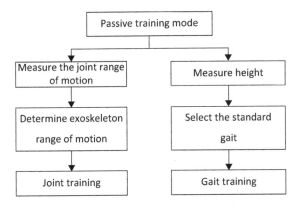

FIGURE 5.11   Passive training methods.

Joint passive training: Statistics shows that among all the patients taking rehabilitation training, joint patients make up a large portion. Joint passive training is for this kind of patients and provides force assistive training for the knee joint and hip joint. The training method is to determine the exoskeleton joint ROM first based on the patients' maximum joint ROM. Then the patient's leg is bound with the exoskeleton, and the joint motion training is implemented under different joints and velocities.

Passive gait training: The height of patient is first measured and the corresponding gait data would be selected from the standard gait database. The inverse kinematics solution and the joint motion data are acquired via the computer. All the servo motors are controlled so that the coordination motion of all the exoskeleton joints could be achieved, which is synchronous to the standard gait. Patients follow the exoskeleton robot to do the standard gait training and recover their motor function gradually and further rectify their walking posture.

The robot control flow is illustrated in Figure 5.12. The two training modes, including the gait training and joint training, are provided by the computer for the doctors. After determining the disease of the patient, the doctor selects the passive rehabilitation mode and sends the motion command to the motion controller in lower-level computer. The controller directly drives the exoskeleton joint motion, and the joint information is fed back by the encoder on the servo motor to achieve the position-loop control for exoskeleton joints. The exoskeleton drives the patient's joint to move, thus achieving the passive gait or joint training.

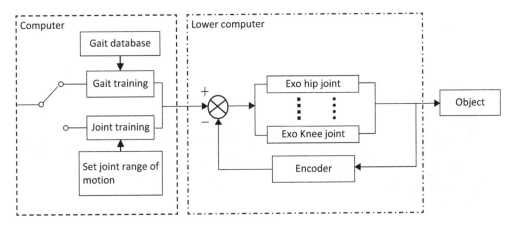

FIGURE 5.12   Passive control strategy.

5.2.2 ACTIVE REHABILITATION STRATEGY

The rehabilitation modes introduced above are further divided into two classes, i.e., the assistive force mode and resistive force mode. The rehabilitation mode is mainly for the patients who had a long time in bed because of stroke or operation. This would give rise to muscle atrophy and disability to perform some basic daily activities. Active rehabilitation training is able to help these patients relieve muscle atrophy, recover muscle contraction, and get used to gait with load gradually. Human–machine interactive forces and sEMG signal are detected in real time to evaluate rehabilitation status. As active training mode consumes more strength, this would prevent muscle spasm and over fatigue during the motion process.

Active control strategy is achieved by human–machine interaction interface. In the later stage of rehabilitation training, muscle contraction is recovered to some extent, but the contraction force is still not enough to drive human joint motion effectively. Thus, exoskeleton is expected to provide force compensation so that the patient is able to move on his own intention with the help of robot.

Based on the analysis in the former chapter, the actual muscle force and joint torque can be acquired through skeletal muscle force model and the collected EMG signal. The force information is used to control the exoskeleton robot and act as the predicted torque of human motion intention. The torque mode is applied to control the exoskeleton. In this process, exoskeleton provides the required torque which acts as the assistive force. The interactive force between human and exoskeleton is detected in real time to evaluate the training efficacy.

The flow chart of active control strategy is illustrated in Figure 5.13. Human–machine interface collects the EMG signal and joint angle. They are integrated together to predict active muscle contraction force and the active torque on the joints. The force provided by exoskeleton joint to human is also predicted and amplified to act as the reference for human motion. Then, the motion driving torque is calculated using inverse dynamics of exoskeleton joint, which is actually the torque provided by exoskeleton to human. The information is used as the input to control the servo motor on exoskeleton joints. The motor works on torque mode and drives the exoskeleton joint to perform force compensation so that the exoskeleton could move with human intention.

5.2.3 PROGRESSIVE REHABILITATION STRATEGY

To achieve effective and suitable physical rehabilitation treatment, personalized progressive rehabilitation strategy is proposed, as shown in Figure 5.14. The strategy is realized by a monitoring system and an active compliance controller, in which the monitoring system determines the rehabilitation mode and rehabilitation system parameters by real-time motion decoding and status evaluation algorithm.

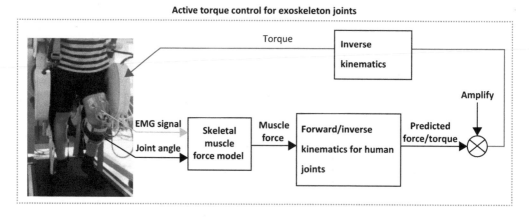

FIGURE 5.13 Active control strategy.

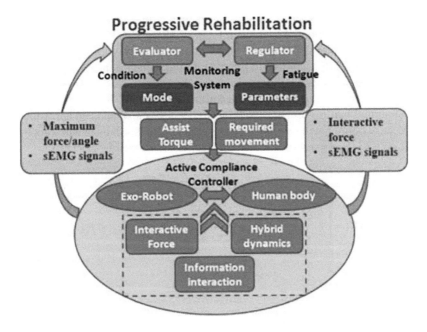

FIGURE 5.14 Progressive rehabilitation strategy.

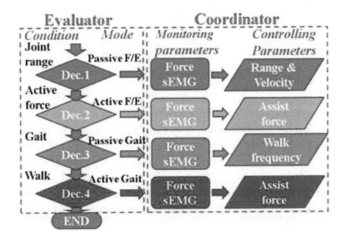

FIGURE 5.15 Updating parameters based on real-time monitoring and evaluation.

The active compliance controller enables the exoskeleton to perform the coordinated motion of human–exoskeleton system by the rehabilitation mode and parameters set by the monitoring system, the pre-developed dynamic model for human–machine system, and the interactive force during the process.

Progressive rehabilitation is achieved by monitoring the patient's condition and updating the parameters of the control system in real time. According to the suggestion of a doctor specialized in rehabilitation of poststroke patients, four commonly used progressive rehabilitation modes are applied: passive flexion/extension (F/E), active F/E, passive gait training, and active gait training with full body weight support, as shown in Figure 5.15. The parameters that determine the assistive torque, movement range, and frequency are decided by a regulator based on interactive force and sEMG signal. Switching between different treatments is done via an evaluator according to the following rules: If the interactive force is bigger than a threshold, F_{sec}, flexion (extension) will be turned into extension (flexion). As shown in Figure 5.15, passive F/E mode will be chosen when human joint ROM is smaller than the set value. Interactive force will be also used to determine the frequency of passive F/E according to Eq. (5.1). In the second step, active force of human joint will be evaluated, and active F/E will be executed if the active force is smaller than the threshold. Assistive force is determined by the sEMG according to Eq. (5.2). In the third step, passive walk is applied if abnormal gait is observed. Walking frequency is also updated according to Eq. (5.1). Finally, active walk training will be implemented if the patient is still unable to walk independently. Similar to the active F/E, the assistive force will also be determined by Eq. (5.2).

$$r = r_0 - k_r F_{int} \cdot \text{sgn}\left(\dot{\theta}\right), \left(\left|F_{int}\right| \le F_{sec}\right), \tag{5.1}$$

$$F_A = \left(F_0 - k_F \int_0^T \frac{F_{sEMG} \cdot \text{sgn}\left(\dot{\theta}\right)}{T} dt\right) \bigg/ l_{fatigue}, \left(\left|F_{int}\right| \le F_{sec}\right), \tag{5.2}$$

$$l_{fatigue} = k_l \left(\tau_{ave} - \tau_0\right) + 1, \tag{5.3}$$

in which r—desired frequency
r_0—set frequency for rehabilitation
k_r, k_F—compensation coefficients
F_{int}—the interactive force
$\text{sgn}\left(\dot{\theta}\right)$—sign function that is related with the direction of rotation
F_A—desired assistive force
F_0—preliminary set assistive force
F_{sEMG}—active human force that is derived from sEMG signal via the method that is described in former sections
T—period of one repetition.

It is reasonable that muscle and mental fatigue will result in time extension of repetitive training in general. Thus, fatigue level, $l_{fatigue}$ is evaluated by Eq. (5.3), where k_l is the fatigue coefficient, τ_{ave} is the average period of three repetitions, and τ_0 is the average period of first three repetitions. F_A will be updated in every repetition. Since fatigue is a relative long-term effect, $l_{fatigue}$ will be updated after every three repetitions.

During the rehabilitation process of all the modes, the structure will automatically transfer from flexion (extension) to extension (flexion) to prevent muscle injuries caused by continuous physical rehabilitation treatment under muscle spasm.

5.2.4 IoT-Based Remote Rehabilitation Strategy

The growing trend of population aging poses many challenges, which have to be dealt with realistically. One of the challenges is the rehabilitation of the elderly, which consumes time, resources, and manpower. The trend of community facilitation of rehabilitation treatment has become popular in recent years [8]. Compared with the traditional local hospital rehabilitation, community-based smart rehabilitation is aimed at providing convenience, effective treatment, adequate interaction, and quick reconfiguration to make the maximum use of the medical resources according to patients' specific requirements possible. Internet of Things (IoT) technology makes it possible [9]. IoT encompasses a set of technologies that enable a wide range of appliances, devices, and objects or things to interact and communicate among themselves using networking technologies [10,11]. Healthcare systems use a set of interconnected devices to create an IoT network devoted to healthcare assessment, including monitoring patients and automatically detecting situations, where medical interventions

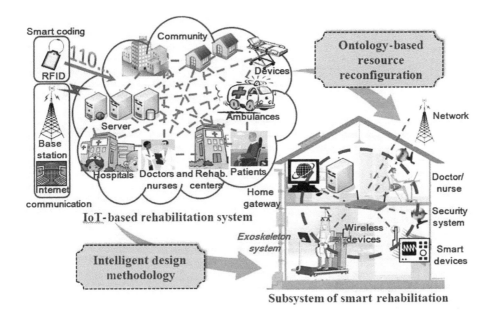

FIGURE 5.16 Prototype of IoT-based smart rehabilitation system. The upper left corner shows that all the medical resources are interconnected with each other in the established system by Ethernet with TCP/IP and each of the devices is allocated a user identification (UID). Automation of design method is applied to build an effective rehabilitation subsystem for a specific patient according to the registered medical resources efficiently, as shown in the lower right corner.

are required [12]. The general system collects information from different sensing devices through a middleware that provides interoperability and security needed in the context of IoT for healthcare. Monitoring devices are connected via wireless networking technology. The monitoring application's front end, which is functionally similar to a network manager, is responsible for storing, aggregating, consolidating, and security alarming.

As illustrated in Figure 5.16, the system is featured with three parts: the master, the server, and the things. The devices of the subsystem are connected to a gateway device by Wi-Fi to form a local area network (LAN), and the subsystem can also communicate with others or the wide area network (WAN) through the gateway device by common TCP/IP Protocol. Meanwhile, the location information is collected by GPS that is integrated in the medical resources. The master represents doctors, nurses, and patients providing specific permissions to the system through end-user devices such as smartphone, personal computer (PC), or tablet. The healthcare application determines the requirement of a rehabilitation system, and it is also regarded as the master. The things include smart IoT devices, patients, and human resources that are connected by WAN, multimedia technology, or short message service (SMS). Furthermore, although normal devices cannot connect to the network itself, they are still commonly used and are essential in current rehabilitation. These devices are included in the smart rehabilitation system and connected to the network by allocating RFID tags. The server is the central part of the system. It is responsible for data recording, data analysis, permission control, rehabilitation strategy creation, subsystem building, and device control.

The operation process is illustrated in Figure 5.17, and it includes three levels, human–IoT rehabilitation system interaction interface, system optimization platform based on intelligent design method, and information and application management platform.

Interaction interface platform: Users input symptom, rehabilitation requirement, and personalized requirements (including cost, treatment time, etc.) into the system through this interface. Meanwhile, system will send the information, such as rehabilitation strategy and status, to users in the form of word, voice, video, or virtual reality.

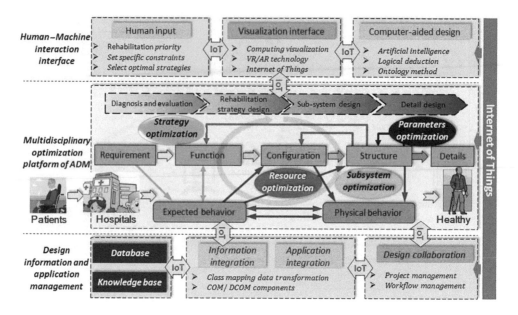

FIGURE 5.17 Schematic diagram of the IoT-based remote rehabilitation system.

Information and application management platform: It is mainly composed of database and expert knowledge base. It collects all the related information (including basic information, service information, location, status, and others) concerning patients, doctors, and devices and stores them in the database. It then acts as the reference for doctors and patients based on all the cases and expert knowledge base. Meanwhile, the data transmission is achieved by network information management, and unified information management of different departments is performed by the process management module.

System optimization platform based on intelligent design method: It is the core part of the smart rehabilitation system. The rehabilitation process can be divided into four stages: diagnosis and evaluation, rehabilitation strategy design, subsystem design, and detailed design, as illustrated in Figure 5.17. When patients first log into the system, their disease symptoms are analyzed, and the treatment requirements are listed. Then, corresponding functions are put forward for further resource allocation. In this process, the patients input the information in the format specifications defined by related ontologies. This is for the purpose that the information is well organized and subsequent analysis can be done more precisely. During the process, the specific rehabilitation activity is extracted from the "Requirement" put forward by the patient, and the mapping relation with "Expected behavior", which means the desired effect, is also established. These activities all belong to the diagnosis and evaluation stage. There are two tasks in the second stage, rehabilitation strategy design stage, which is also the most important stage. One is the generation of prescription. It is done first by the system based on the numerous cases stored in the database to produce the preliminary rehabilitation strategy. Then it will be checked by doctors from different departments through the consultation. Detailed steps will be illustrated later in this section. The other is the allocation of medical recourses for a specific patient. It is evident that there is gap between the "Expected behavior" (the desired treatment effect) and the "Physical behavior" (the actual therapeutic effect). This is where optimization happens. The third stage deals with conflicts that arise from meeting the requirements of various patients' rehabilitation strategies. Thus, the optimization first takes place in the "Structure" of the subsystem to make some minor modification. If the changes in the subsystem cannot solve the problems, then the reconfiguration will happen in the "Configuration" or even the "Function" model to have them rebuilt again. The last stage, the detailed design stage, determines all the parameters and corresponding parametric optimizations.

5.3 CLINICAL REHABILITATION EXPERIMENTS

5.3.1 ZERO-LOAD CHECK OF EXOSKELETON ROBOT

To test the performance of the robot system, the exoskeleton robot undergoes a long run based on the preset program. As illustrated in Figure 5.18, self-check of the robot is first performed before experiments. Joints rotate one by one to calculate the ROM and determine the working space of the system.

Then, the joint motion ranges are set, and the position information of each joint is read from the encoder of the servo motor and transformed into the practical joint angle, so the theoretical value can be compared with the practical position, which determines the control accuracy of the system. Figure 5.19

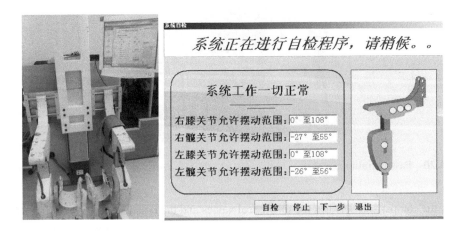

FIGURE 5.18 Self-check of the robot system.

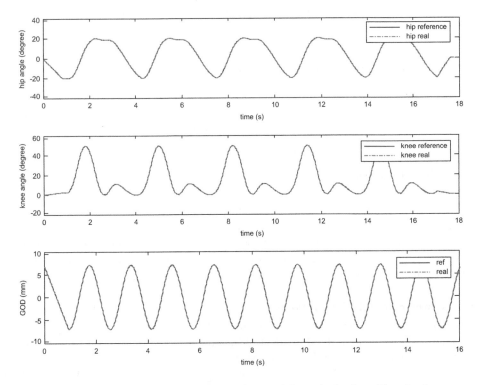

FIGURE 5.19 Comparison between the practical position and theoretical value with no load.

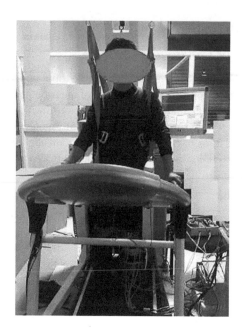

FIGURE 5.20 Passive training.

illustrates the comparison between the theoretical values and the practical positions of hip joint, knee joint, and the supporting mechanism of the robot system. After the system works under the training mode for a period of time, the position data of exoskeleton joint is recorded with the sampling interval of 50 ms. Thus, the motor position response curve can be compared with theoretical curve. The two groups of data agree well, indicating the exoskeleton robot system has a high response speed and control accuracy.

5.3.2 Application Experiment of Exoskeleton Rehabilitation Robot

Before the exoskeleton robot is used in clinical applications, debugging of various training modes should be done to test the training efficacy. It is first tested on healthy people as illustrated in Figure 5.20. The subject with the height of 170 cm and the weight of 65 kg is bound with the exoskeleton.

5.3.2.1 Joint F/E Training

First the ROM is set for each joint. Reciprocating motion is performed for human legs driven by exoskeleton joints. As illustrated in Figure 5.21, the knee joint ROM is 0°–60°, and hip joint ROM is 0°–15°. The period of motion is 6.5 s. When loads are present, exoskeleton joint follows well the theoretical values. Human weight is loaded on the exoskeleton with little influence on system operation. The performance is almost the same as that without any load, indicating that the exoskeleton has a good loading capacity.

5.3.2.2 Lower-Extremity Gait Training

Similarly, the passive gait mode can be selected to conduct the rehabilitation training. First, set the gait period as 8 s. The hip joint ROM is −18° to 18°, and knee joint ROM is 0° to 45°. The variation of center of gravity is −7 to 7 mm. Human is driven by exoskeleton to do the gait training with the data recorded as illustrated in Figure 5.22. It can be inferred that the exoskeleton is able to drive human motion easily with a fast system response time.

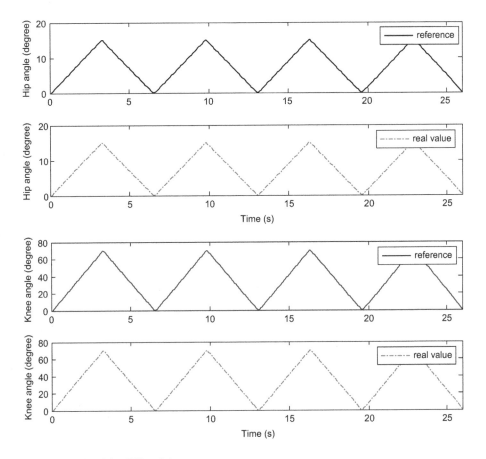

FIGURE 5.21 Passive joint F/E training.

5.3.2.3 Active Muscle Force Training

Active muscle force training is a kind of training mode in which rehabilitation subjects take an active role. Human–machine interaction interface (gasbag, EMG DAQ instrument, and other devices) is adopted in the training process. Impedance is provided by the exoskeleton robot to the patient. Subjects could raise or hold back the leg to generate active contraction force to overcome the impedance of exoskeleton. Through continuous raising and holding back of legs, muscle contraction force can be strengthened. The training modes include isometric contraction training and isokinetic contraction training (Figure 5.23).

1. **Isometric contraction training**: While doing isometric contraction training, the exoskeleton's joint angle is fixed. The gasbag is bound with human leg, and human joints are fixed. When the training starts, set the hip joint and knee joint of exoskeleton as 30° and 45° so that human legs are fixed. Then, the gasbag is charged, and F/E of calf is repeated to train the thigh muscles. In this process, the gasbag pressure and the EMG signal of each muscle are recorded, as illustrated in Figure 5.24. Referring to the figure, a group of antagonistic muscles, including the quadriceps femoris, biceps femoris, semitendinosus, and semimembranosus, are responsible for the extension and flexion of knee joint, respectively. When human calf extends forward, the EMG signal of quadriceps femoris is stronger. When calf flexes backward, the EMG signals of biceps femoris, semitendinosus, and semimembranosus are stronger. The muscle force can be calculated by force models to represent the training efficacy, as illustrated in Figure 5.25.

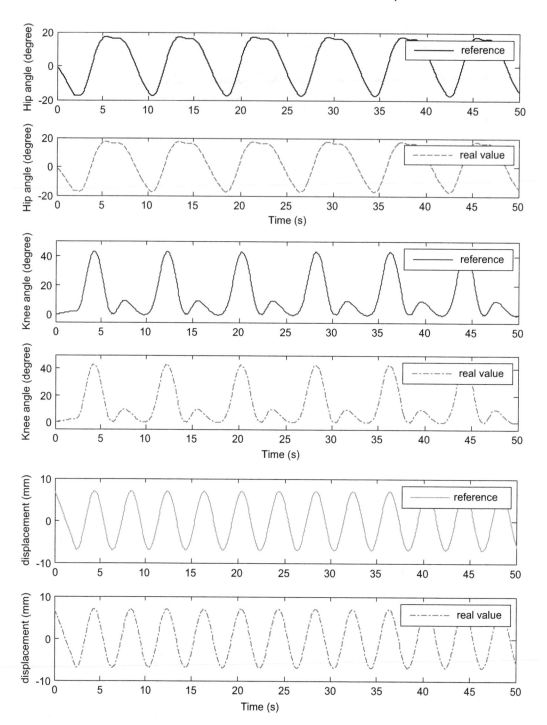

FIGURE 5.22   Passive gait training.

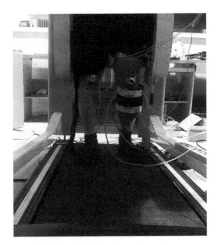

FIGURE 5.23 Active muscle force training.

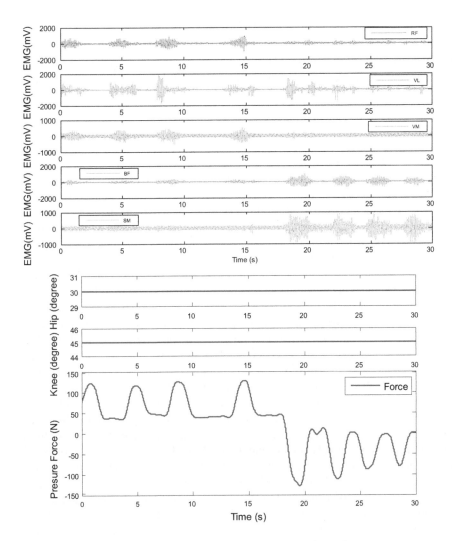

FIGURE 5.24 EMG signal, joint angle, and gasbag interactive force of muscles.

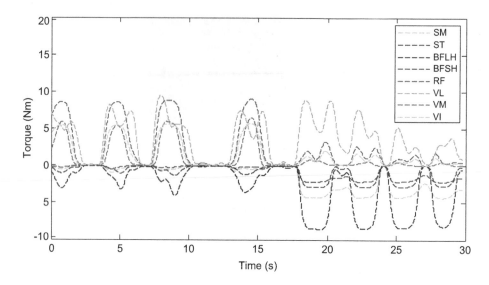

FIGURE 5.25   Active torques generated by each muscle contraction.

2. **Isokinetic contraction training**: Here, the training mechanism is the same as the isometric contraction training, except that exoskeleton joints move with a certain velocity. The bound leg of the subject follows the motion of the exoskeleton joint. When the leg extends forward, muscle contracts actively against exoskeleton joint motion. The interactive force is recorded by the gasbag (Figure 5.26).

5.3.2.4   Active Control Training

Active control training aims at controlling exoskeleton robot to move based on human motion intention. Moreover, exoskeleton will provide active assistive force to human joints. Based on the active control strategy, human–machine interface should be applied and the motor should work in the torque mode. First, human EMG signal is collected by myoelectric apparatus. The required torque for human joint motion is then predicted using the muscle force model and is sent to the servo motor on the exoskeleton joint as control signal. The motor provides corresponding torque for human joint and makes it possible for the joint to move in the labor saving mode. Thus, the active control of exoskeleton robot can be achieved. On the other hand, the interactive force information is collected using the human–machine interface to detect the value of assistive force provided by exoskeleton and to observe the training efficacy. At present, this kind of training mode has been achieved. As illustrated in Figure 5.27, human knee joint is bound with exoskeleton joint. The electromyographic electrodes are placed on rectus femoris and biceps femoris to collect the EMG signals of the two muscle groups, and joint motion intention can be predicted to represent the required torque of joint motion. The interactive force information is collected through gasbag force sensor to detect the training effect.

During the experiment, human knee joint extends forward or flexes backward based on the subject's intention. Exoskeleton is used to do active muscle force compensation training. Referring to the feeling of the subject, when human tends to move backward, the EMG signal of biceps femoris is detected. Exoskeleton responds quickly and drives the calf to move backward to provide assistive force for human calf. Similarly, when human extends forward, exoskeleton will also provide assistive force for the calf. Because EMG signal is generated 200 ms ahead of muscle contraction, human will only consume very little energy. Thus, the active control training of human joint is achieved corresponding to the original research target. The data recorded in the experiments is illustrated in Figure 5.28, including the EMG signals of rectus femoris and biceps femoris, predicted motor control signal, and the interactive force between human and exoskeleton. Referring to the EMG

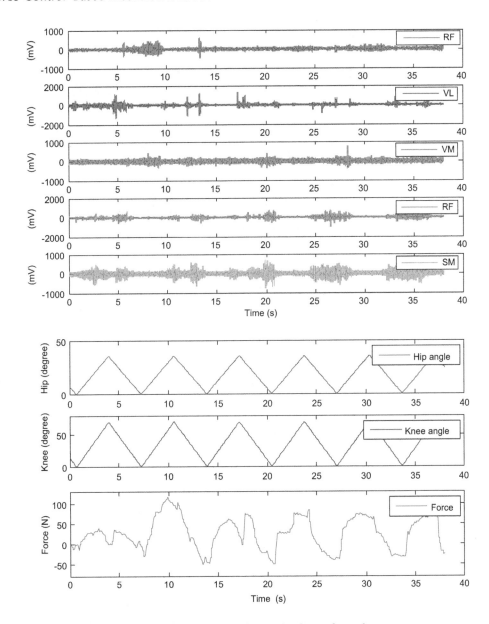

FIGURE 5.26 EMG signal, joint angle, and gasbag interactive force of muscles.

signal in the figure, when calf extends forward, the EMG signals of the two muscles are generated one after the other without disturbing each other as rectus femoris and biceps femoris are a group of antagonistic muscles. This is the prerequisite when we use EMG signal to perform active control. The predicted control voltage signal is illustrated in the third figure. Compared with the detected interactive force, the trends of the two signals are almost the same. The interactive force signal follows the predicted control single well, indicating that the required force for motion comes mainly from the supporting force from the exoskeleton. The force provided by human is small. Thus, the exoskeleton provides the assistive force correctly. There is another phenomenon that the predicted control voltage signal of calf flexion is larger than that of calf extension. This is mainly due to the gravity of the leg. Thus, the experiments prove that the active control training mode reaches the target results. It lays a foundation for clinical application in the future.

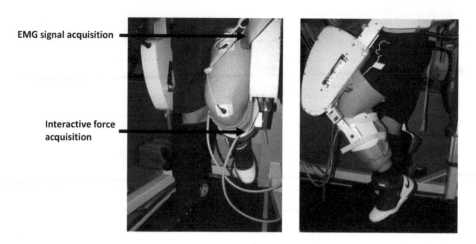

FIGURE 5.27   Active control training.

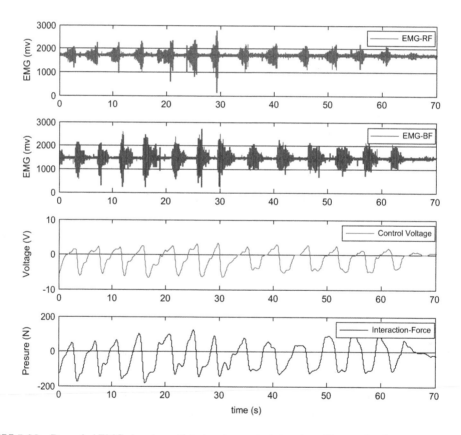

FIGURE 5.28   Recorded EMG signal, predicted motor control signal, and interactive force.

5.3.3   EXPERIMENT DEVICE AND PATIENT SELECTION

Preliminary clinical experiments were carried out to evaluate the effect of the proposed lower-extremity rehabilitation system in clinical trials. A clinical trial on rehabilitation of poststrokes was carried out at Shanghai Sixth People's Hospital (Shanghai, China), a general hospital specialized in rehabilitation of poststrokes. The subjects were a 54-year-old man 2 months after left-sided stroke (S1), a 30-year-old lady 1 month after left-sided stroke (S2), and a 68-year-old man 2 years after right-sided stroke (S3). The joint ROMs were respectively 0°–80°, 0°–103°, and 0°–92°; the peak active joint forces measured by the exoskeleton system were respectively 36, 60, and 47 N for flexion and 65, 52, and 62 N for extension with the joint angle of 60°.

The bed-type lower-extremity exoskeleton robot is selected as the experimental device. Other instruments include sEMG and multi-source biosignal-based neurofuzzy network controller, haptic-based human–machine interface, and IoT-based intelligent rehabilitation system.

5.3.4 AIM, PROCESS, AND METHOD OF CLINICAL EXPERIMENT

There are three goals of clinical experiments: first, to prove the effectiveness of the proposed evaluation algorithm in the progressive rehabilitation treatment mode; second, to evaluate the clinical performance of the exoskeleton robot rehabilitation system on stroke patients; and third, to evaluate the feasibility of IoT-based intelligent rehabilitation system through simulation.

To verify the effectiveness of real-time evaluation algorithm, the real-time detection and evaluation experiments were implemented under active F/E mode. In this process, subjects are required to perform active F/E rehabilitation experiment with assistive force using the lower-extremity exoskeleton robot. The duration of each group of experiments is 2 min, and there are totally five groups. Meanwhile, human–machine interactive force, fatigue evaluation degree, and the value of assistive force are monitored in real time.

Based on the proposed progressive rehabilitation strategy, the rehabilitation process includes passive F/E mode, active F/E mode, passive gait mode, and active gait mode. In clinical rehabilitation, subjects are required to focus their attention and take part fully in every stage of the rehabilitation training to maximize the rehabilitation efficacy. Meanwhile, common physical therapy means, such as low-frequency electric stimulation and infrared physiotherapy, are applied to relieve the discomfort during physical rehabilitation training, improve blood circulation, and avoid inflammation. Similar cases are selected as references to verify the performance of the rehabilitation system.

To verify the effectiveness of the IoT-based intelligent rehabilitation system, we use the developed intelligent rehabilitation system to generate prescription and compare it with that given by doctors to verify the similarity and effectiveness. In the database, we include 57 cases in which patients are with different diseases and corresponding rehabilitation strategies. New patients who have not been diagnosed will receive treatment in 21 hospitals and 18 rehabilitation centers. Besides, information about doctors, medical staff, and equipment, such as continuous passive motion (CPM) devices, electronic stimulator, high-frequency-treatment apparatus, electromyography, and exoskeleton robot, is also available. The system will optimize the configuration of all the resources with the consideration of all the requirements of the patients and the limitations as a whole, and after the interaction with the master, the final solution will be determined.

5.3.5 EVALUATION INDEX AND STATISTICAL METHOD

As for the real-time monitoring and evaluation experiment, the fatigue evaluation value is compared with training time and human status to see if they are compatible with each other, and it is verified whether the assistive force changes with fatigue grade.

For clinical rehabilitation experiment, the evaluation indices include joint ROM, muscle contraction force, and the gait status changing with the rehabilitation process. Each index is measured three times after every rehabilitation step, and the average value is selected as the effective value. All the untoward reactions are recorded during the rehabilitation process.

For the IoT-based intelligent rehabilitation system, the revision rate of the prescription is calculated by Eq. (5.4):

$$\phi = \frac{\sum \left| \dfrac{\phi_r^i - \phi_0^i}{\phi_{op}^i} \right|}{n}, \qquad (5.4)$$

in which ϕ_r^i—ith revised value of the prescription
ϕ_0^i—ith original value
ϕ_{op}^i—optional number of ith parameter
n—number of all the parameters.

The average treatment cost, distance, and treatment performance of all the patients are compared after the system reconfiguration.

5.4 EXPERIMENTAL RESULTS AND ANALYSIS

5.4.1 CLINICAL EXPERIMENTAL RESULTS AND CASES

A clinical trial on rehabilitation of poststrokes was carried out at Shanghai Sixth People's Hospital (Shanghai, China). Figure 5.29 illustrates the photos of clinical rehabilitation experiments.

Figure 5.30 shows the results of parameters updated during active F/E rehabilitation according to (2) and (3). The assistive force is updated with the active force and fatigue rate, while the fatigue rate is changed with the average period of flexion and extension.

Figure 5.31 shows the results of clinical trial. The passive F/E training of the three subjects lasted for 14, 4, and 8 days, respectively, according to their joint ROM. The joint ROM is improved from 80° to 95° for S1, 103° to 103° for S2, and 92° to 99° for S3. The active flexion force is improved from 35 to 50 N for S1, 60 to 148 N for S2, and 47 to 50 N for S3, while the active extension force is improved from 65 to 90 N for S1, 52 to 115 N for S2, and 62 to 66 N for S3, in the second stage. After three weeks' gait training process, S1 and S2 were able to walk independently. The pace values were about 0.2 m/s and 0.8 m/s. The subjects' self-report on pain and discomfort level did not show any significant increase during therapy sessions.

In the IoT-based intelligent rehabilitation system experiments, the average value of the revision rate of the prescription is 7.51%. Figure 5.32 is the proposed intelligent design method based on different patients' requirements and the rehabilitation strategies after reallocation of medical resources.

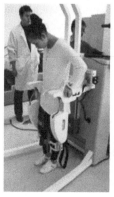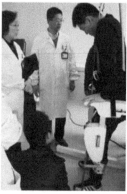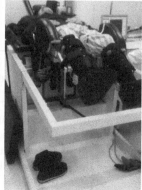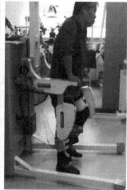

FIGURE 5.29 Clinical rehabilitation photos.

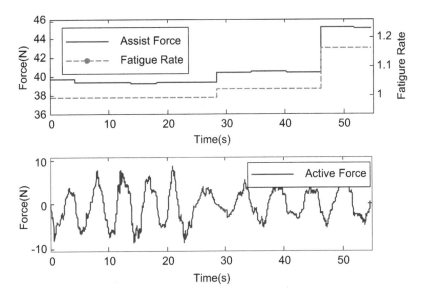

FIGURE 5.30 Updating parameters during active F/E; the figure below is the active force; the figure above shows assist force (solid line) and corresponding fatigue rate (dashed line).

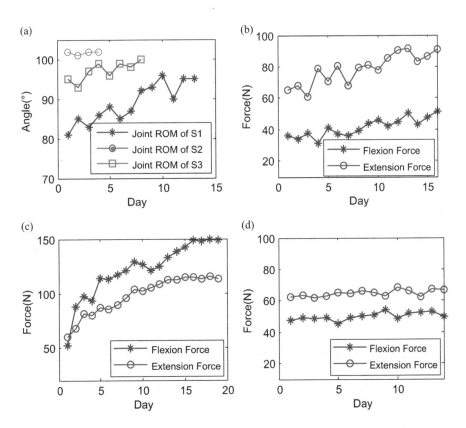

FIGURE 5.31 Evaluation during training process. (a) Joint ROM of the three subjects, (b) active joint force of Subject 1 (S1), (c) active joint force of Subject 2 (S2), and (d) active joint force of Subject 3 (S3).

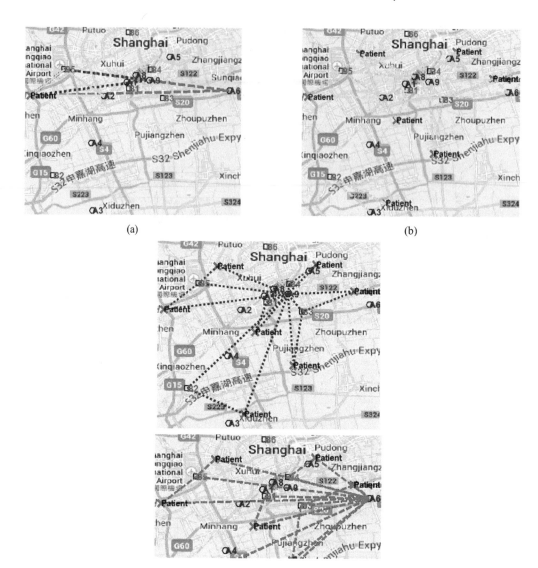

FIGURE 5.32 (a) One patient with different treatment requirements. (b) Different patients with shortest distance. (c) Different patients with lowest cost. (d) Different patients with best treatment resource. The patient location is represented by a cross, hospital by a circle, and the rehabilitation center by a black rectangle. The lines connecting patients, hospital, and rehabilitation centers are the chosen paths. A1: Shanghai Zhongshan Red Cross Hospital, A2: The Sixth People's Hospital of Shanghai, A3: The Fifth People's Hospital of Shanghai, A4: Huadong Hospital, A5: Shanghai East Hospital, A6: Shuguang Hospital, A7: The Third People's Hospital of Shanghai, A8: Ruijin Hospital, and A9: The Nineth People's Hospital of Shanghai.

The optimized results with different considerations are compared with non-optimized results. The results are shown in Figure 5.33. During the preliminary experiment, the distance is 49.08% shorter in average, and the cost is 53.14% lower in average, whereas the treatment resource is 55.56% better in average. It demonstrates that appropriate reconfiguration of the medical resources can improve the performance of the rehabilitation system, providing convenience to the patients, and increase the utilization of the medical resources.

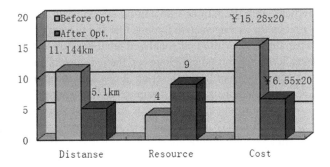

FIGURE 5.33 Comparison between the optimized results with different considerations and the pre-optimized results. The dark color bar is the average value before optimization, and the light color bar is the average after optimization.

5.4.2 RESULTS' ANALYSIS

At present, the exoskeleton robot system has been put into clinical application in Shanghai Sixth People's Hospital (Shanghai, China). Users are mainly patients with lower-extremity joint diseases. Different training modes are selected for different users. As illustrated in Figure 5.34, a patient with joint disease is taking rehabilitation training under the guidance of doctors. The corresponding strategy is determined with the aim of strengthening his muscle contraction force. It works on the active/passive training mode with the aid from the exoskeleton robot. Acceptable rehabilitation efficacy has been achieved. Because of the time limitation, EMG-signal-based active compensation training mode has not been applied on patients. Although practically EMG signal of patients is slightly different from that of normal people, the frequency and intensity can also reflect muscle activation degree and represent the muscle status. Our research group will continue to study intensively about the clinical research on exoskeleton robot based on the above research to reach a better efficacy and lay a foundation for the industrialization of the rehabilitation robot.

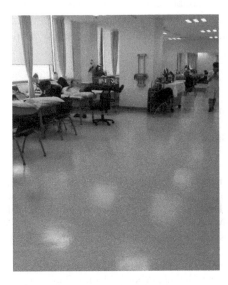
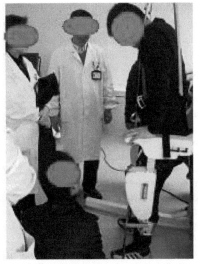

FIGURE 5.34 Patient is doing rehabilitation training under doctor's guidance.

Experiments also indicate that the fatigue rate can be evaluated in real time by Eq. (5.3). The assistive force is higher when the average active force is low and the subject is tired, and vice versa. The control strategy is capable of providing personalized rehabilitation and preventing further injuries or overfatigue during active rehabilitation. However, the parameters and actual fatigue level are to be determined more accurately according to a series of research in future work.

Results of clinical research demonstrate that the passive F/E training can provide continuous passive motion. The active F/E training can help muscle recover for a poststroke patient. The effect is not so remarkable for S3, and it may result from lack of exercise for a long time and muscular atrophy of the patient. Compared with traditional gait training, the exoskeleton-assisted treatment is convenient for physical therapist and meanwhile effective for patient. Another key factor to consider is the safety of robotic training. Based on the findings of the clinical trial, no adverse events are observed, and the repetitive robotic exercises did not result in significant fatigue or discomfort as reported by the subjects.

In traditional rehabilitation treatment, CPM is usually adopted to do F/E training. For patients with short illness time, normal joint ROM can be recovered after a 15-to-30-day rehabilitation training. Passive F/E mode of the exoskeleton robot has the same mechanism; thus, the rehabilitation efficacy is almost the same.

Nowadays in China, there are few muscle force recovery trainings in traditional treatment. Patients have to take rehabilitation training by themselves, such as the F/E exercise, gait training, and moderate mechanical training. Formal medical equipment for muscle force recovery is in short.

For traditional treatment method, there are many subjective factors that influence muscle force recovery. Some patients take the exercise frequently and recover in a short time, while others lack necessary training, leading to a long recovery period. Referring to the muscle force recovery treatment experiment using exoskeleton, it provides safe and quantized muscle force rehabilitation training with good performance. It is becoming one of the effective methods to recover muscle force.

Traditional gait training is always on the ground, step, or treadmill, with the help of crutch, guard bar, or other weight-reducing devices, and is monitored by medical staff. Compared with traditional gait training, exoskeleton-aided gait training is able to provide similar clinical training efficacy but largely decreases the work load of medical staff and is convenient for patients to do self-training.

In the clinical experiments, a whole process log recording and observation are implemented to avoid safety problems in the exoskeleton-aided rehabilitation training. There has not been any obvious untoward reaction or fatigue during and after the rehabilitation training. Meanwhile, the situation is also good for healthy subjects. Thus, it can be accepted that the safety property of the exoskeleton rehabilitation system is satisfactory.

REFERENCES

1. Hayashi, T, Kawamoto, H, Sankai, Y. Control method of robot suit HAL working as operator's muscle using biological and dynamical information, *IEEE/RSJ International Conference on Intelligent Robots and Systems*, Edmonton, AB, 2005, pp. 3063–3068.
2. www.cyberdyne.jp/English/index.html/HAL-5 homepage, active exoskeleton project under the guidance of Prof. Sankai.
3. Riener, R, Lunenburger, L, Jezernik, S, et al. Patient-cooperative strategies for robot-aided treadmill training: First experimental results. *IEEE Trans. Neural Syst. Rehabil. Eng.*, 2005, 13(3): 380–394.
4. Veneman, J F, Kruidhof, R, Hekman, E, et al. Design and evaluation of the LOPES exoskeleton robot for interactive gait rehabilitation. *IEEE Trans. Neural Syst. Rehabil. Eng.*, 2007, 15(3): 379–386.
5. Kong, K, Jeon, D. Design and control of an exoskeleton for the elderly and patients. *IEEE/ASME Trans. Mech.*, 2006, 11(4): 428–432.
6. www.googoltech.com.cn/webnew/dispro.php?findid=202&flord=prol53l54.
7. Quan, S. *Rehabilitation Estimation*. Beijing, China: Beijing, People's Medical Publishing House, 2010 (in Chinese).
8. Dohler, M, Ratti, C, Paraszczak, J, et al. Smart cities. *IEEE Commun. Mag.*, 2013, 51(6): 70–71.

9. Li, X, Lu, R, Liang, X, et al. Smart community: An internet of things application. *IEEE Commun. Mag.*, 2011, 49(11): 68–75.

10. Atzori, L, Ieraa, A, Morabito, G. The internet of things: A survey. *Comput. Netw.*, 2010, 54(15): 2787–2805.

11. Chui, M, Löffler, M, Roberts, R. The internet of things. *McKinsey Quarterly*, 2010, 2(2): 1–9.

12. Tarouco, L M R, Bertholdo, L M, Granville, L Z, et al. Internet of Things in healthcare: Interoperatibility and security issues, *Proceedings of the 2012 IEEE International Conference on Communications (ICC)*, Ottawa, 2012.

6 Bionic Design of Artificial Muscle Based on Biomechanical Models of Skeletal Muscle

Skeletal muscle has long been recognized as the best and most effective biologic actuator [1]. For a long time, bionic design of skeletal muscle has been the research hotspot over the globe. Scholars have agreed that once skeletal muscle bionics is achieved, it would be promising that complex diversity movements, such as running as cheetah, swimming as dolphin, and even flying as sparrow, can be realized [2]. Moreover, bionic techniques for skeletal muscle also promote the researches on humanoid robot, achieving the simulation of complex human body movement, such as walking in complex environment, complicated and accurate operation manipulation, fruit picking in the garden, etc. All these activities are hard to achieve by normal actuators, such as electric motor or hydraulic actuator [3].

From 1930s, scholars have devoted themselves on the research of skeletal muscle, proposing a series of skeletal muscle models to describe its mechanical properties [4–13]. All these lay the theoretical foundation for studies on artificial muscle (AM). However, skeletal muscle bionics is not a blind simulation of skeletal muscle but is the study on comprehensive considerations of bionic design goals, bionic feature recognition, and technical realization. Moreover, there are muscle property differences between different species and different individuals of the same species. Thus, the first step of skeletal muscle bionics is to solve the problem of bionic design methodology and design principle, i.e., how to guide bionic design. The second step is the selection and processing of bionic materials, i.e., how to realize bionic design. However, the biologic mechanical property of skeletal muscle is too complex that there has not been one driving device or material that is able to simulate skeletal muscle property effectively [14,15]. Numerous attempts have been made on bionic muscle researches, such as conventional electric motor, hydraulic actuator [16–20], pneumatic AM actuator [3], and some intelligent actuation materials [21–26], like piezoelectric ceramics (PZT), electropolymers, and shape memory alloys (SMAs). However, the skeletal muscle bionics under microscale and nanoscale (artificial molecular motor actuator) is hard to realize because of the limitation on microtechnology, nanotechnology, and biomimetic materials. Skeletal muscle bionics under macroscopic scale is always with low control accuracy, mismatching with skeletal muscle dynamics and low power-to-mass ratio because of the shortcomings of large volume and low power-to-mass ratio [14] of conventional actuation devices (electric motor and hydraulic and pneumatic actuators). Moreover, one single intelligent actuation material, such as PZT, electropolymers, also cannot achieve the skeletal muscle bionics due to the immutable limiting factors, like actuation voltage and environment. Thus, most of the bionic designs stay in the preliminary driving stage or the conceptual stage.

The researches on skeletal muscle bionics include the comprehensive research, recognition on the biologic features of skeletal muscle, and extraction and development of appropriate bionic models. While designing AM after selecting appropriate bionic materials, the shortcomings of the materials should also be overcome. Further research on actuation properties of bionic materials should be done. Thus, the research on AM is a multidisciplinary study including biology, mechanics, bionics, and materials.

Compared with other actuation devices and materials, SMA has many properties that are similar to skeletal muscles, such as flexibility, large power density, large output force, etc. [27].

Besides the actuation function, SMA also has the function of self-sensing, i.e., detecting self-length variation by observing self-resistance changes. Besides, compared with the rigorous actuation voltage (larger than 1,000 V) of electropolymer, actuation of the SMA could be achieved with the voltage of 5 V. Thus, SMA is better and more feasible in achieving skeletal muscle bionics. Thus, SMA is selected as the main actuation unit in this book. However, there are many unfavorable factors limiting its application in skeletal muscle bionics. These are what we have to face and solve in AM design:

a. Low strain and low response speed of SMA. Compared with the strain capacity of skeletal muscle (20%–40%), the largest strain capacity of SMA is only 10%. Besides, the response time of SMA is largely limited by the phase transformation speed of SMA and the temperature change speed. Thus, how to improve the strain capacity and phase transformation speed of SMA has to be considered.

b. Self-sensing property of SMA. SMA has the self-sensing property which is similar to skeletal muscle, i.e., feeding back the length of SMA by resistance. However, resistance change of SMA is affected by various factors, such as temperature, pressure, material composition, etc. Developing effective self-sensing model is the key to achieving AM integrated actuation and sensing.

c. Hysteresis characteristics of SMA. The inherent nonlinear saturated hysteresis characteristic of SMA badly limits the actuation speed and accuracy of SMA and even results in the instability of the actuation system. All these limit the bionic application of SMA. Moreover, the hysteresis characteristic is also affected by pressure and driving frequency, presenting complex dependence on strain and frequency. Thus, eliminating hysteresis influence of SMA is the key to achieving AM driving application.

Based on the above analysis, four aspects are selected to be discussed in detail in the related field, including the bionic design methodology, skeletal muscle structure and models, AM, and key techniques of SMA artificial muscle (SMA-AM).

6.1 BRIEF INTRODUCTION OF SKELETAL MUSCLE BIONICS

Bionic design aims to solve the problems in engineering system by studying the biological system. Bionic design has large influence on sustainable design and innovative design. Since ancient times, there have been numerous cases of bionic design. Human ancestors used fishing net by imitating cobweb. In industrial ages, humans created many innovative buildings and mechanical objects by imitating the structures of animals and plants, such as airplane and various humanoid robots. Although there have been many bionic design cases, few bionic design methodologies have been proposed. This is because there are strong subjectivities in bionic design. The unification of bionic design methodologies is largely limited by biodiversity. Thus, the research on bionic design theories aims to develop systematic bionic design theory to guide and evaluate bionic design.

6.1.1 Bionic Design Concept Evolution

Bionic design is the application of bionics to the field of design. It develops together with that of bionics. Early in 1960, the first bionics meeting was held in Ohio, and such design was named as "bionics". During this period, bionic design was to copy what existed in nature. In 1991, United States Air Force Research Office proposed the definition of "biomimetics", proposing that the aim of bionics is to provide biological aid for material design and processing.

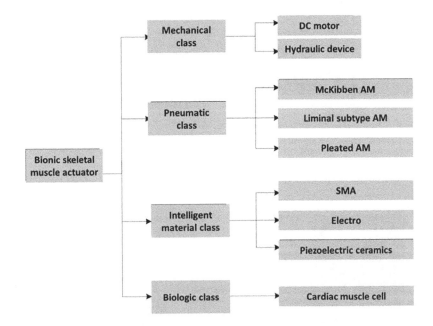

FIGURE 6.1 AM classification.

The aim of AM research is to simulate the structure and function of skeletal muscle and further simulate the flexible and agile movement of animals [28]. From the 1940s, US and Japan started to study AM and applied it to military investigation and transportation. Based on the differences on actuators, AM can be divided into four classes—the mechanical class, pneumatic class, intelligent material class, and biological class—as illustrated in Figure 6.1. The application status will be discussed as follows.

6.1.1.1 Mechanical AM

Mechanical AM refers to the artificial muscle actuator based on electric motor and hydraulic driver. They have the advantages of high accuracy, easy control, fast response speed, and large output force, making them the most widespread and mature actuators. The research on robots based on electric motor and hydraulic actuator has also become mature, and these robots have extensive applications, for example, spraying robots, welding robots, etc. However, these robots are unable to accomplish tasks which seem to be quite easy for human, such as screwing, toy assembly, apple picking, etc. The key reason is that the mechanical actuator is of high stiffness, making them capable of moving only in specific and known environments and free spaces. They do not have the flexible motion characteristics like muscle which is able to adapt to unknown environment.

From the 1980s, the Leg lab in Massachusetts Institute of Technology has been devoted to the bionic research on conventional actuator based skeletal muscle and its motion characteristics. They connected the electric motor and hydraulic actuator in series to achieve the simulation of skeletal muscle. Spring increases the flexibility of the mechanical actuator, environment adaptability, and energy storage characteristics. This kind of actuators has been named as series elastic actuator (SEA) [29], as illustrated in Figure 6.2.

The Leg group in MIT has designed multiple bionic robots to achieve the running and jumping simulation of macrofauna using the SEA. As illustrated in Figure 6.3a, Leg group developed a hydraulic SEA-based Uniroo bionic robot to mimic jumping of kangaroo. There is a stainless steel coil spring placed on the ankle joint of this bionic robot, achieving the storage and instant release of energy. Uniroo is able to mimic the lower-extremity jump of kangaroo well. Besides, Professor Hugh Herr in MIT Media lab developed the active ankle prosthesis and orthosis using the electric

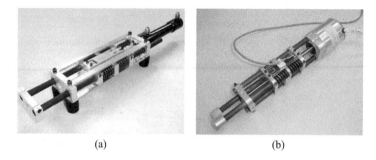

FIGURE 6.2   (a) Electric motor with SEA; (b) hydraulic drive with SEA.

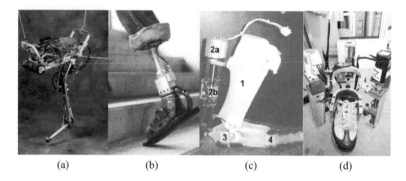

FIGURE 6.3   (a) MIT Uniroo Robot; (b) MIT active ankle prosthesis; (c) MIT active ankle orthosis; (d) SJTU ankle exoskeleton.

motor SEA from the bionic perspective [14,30–32]. Series spring not only achieves the gait actuation of ankle and foot and the energy storage bionics, but also increases the instantaneous motor power by 1.4 times [33]. Professor Yuehong Yin in Shanghai Jiao Tong University developed a three-DOF (degree of freedom) active ankle–foot exoskeleton based on the bionic design of ankle skeletal muscle. The group used three servo motors to achieve the introversion and ecstrophy, and the exoskeleton motion was driven by acquiring the electromyography (EMG) signal of calf skeletal muscles [19].

So far, the most advanced bionic robot might be the ASIMO developed by Japan Honda Corporation [34]. The height of this robot is 1.3 m, and the weight is 52 kg. The multi-DOF motion is achieved by servo motors. There are also flexible damping materials connecting electric motor and driving joint. The structure has the similar functions of buffer and energy storage as the above SEA, as illustrated in Figure 6.4. Boston Dynamics used hydraulic actuators to develop the BigDog, simulating quadruped locomotion of dogs with the speed of 4 km/h. It also uses springs to simulate the functions of buffer and energy storage of skeletal muscle [35].

Using the conventional electric motor and hydraulic actuator, the advanced bionic robots, such as ASIMO and BigDog can be developed, achieving the partial simulation of AM, but the inherent shortcomings of conventional actuators still form the bottleneck of the development of bionic robots. First, although the stiffness of electric motor and hydraulic actuator can be effectively decreased with series springs and dampers, actuation devices such as the SEA are still large in stiffness and size with a complex structure when compared with biological skeletal muscle. Besides, the force-to-weight ratio is much less than that of the biological skeletal muscle, making it hard to realize the simulation of flexible motion characteristics. Second, electric motor and hydraulic actuator are often used in the successive and repeated rotary devices. To realize non-successive and complex contraction motion of skeletal muscle, a more complex transfer mechanism is needed. Third, compared

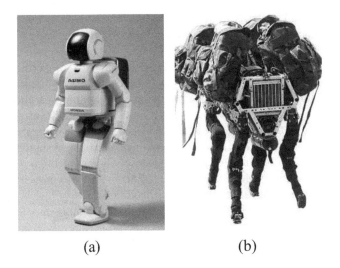

(a)   (b)

FIGURE 6.4   (a) ASIMO; (b) BigDog.

with the integrated properties of actuation, sensing, and energy storage of skeletal muscle, electric motor and hydraulic actuator have only the actuation function. The feedback function can only be achieved by adding sensors. Thus, scholars home and abroad all concentrate on the research of new actuators, hoping to realize the bionic simulation of the structure and function of skeletal muscle.

6.1.1.2   Pneumatic AM

The actuation source of the pneumatic AM is air. Pneumatic AM is so far the most studied bionic actuator of muscle. It can be divided into several classes based on different structures, but their main structure and actuation mechanism are almost the same. Pneumatic AM is always composed of rubber capsules which are easily deformed and the supporting mesh which limits the deformation. The rubber capsule and mesh support are connected by connectors in both ends. When the pneumatic AM is inflated, the rubber tube becomes bloated and abuts to the mesh support. Rubber tube contracts in the axial direction because of the limitation of mesh support. When the inflating pressure decreases, the pneumatic AM recovers to the original length due to the restoring force of rubber tube and the external load. The extension and contraction states are illustrated in Figure 6.5.

Among all the existing pneumatic AMs, McKibben is the most classic and widely applied one. Compared with conventional mechanical actuator, pneumatic AM has the advantages of clean, good dynamic properties; low friction; no creep phenomenon; etc. Moreover, pneumatic AM is one-way driven with high force-to-weight ratio and flexible structure, which are all similar to biological skeletal muscles. Thus, it has always been one of the main types of skeletal muscle bionic research.

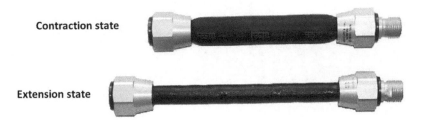

FIGURE 6.5   Different states of pneumatic AM.

The bionic robot lab in University of Washington has concentrated on the bionic properties and applications of pneumatic muscle for the last two decades [3,36–39]. Based on the static model of McKibben, it can only partially simulate the force–length relation of skeletal muscles but is unable to simulate the force–velocity properties compared to the mechanical properties of skeletal muscles. This is due to the fact that the damping of pneumatic muscle is small while that of skeletal muscle is large. Thus, the pneumatic muscles simulate the damping by adding a parallel hydraulic damping cylinders. Besides, two parallel springs are used to simulate the nonlinear property and energy-storage buffer function of tendon. The resultant AM is illustrated in Figure 6.6. The improved pneumatic muscle–tendon system achieves the approximate mechanical simulation of skeletal muscle, while the structure also becomes complex. Japanese scholar Norihiko Saga did some bionic mechanical property analysis of McKibben muscle [40,41], which was proven to have acquired the similar bionic results of mechanical properties of skeletal muscle.

Besides the properties of flexibility and linear actuation, pneumatic muscle is also able to store and release energy and absorb the motion shocks. These properties which are similar to those of skeletal muscles make it flexible to be applied in the actuation of bionic and rehabilitation robots. In the field of bionic robot, a pneumatic muscle-based four-DOF climbing robot named ROBIN was developed by Vandebilt University in US [42], as illustrated in Figure 6.7a. Each DOF of the robot is in the form of muscle-dragging, simulating the motion pattern of gecko with the ability of moving forward, backward, and turning around on the vertical plane. A six-foot robot named AirBug was developed by Karlsruhe University in Germany, simulating the insects. The weight of

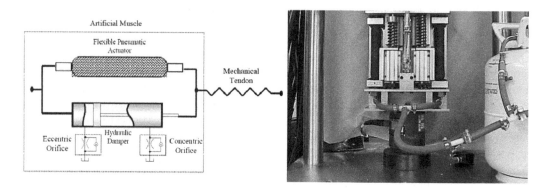

FIGURE 6.6   Pneumatic AM in University of Washington.

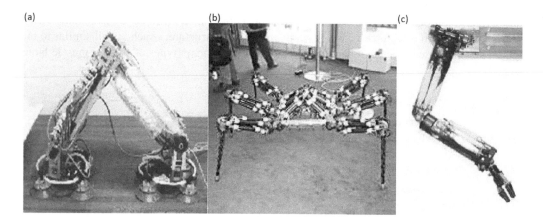

FIGURE 6.7   (a) Vandebilt ROBIN; (b) Karlsruhe AirBug; (c) Washington upper limb bionic robot.

the robot is 20 kg and is driven by eight pneumatic muscles, as illustrated in Figure 6.7b. Simulation of human muscle groups can also be achieved by pneumatic muscles, as illustrated in Figure 6.7c. The upper-limb bionic robot developed by University of Washington simulates the muscle groups of the elbow joint and wrist joint using multiple paralleled pneumatic muscles. It cannot be achieved by conventional actuators.

In the field of rehabilitation robotics, the properties of pneumatic muscle similar to skeletal muscle are also applied. Three paralleled McKibben pneumatic muscles were used to develop the wearable ankle exoskeleton robot in Harvard University [43], as illustrated in Figure 6.8a. It can be applied in the rehabilitation and assisted walking for patients with the problem of foot drop. The three pneumatic muscles are able to simulate the musculi tibialis anterior, extensor longus pollicis, and musculus extensor digitorum longus, achieving the dorsiflexion and ecstrophy of human ankle. University of Michigan developed an active ankle orthosis with two McKibben pneumatic muscles [44,45], as illustrated in Figure 6.8b. The weight of the orthosis is 1.6 kg, without including the controller and air compressor. It provides the maximum flexion torque of 70 Nm and dorsiflexion torque of 38 Nm.

Although the pneumatic AM has many properties similar to skeletal muscle, such as flexibility and high power-to-weight ratio and there have been numerous bionic designs of pneumatic AM, its shortcomings limit its bionic application. First, high-pressure holder is needed to provide energy for pneumatic AM. The heavy holder largely decreases the power-to-weight ratio and limits the application range and activity space. To realize the portable application of pneumatic muscles, a mini air bottle is used to develop a portable ankle orthosis [46,47], as illustrated in Figure 6.9. But it didn't

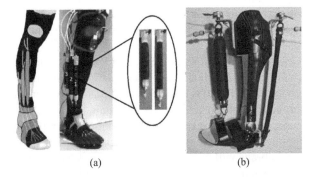

(a)   (b)

FIGURE 6.8   (a) Ankle exoskeleton by Harvard University; (b) ankle exoskeleton by University of Michigan.

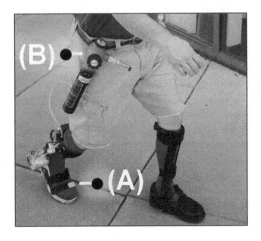

FIGURE 6.9   Portable ankle orthosis.

solve the problem thoroughly. Second, there will be large noise in the driving process of pneumatic muscle. Moreover, the inherent nonlinear property makes it hard to be controlled accurately. All these factors largely limit its bionic application.

6.1.1.3 AM with Smart Material

Because of the insurmountable limiting factors of conventional mechanical and pneumatic actuators, scholars all over the world are searching for smart bionic materials, hoping to achieve the bionic simulation of the structure and function of biological skeletal muscles. Among the existing intelligent bionic materials, the most representative ones are electroactive polymer (EAP) and SMA.

6.1.1.3.1 Electroactive Polymer (EAP)

EAP is a new type of functional material which can efficiently conversion of electric and mechanical energy. As early as one century ago, the actuation property of EAP has been discovered. In an electric field, the length and volume of the EAP can vary within a wide range. According to energy transformation mechanism, EAPs can be divided into electronic and ionic EAPs [2], as illustrated in Table 6.1. Electronic EAP is composed of dielectric elastomer, ferroelectric polymers, electrostrictive elastomer, and electret. Electric field is the driving source of electronic EAP, and the deformation can be maintained under DC. This can be used in the development of bionic muscle and robot driving. Besides, these materials have a high power density and are able to run in the open air environment. However, their actuation voltage is too high, limiting their application prospect. Different from electronic EAP, ionic EAP is driven through diffusion of ions in the electrolyte. Ionic EAP has many types, such as conductive polymer, ion exchange membrane, metal composite, carbon nanotube, and ionic polymer gel. The actuation voltage can be 1–2 V. However, the requirement of actuation environment is strict as the driving carrier must be the electrolyte. Thus, humid environment must be ensured.

For a long time, because of the various properties which are similar to skeletal muscle, EAP has always been one of the most important smart materials for bionic research on skeletal muscle. Ionic polymer–metal composite (IPMC) is a typical smart material of ionic EAP. It is composed of cation-exchange membrane and noble metal, such as platinum, through chemical plating. IPMC can be actuated in low voltage. When there is DC in IPMC membrane, it will bend to the positive direction as illustrated in Figure 6.10a, and the bending degree is proportional to the voltage magnitude. When there is AC, the membrane will wag. Its displacement is related to the voltage amplitude and frequency. IPMC has the advantages of low actuation voltage and fast response, making it popular

TABLE 6.1

Advantages and Disadvantages of the Two Kinds of EAP

EAP Types	Advantages	Disadvantages
Electronic EAP	• Fast response time (millisecond) • Deformation can be maintained under DC • Large driving force • Higher energy intensity • Long-time run at room temperature	• Extremely high driving voltage (100 MV/meter) is needed, 20 MV/meter for ferroelectric polymers • Has no relation with voltage direction. Only one-way driving can be achieved
Ionic EAP	• Two-directional driving can be achieved based on voltage direction • Low-voltage driving • Some ionic EAP has special double stability	• Electrolyte is needed • Extremely low electromechanical efficiency • Slow response speed • Small driving force • Deformation can't be maintained

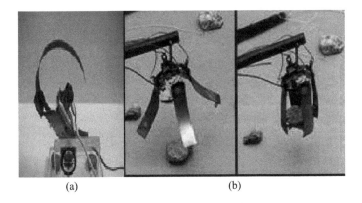

(a)   (b)

FIGURE 6.10   (a) IPMC actuator; (b) stone grabbing of EAP-based bionic hand.

among researchers. IPMC can be used in the holding device research of micro robot and the actuation of bionic insects or fishes. Its application is very promising. Figure 6.10b illustrates the bionic hand based on IPMC. It can be used to simulate the grabbing activity of fingers. The grabbing manipulation can be achieved by applying voltage to the bionic hand.

Dielectric elastomer is the representative type of electronic EAP materials and is also the most notable EAP actuation material among researchers. It has the advantages of flexibility, less noise, etc. (Figure 6.11). Thus, it has been applied in many bionic muscle studies [22,23,48]. Stanford Research Institute (SRI) developed a two-DOF cylindrical spring roll actuator using the dielectric elastomer. Its size is the same as the finger with the driving stress of 8 MPa, which is 30 times that of skeletal muscle. The actuator deforms under high voltage (5.5 kV). The force generated by the deformation is able to raise objects with the weight of 1 kg, as illustrated in Figure 6.12. Based on the actuator, SRI also developed a six-leg bionic robot called FLEX2. Its gait is similar to living things with the speed of 315 cm/s, as illustrated in Figure 6.12a. To apply the bionic feature of EAP further, some scholars developed artificial skeletal muscle with similar shape and strain as real skeletal muscle using the dielectric elastomer, as illustrated in Figure 6.12b. The simulation of biceps brachii has also been done, which is expected to be applied in the field of rehabilitation.

As a polymer, EAP can be easily shaped as required. Various EAP bionic actuators have been produced. However, EAP actuator still has the disadvantages of low actuation efficiency and weak robustness. Moreover, most EAP materials are still at the leading edge research stage. Commercialization has not been achieved. The harsh actuation requirements (extremely high voltage or liquid environment) also limit its bionic applications.

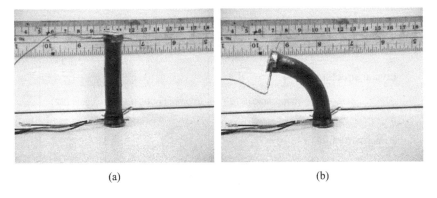

(a)   (b)

FIGURE 6.11   (a) Static states; (b) high-voltage driving state (5.5 kV).

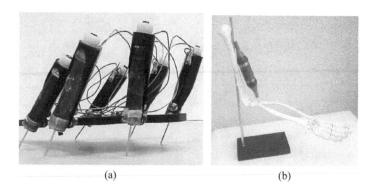

(a)   (b)

FIGURE 6.12   (a) FLEX2; (b) EAP artificial skeletal muscle.

6.1.1.3.2 Shape Memory Alloy (SMA)

SMA is a special metallic material. Different from normal metallic material which will generate permanent set with stress, SMA can recover to the original shape after being heated to certain temperature when plastic deformation occurs [49]. SMA is able to absorb and consume mechanical energy under certain mechanical repetitive loading, showing good damping function. These properties are closely related to its unique crystal structure. SMA is mainly composed of two bulk phases: the martensite in low temperature and austenite in high temperature. Each bulk phase has totally different crystal structure, and thus totally different material properties. Besides, there is also R-phase in some SMA, as illustrated in Figure 6.13. Austenite has body centered cubic structure, while martensite has face centered cubic structure. From the perspective of microscopic crystallology, the essence of SMA actuation is caused by the mutual transformation of SMA crystal lattice, i.e., the martensitic transformation. In this process, the lattice atom will move in a highly ordered way. The macroscopic deformation of SMA is achieved by the collective motion of numerous lattice atoms.

SMA has two unique material properties: the shape memory effect and superelasticity [49]. Shape memory effect refers to the phenomenon in which after SMA deforms in low temperature, it can recover to the original shape through heating, similar to the behavior of memory. Superelasticity refers to the phenomenon in which under the same temperature, the deformation of SMA can be 10% in the state of stress cycle loading. It is much larger than that of normal alloys. The experimental results of the two properties are illustrated in Figure 6.14 [50]. Based on these, SMA has wide application as smart actuator.

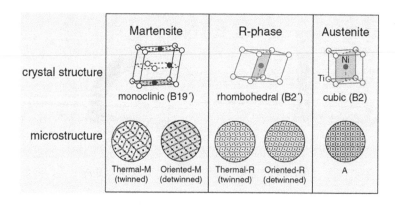

FIGURE 6.13   Nitinol crystal structure and microstructure of each phase.

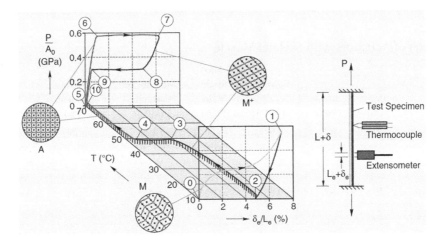

FIGURE 6.14 Experimental results of SMA shape memory effect (0–5) and superelasticity (5–10).

SMA has many properties which are similar to those of skeletal muscle, such as high power density, large output force, flexibility, one-way contraction, etc. Besides the actuation function, SMA also has the function of self-sensing. Moreover, the actuation of SMA is simple, which can be achieved through low-voltage heating. Thus, SMA is not only used as actuator, sensor, and buffer, but it is also an excellent choice for skeletal muscle bionic material. For the last few decades, related research has been carried out extensively, hoping to achieve flexible actuation of exoskeleton or robot by using SMA AMs [51–55].

The most representative research product is the bionic hand driven by SMA. It was developed by H. Asada in MIT [54], as illustrated in Figure 6.15a. Matrix arrangement and coordinated control are applied in this bionic hand. As many as 16 hand action patterns can be achieved through SMA driving. It is hard to be accomplished when using conventional driving method. Moreover, SMA was set as braid by A. Price in the University of Toronto [53] and applied on two-DOF bionic upper-limb driving, as illustrated in Figure 6.15b. The comparison of SMA and other actuators is illustrated in Table 6.2. While SMA is a bit lower than skeletal muscle in strain, velocity, and power, it is much better than skeletal muscle in other aspects. Particularly, the force-to-weight ratio of SMA is much higher than that of skeletal muscle. Thus, SMA is promising to realize the integrated AM with large output force, large power density, and the

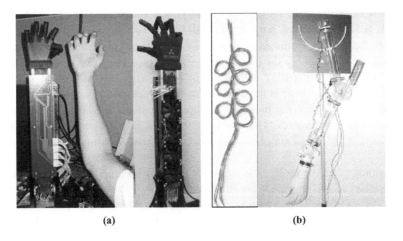

(a)   (b)

FIGURE 6.15 (a) Bionic hand driven by SMA; (b) bionic upper limb driven by braid SMA-AM.

TABLE 6.2

Comparison of Actuators with Skeletal Muscle

Driving Method	Strain (%)	Stress (MPa)	Power Density (J/g)	Max Strain Rate (%/s)	Modulus of Elasticity (MPa)	Driving Efficiency (%)	Relative Velocity (Complete Period)
Skeletal muscle	**20**	**0.1**	**0.041**	**>50**	**10–60**	**20**	**Medium**
Dielectric elastomer	25	1.0	0.1	>450	0.1–10	60–90	Med.–Fast
IPMC	0.5	3	0.004	3.3	50–100	1.5–3	Med.–Slow
Electromagnetic actuator	50	0.1	0.003	>1,000	NA	>80	Fast
PZT	0.2	110	0.013	>1,000	25,000	>90	Fast
SMA	**10**	**700**	**>15**	**300**	**9,000**	**<10**	**Slow**

"actuation–sensing–structure" function. Von Howard Ebron in the University of Dallas (Texas, USA) developed a strong AM with the driving force of alcohol and hydrogen using different heating methods [52]. It was introduced in *Science* in 2006. It can transform chemical energy into heat, leading to SMA contraction. When the temperature decreases, it also relaxes. The raising ability of the AM is 100 times that of normal skeletal muscle. It can be used to develop better artificial limbs or exoskeleton robots, providing fire fighters, soldiers, or astronauts with super power.

6.1.2 BID Bionic Design Methodology

As the important component of animal motor system, skeletal muscle integrates actuation, sensing, and energy storage. Evolution makes skeletal muscle not only able to meet actuation requirements of all the animals under different motion status and environments, but also have incomparable features over any other actuators, such as flexibility, large power density, high actuation efficiency, etc. Thus, bionic design of skeletal muscle has always been the hotspot. However, there are two challenges of bionic design of skeletal muscle, i.e., bionic design methodology and technical realization.

Biologically inspired design (BID) aims to solve engineering problems based on biological inspirations. BID is the guiding mark for innovative design and sustainable design. Although there have been numerous BID bionic cases, how to apply BID systematically into bionic design and develop a repeatable and ponderable bionic design methodology is still a problem in the design field. There are two parts in the BID method: the biological system identification (BSI) and engineering system realization (ESR). The existing BID methods mainly deal with the BSI process. It belongs to conceptual design, the aim of which is to select biological target based on engineering problems and avoid cognitive bias. However, the bionics of complex organism (the skeletal muscle for example) belongs to multi-objective bionics. The problems faced include not only avoiding cognitive bias, but also organism analysis and simplification, multi-objective coordination bionics, and technical realization.

BID methodology and the evaluation criterions of bionic degree (BD) are proposed systematically. The processes of BSI and ESR are illustrated in detail. Based on the BID method, identification and modeling of the bionic features of skeletal muscle system is also done after the deep analysis of the structure, function, and mechanical properties of skeletal muscle. It lays a foundation for further research.

6.1.2.1 Framework of BID

Aiming at the bionic design and realization of complex organism (skeletal muscle), BID is proposed to guide the bionic design process. There are two parts in the BID method: the BSI and ESR. The BSI process belongs to conceptual design, which is composed of concept selection and sub-conceptual design. The ESR process includes embodiment design and detail design, and iteration and learning. The detailed framework is illustrated in Figure 6.16.

The first step is concept selection. It solves the engineering problems through bionic methods. The detailed Requirement (R) of the engineering problem has to be determined first. Generally, conventional engineering design undergoes the conceptual design process including function division and configuration determination after the target requirements are clear. However, for bionic design, its inspiration comes from living creatures; the design process comes directly to the mapping stage after the target requirements are determined. We call this process as concept selection, i.e., mapping the target engineering problem to appropriate creatures to get the biological configuration correctly, which is the target morphology (M) provided by nature. For example, scholars got the inspiration from dung beetle when it shapes the feces into a sphere without getting stuck to it. Setting the dung beetle as the target morphology (M), the problem of earth getting stuck in tunnel excavator and agricultural machinery is solved [55]. However, the evolution of creatures in the past millions of years has formed the biodiversity in nature. Every species has its unique structure, function, and operating mechanism. Thus, M largely depends on human experience and knowledge (H), i.e., the cognitive level of structure, function, and operating mechanism of the creatures in nature. From the perspective of design methodology, bionic design is a typical interdisciplinary problem concerning engineering and biology. Thus, how to extract solutions for engineering problems from the perspective of biology is of great significance. Thus, methods, such as database search, natural language, etc., are selected to eliminate the cognitive bias toward the creatures in the conceptual selection stage. Moreover, as for the bionics of complex organism (skeletal muscle) and its engineering realization (artificial muscle), the determination of M is the iteration and evaluation process of human (H) based on creature cognition. Thus, the expected behavior (B_E) of engineering products is determined together by R, M, and H. BID is a unique iterative process as illustrated on the left side of Figure 6.16. Take the bionic design of AM as an example; R includes large force-to-weight ratio, high integration degree, versatility, etc. Skeletal muscle is the bionic object.

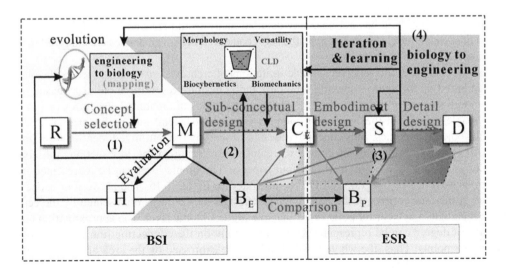

FIGURE 6.16 Framework of BID.

Second, sub-conceptual design. Because of the structure complexity, M cannot be applied in bionic design directly. Thus, one needs to map M to the field of engineering to acquire appropriate engineering configuration (C_E). In essence, this process belongs to a special conceptual design process of conceptual selection as discussed above, so we call it sub-conceptual design. How to analyze and simplify the structure, function; and operation mechanism; propose an appropriate biological model to guide bionic design; and develop BD evaluation criteria are the problems which have to be solved. To clarify the design principles for bionic design stages, four bionic aspects are proposed in the sub-conceptual design stage: the morphology, versatility, biomechanics, and biocybernetics. The bionics of most creatures (including animals and plants) includes morphology and versatility. Biomechanics and biocybernetics are mainly applied in more complex beings (animals and human beings). The process of sub-conceptual design is illustrated in Figure 6.16. Taking the bionic design of AM as an example, basic knowledge about skeletal muscle is its spindle structure and one-way contraction function. Through further analysis, it is found to also have highly integrated active/passive structures, self-sensing function, and unique mechanical properties. Thus, in-depth analysis has to be made on the structure, function, and operation mechanism of skeletal muscle, thus determining the parameters based on the practical bionic targets to achieve maximum simulation of skeletal muscles.

Third, embodiment design and detail design. Based on the development of C_E, the structure (S) and details (D) are refined in the stages of embodiment design and detail design. The design process (as illustrated on the right side of Figure 6.16) is similar to the later stage of conventional engineering design; i.e., it is also composed of embodiment design and detail design. Physical behavior (B_P) is determined by C_E, S, and D. B_P and B_E are compared to assess the bionic efficacy. There are also three local optimization processes in this stage, i.e., the topological optimization among C_E, B_E, and B_P; the structural optimization among S, B_E, and B_P; and the detailed optimization among D, B_E, and B_P.

Fourth, iteration and learning. As bionic design depends largely on human experience and the cognitive level to the bionic target (the corresponding creature), iteration is necessary to find out the appropriate bionic design scheme. When B_P does not meet the design requirements, designers can change the engineering configuration by structural modification or redo the sub-conceptual design. If the requirements still cannot be met, one can even select other creatures as the biological target.

Up to present, BID methods have been explained in detail by the above steps.

6.1.2.2 Sub-Conceptual Design Principles

Compared with other stages, sub-conceptual design is a critical stage in the bionic design of complex organism, but there has not been any detailed analysis and research on it. Taking the bionic design of skeletal muscle as an example, the sub-conceptual design principles are analyzed in detail in this section.

Many bionic cases are relatively simple imitations of creatures' structures, such as the medical syringe based on mosquito's sucking tube [56] and adhesion-preventing moldboard based on the non-smooth surface of dung beetle [55]. The simple bionics of creatures' structures or functions has a single target, but the bionics of complex organism (skeletal muscle for example) belongs to multi-objective bionics. Sub-conceptual design process is the optimized identification process of multi-objective properties of complex creatures. Referring to the last section, sub-conceptual design process can be divided into four aspects. The bionic level can be represented by the Comprehensive Level Diagram (CLD), as illustrated in Figure 6.16. The above four aspects are located at the four corners of the rectangle. The design start point is represented by the centroid of the rectangle. Each corner point represents the highest bionic level. The approximation level of the highest degree can be represented by the level point on the connecting line between centroid and corner points. Thus, the whole bionic level can be expressed by the area of the quadrilateral formed by the four level points.

Ideally, the red region should fill the entire rectangle. CLD represents the multi-objective property of the sub-conceptual design of complex creatures clearly.

The nature of bionics is a multi-objective optimization process. Limited by feasibility and cost, the highest level of bionics in CLD may not be the best choice. Thus, the bionic level and engineering feasibility should be balanced. The four aspects are stated as follows:

1. **Morphology**: Long-time evolution provides creatures with highly integrated and multi-level morphologies. Thus, the morphology here is a generalized concept, not only including the shape under macroscopic scale, but also including shapes under mesoscopic scale and microscopic scale. Taking skeletal muscle as an example, under macroscopic scale, it is spindle shaped and connects to skeleton through tendon. Under mesoscopic scale, there are many muscle fibers and connective tissues. Under microscopic scale, sarcomere is the basic contraction unit of skeletal muscle. Morphological bionics should consider both the morphologies under different scales and the bionic target. Besides, morphological bionics is not the simple imitation of creature structure. Instead, creative bionics should be achieved in solving practical problems. Technical feasibility should also be considered. Typical bionic cases include the functional surface based on lotus leaf, compound eye, and gecko foot.

2. **Versatility**: Long-time evolution provides creatures with unique multi-functional properties. The more complex the creature, the more obvious its multi-functional properties are. Skeletal muscle not only has the function of active contraction, but also has features like self-feedback, self-recovery, energy storage, and buffer. Thus, skeletal muscle can be regarded as the multi-functional actuator integrating actuation, sensing, and energy storage. The multi-functional property is closely related to its unique structure. Its multi-functional property provides skeletal muscle with much better properties than any other artificial actuator, such as force-to-weight ratio and integration level.

3. **Biomechanics**: Another bionic key point for complex creatures (especially animals) is the biomechanical property. Biomechanics applies classic mechanical theory to analyze creature and physiological system and explains creatures' activities. It is the foundation to understand biological system. For example, statics is applied to analyze the force value and characteristics of the joints and muscles in musculoskeletal system, while dynamics is used to describe human gait and biological fluid mechanics to study cardiovascular system. Biomechanics explains what makes creatures different from other non-living things. Moreover, different mechanical features will be presented under different states (health or disease for example). The study on biomechanics not only helps to understand the functions and physiological features of creatures, but also helps to develop bionic guiding principles for bionic design; i.e., bionic design should meet the biomechanical properties of creatures.

4. **Biocybernetics**: Complex creatures (especially animals) have a strong ability of environment adaption and learning. This property is not only determined by the structure of creatures, but is also more closely related to biocybernetics. Biocybernetic system is a multilevel control system. For skeletal muscle, the low-level control is achieved by the multi-closed-loop feedback control system composed of actuation unit (muscle fiber), sensory unit (proprioceptor), and motoneuron. High-level control system is the central nervous system. The multilevel control strategy meets the control principle of decentralization and concentralization well. For example, when human breathes normally, brain will not intervene the skeletal muscle contraction in respiratory system, but when the breathing rate needs to be changed, brain will change its contraction frequency and amplitude. Biological control belongs to the domain of optimum control and adaptive control. It is the result of long-time revolution. Limited by cognitive and technical levels, only partial biocybernetics can be achieved by engineering (such as neural network algorithm).

Note that the above four aspects are not completely independent of one another but have some coupling properties. For example, different morphologies lead to the differences in functions and mechanical properties. The bionics of the above four aspects under different scales (macroscopic, mesoscopic, and microscopic scales) will be different because of the differences in bionic target, cognitive level, and technical level. How to analyze the differences and propose appropriate bionic design principles has to be solved in bionic design. Based on the above analysis, in this book, the guiding principles for sub-conceptual design are proposed:

1. **Biological system identification should be maximized and feasible**. A too complex biological system identification will not be achieved because of technical limitations. Simply imitating a biological system is not only impossible (even the smallest skeletal muscle has very complex structure), but also meaningless (there are many properties which are not required in AM design, such as the process of metabolism). On the contrary, a too simple biological system identification will lead to cognitive bias because of the lack of main characteristics and also decrease the BD (for example, regarding skeletal muscle simply as a spindle is far from enough). The relationships among BSI, ESR, and BD are illustrated in Figure 6.17. Thus, the principles of maximization and feasibility should be followed in biological system identification, i.e., to maximize the identification degree to extract biological features and meanwhile fully consider the feasibility. Only when the relation between BSI and ESR is balanced, the BD can be maximized.

2. **Bionic material selection should follow the principle of optimization and compensability**. Bionic material selection is essential to realize bionic design, as the material is the foundation to realize all the functions. It is hard to achieve high-level bionics of complex creatures with conventional materials. Bionic material selection should approximate the multi-objective properties. For skeletal muscle, smart materials, such as EAP and SMA, can not only simulate the flexibility of skeletal muscle, but also have actuation and sensing properties which are similar to skeletal muscle. From this perspective, they are much better than pneumatic AM and conventional motors. Also, the limitations of material itself should also be considered. Actuation conditions of EAP are harsh, and SMA has disadvantages such as small strain and nonlinear properties. Thus, bionic material selection should follow the principles of maximizing multi-objective properties and the feasibility to compensate the limiting factors.

3. **Bionic design should follow the principle of priority and concurrency**. For the multi-objective bionics, the principle of concurrency should be followed. The primary and secondary sequences should also be considered based on the bionic requirements. For bionic design of skeletal muscle, targets include structure (large force-to-weight ratio, high integration level, and flexibility), function (actuation, self-sensing, energy storage), and biomechanical properties. Among them, biomechanical properties are the primary bionic targets.

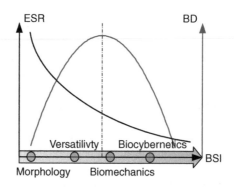

FIGURE 6.17   Relationships between BSI, ESR, and BD.

6.2 SKELETAL MUSCLE CHARACTER IDENTIFICATION AND MODELING

BSI is the first step of bionic design. If we define an artificial actuator as artificial skeletal muscle, we have to clarify what different types of skeletal muscles have in common and what unique structures, functions, and mechanical properties make them different from other actuators. The simulation of these properties is the main aim of skeletal muscle bionic design. However, the properties of skeletal muscles of different vertebrates can be radically different from each other. The skeletal muscle of the same species may not be the same either, but its basic composition, actuation mechanism, and mechanical properties are identical. The method applied in this section is to analyze the complex structure and function properties of skeletal muscle and extract simple and correct structural and functional models. Moreover, as for the mechanical property of skeletal muscle, we developed the modified 4M model of skeletal muscle through the further simplification of the originally proposed 4M model and the mechanical data of different vertebrates. Then, the guiding principles for the bionic design of skeletal muscle are determined.

6.2.1 BIOLOGICAL CHARACTER IDENTIFICATION OF SKELETAL MUSCLE

6.2.1.1 Structure and Function Properties of Skeletal Muscle

From the perspective of structure, skeletal muscle is mainly composed of muscle fibers and connective tissues. Each fiber includes numerous parallel myofibrils. Each myofibril consists of numerous sarcomeres in series. Each sarcomere is made up of thick myofilaments and thin myofilaments. Among them, thin filament is composed of actin, and thick filament is composed of myosin (molecular motor). Skeletal muscle contraction is the macroscopic phenomenon of collective operation of numerous molecular motors. Detailed introduction can be found in Section 1.2. Muscle fiber is the contractile element (CE), and connective tissue is the parallel elastic element (PE). There is also series element (SE) in skeletal muscle, referring mainly to titin in sarcomere. Each skeletal muscle connects to skeletons via tendon. Thus, the detailed skeletal muscle–tendon system can be illustrated in Figure 6.18. In a simple sense, we regard the skeletal muscle–tendon system as skeletal muscle system.

Referring to animal experimental data [57], the elastic force of PE is small when the length of skeletal muscle is shorter than the resting length. When the length is larger than the resting length, the passive force will increase exponentially. Resting (slack) length is the length of skeletal muscle at which the isometric force is the largest. Thus, when the length is smaller than the resting length, PE can be neglected for skeletal muscle modeling and bionic design, but when the length is larger, it has to be taken into account. The parallel elastic structure of skeletal muscle not only ensures the energy storage and release in the process of muscular contraction, but also prevents the sprain of muscle fibers. Besides, when compared with tendon, the properties of passive elasticity and energy storage of SE can be neglected [58]. Thus, the skeletal muscle–tendon system can be further simplified as illustrated in Figure 6.19.

From the perspective of function, skeletal muscle is a multi-functional biological actuator. Its functions can be divided into three classes: actuation, self-sensing, and energy storage. The multi-functional

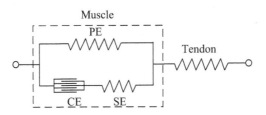

FIGURE 6.18 Skeletal muscle–tendon system.

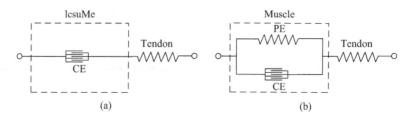

FIGURE 6.19 Simplified figures of skeletal muscle–tendon system when the length of skeletal muscle is (a) smaller than resting length; (b) larger then resting length.

property of skeletal muscle is closely related to its unique structure. As described in the last section, the actuation function of skeletal muscle comes from muscle fiber, and the sensing function originates from the proprioceptor inside muscle. Skeletal muscle is controlled by motoneuron. To function appropriately, motoneuron has to send action potential in appropriate timing and change the firing frequency based on motion and muscle loading. The real-time adjustment of firing frequency depends on the real-time feedback to central nervous system from the proprioceptors inside skeletal muscle.

The proprioceptors of skeletal muscle can be divided into two kinds, the Golgi tendon organ (GTO) and muscle spindles. GTOs are located in the connecting part of skeletal muscle and tendon and interact with tendon fibers. When muscle contracts, GTOs can detect the force change of motor units sensitively. Thus, GTOs can be regarded as the force sensors integrated inside muscle. Muscle spindle is a special kind of muscle fiber integrated inside muscle. It is wrapped by spindle capsule. Thus, it is also called as intramuscular spindle. Other muscle fibers are called as outer muscle spindles. They are parallel to each other. There are two kinds of intramuscular spindles: the nuclear bag type and nuclear chain type. Nuclear bag is able to detect the change rate of skeletal muscle length and velocity, while nuclear chain is able to detect the length of skeletal muscle. Thus, muscle spindle can be seen as the displacement sensor integrated inside the muscle. The properties of muscle spindle make it significant in reflection response, proprioception, and motion and position control. The functional unit of skeletal muscle is called motor unit. One motor unit is composed of one motoneuron and all the muscle fibers dominated by this motoneuron. This functional unit and the proprioceptors consist of the complete force and displacement double-closed-loop control of skeletal muscle, as illustrated in Figure 6.20.

The energy storage capacity of skeletal muscle depends on the connective tissue and the special viscoelastic structure of tendon. The connective tissue is in series with tendon. It stretches when skeletal muscle contracts actively or passively, generating tension and storing elastic potential energy at the same time. When muscle relaxes, elastic body rebounds, and the stored elastic potential energy is released. The function of connective tissue and tendon not only decreases energy consumption and increases power efficiency, but also prevents muscle from getting injured.

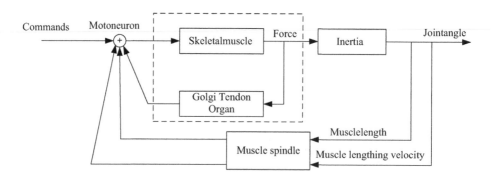

FIGURE 6.20 Actuation-and-sensing–integrated control diagram of skeletal muscle.

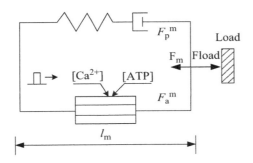

FIGURE 6.21 Simplified structure of skeletal muscle [67].

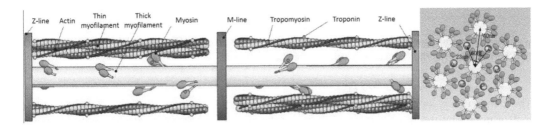

FIGURE 6.22 Composition of sarcomere.

6.2.1.2 Biomechanical Property of Skeletal Muscle

The imitation of mechanical properties is the key in the bionic design of skeletal muscles. The mechanical property of skeletal muscle can be described by the mechanical properties of isometric contraction and isotonic contraction [4]. The property of isotonic contraction refers to the contraction properties when the tension of skeletal muscle is fixed and that of isometric contraction refers to the contraction properties when the length of skeletal muscle is fixed. The 4M model describes the contraction force and velocity properties under different microscopic and macroscopic factors [59–63]. Using 4M model as the basis, we can modify it after analyzing the mechanical properties of skeletal muscle and combining existent skeletal muscle data to guide the design of AM.

The modeling objective of 4M model is single sarcomere. It uses the mechanism of nonequilibrium statistical mechanics and is based on the spatial structure of molecular motor, the collective operation mechanism, and characteristics of series and parallel connections of sarcomere. It is a biomechanical model of skeletal muscle developed from microscopic to macroscopic scale.

The loading, ATP concentration, and action potential (represented by $[Ca^{2+}]$) are all fully considered in this model. The modeling configuration is illustrated in Figure 6.21. Sarcomere is the basic unit of skeletal muscle contraction. The structure of single sarcomere is illustrated in Figure 6.22. Molecular motor is the source of muscular contraction [63]. It produces work periodically, featuring complex chemical status through conformational changes. The collective operation of large amount of molecular motors leads to the relative sliding of thick and thin filaments and generates muscular contraction [64].

6.2.1.2.1 Isometric Contraction Properties

The active force is produced by the collective working of numerous molecular motors. The total force F generated by skeletal muscle comprises the active force F_a and the passive force F_p:

$$F = F_a + F_p. \tag{6.1}$$

Based on the 4M model, active force can be expressed by the following equation:

$$F_a = \frac{A\alpha\beta n_0 k_c}{s} \int_0^L x\rho(x,t)dx,$$ (6.2)

where a is the overlap degree between thin and thick filaments and β is the activation degree of sarcomere. If $a = 1$, the muscle contracts at tetanic state. k_c is the elasticity coefficient of molecular motor. An_0/s represents the total number of molecular motors in the muscle. The term $\int_0^L x\rho(x,t)dx$ represents the average displacement of molecular motor on thin filaments, which can be considered as a constant [63]. When skeletal muscle is passively pulled under resting state, it can be described as a nonlinear viscoelastic body [65]. The passive force is produced by the viscoelastic tissue of skeletal muscle, which satisfies the following equation:

$$F_p = k_m \Delta l + \gamma l,$$ (6.3)

where k_m is the nonlinear elasticity coefficient and γ is the drag coefficient of PE. Δl is the contraction length, and l is the contraction velocity of the muscle.

6.2.1.2.2 Isotonic Contraction Properties

The contraction velocity of sarcomere, i.e., the relative sliding velocity of thick and thin filaments, is determined by the transition speed of molecular motor among different chemical states. The transition speed is determined by load capacity and [ATP]. Based on the 4M model, the contraction speed of sarcomere is

$$v = \frac{1}{N}\sum_{i-1}^{N} V_i = \frac{1}{N}\sum_{i-1}^{N} LJ_i,$$ (6.4)

where $vi = LJi(x)$ represents the movement speed of molecular motor in state i. N is the number of all the chemical states of molecular motor. Figure 6.23 illustrates the relationships among the load capacity of molecular motor, [ATP], and contraction speed of sarcomere. Moreover, the length of muscle fiber is approximately equal to the largest length of myofibril, i.e., the length summation of all the sarcomeres. Thus, the contraction velocity of skeletal muscle is equal to the equivalent speed determined by all the serial sarcomeres. The relationship between contraction velocity and load capacity is that they are inversely proportional to each other, as illustrated in Figure 6.23. It is consistent with the macroscopic scale force–velocity relation expressed by Hill equation.

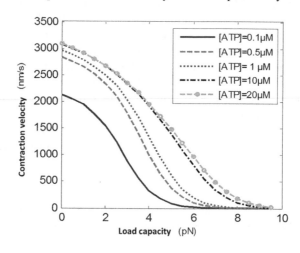

FIGURE 6.23 Relationship between load capacity and contraction velocity.

6.2.2 Contraction Property Modelling of Skeletal Muscle

Based on the analysis in the above section, muscular contraction is affected by multiple factors and presents complex biomechanical properties. 4M model describes macroscopic biomechanical property of skeletal muscle from the microscopic perspective of molecular motor; thus, it is of good generality. However, there are too many biological parameters in this model. Hence, it cannot be applied in AM design directly. To overcome this difficulty, the modified 4M model is proposed from two perspectives, i.e., isometric contraction and isotonic contraction, to guide AM design based on skeletal muscle properties and experimental data of various vertebrates.

6.2.2.1 Isometric Contraction Modeling

Isometric contraction property refers to the property when skeletal muscle is under the fixed length (when the contraction velocity is zero). Referring to Figure 6.19, skeletal muscle is composed of CE and PE. Under the condition of isometric contraction, the mechanical properties of the two parts are totally different.

6.2.2.1.1 Contractile Element (CE)

CE is composed of muscle fibers and is the main component of skeletal muscle and also the key point in 4M model analysis. Cook found that CE can be treated as a force generator with paralleled damping [66]. Referring to Eq. (6.2), the active force is determined only by the overlap degree between thin and thick filaments and the activation degree of sarcomere, and the overlap degree can be measured by the length of sarcomere. Thus, the active force of skeletal muscle can be described by the function concerning muscle length and activation degree. Besides, based on the experimental results obtained by Gordon, the force–length curve is approximately parabolic, i.e., the force increases first and then decreases, reaching its maximum at the resting length. Thus, the active force of skeletal muscle can be described as

$$\frac{F_a}{F_0} = \beta \left[a \left(\frac{l}{l_0} \right)^2 + b \left(\frac{l}{l_0} \right) + c \right], \tag{6.5}$$

where l_0 is the resting length and F_0 is the maximum isometric contraction force under resting length. l is the real-time length of skeletal muscle, and F_a is the real-time active contraction force. β is the activation degree of skeletal muscle, and $\beta \in [0, 1]$. $\beta = 1$ indicates that muscle is in the tetanic state, while $\beta = 0$ indicates that the skeletal muscle is not activated (the passive state). Parameters a, b, and c can be measured through skeletal muscle data of mouse [67], frog [68], cat [69], or human [70]. Detailed parameters are illustrated in Table 6.3.

Based on Eq. (6.5), the active force–length relationship in the tetanic state and isometric contraction is illustrated in Figure 6.24 (note that to get easy comparison, the experimental results are all normalized). The four vertebrates prove the parabolic feature of isometric muscular contraction, but as the species are different, the widths of the curves have clear difference. Among them, the driving range of human skeletal muscle is the smallest, while that of frog and mouse is large. Moreover, skeletal muscle of cat can still generate contraction force when the length is far from the resting length.

6.2.2.1.2 Passive Element

The passive elements are divided into the parallel element (PE) and the series element (SE). As SE is much weaker than PE in deformation and energy storage, here the passive element refers to PE only, which is the connective tissue. Based on the analysis in Section 6.3.1.2, muscle force is mainly provided by PE when skeletal muscle is inactivated ($\beta = 0$). At this time, skeletal muscle can be described as a nonlinear viscoelastic body satisfying Eq. (6.3). Experiments show that PE has small nonlinear damping [71]. Moreover, based on Section 6.3.1.1, PE works outside the resting length, and the output force increases exponentially. Thus, Eq. (6.3) can be simplified into

$$\frac{F_p}{F_0} = \begin{cases} 0 & \text{for } l < l_0 \\ k_1 \left(\dfrac{l}{l_0} \right)^{k_2} & \text{for } l \geq l_0 \end{cases}, \tag{6.6}$$

where l is the real-time length of skeletal muscle; F_p is the real-time passive force; k_1 and k_2 are the passive force model parameters, and they are acquired from the skeletal muscle data from frog [68], cat [69], and human [70]. Detailed parameters are illustrated in Table 6.4.

TABLE 6.3

Active Force–Length Data under Isometric Contraction

Vertebrate	a	b	c	l_0 (mm)	F_0 (N)	
Mouse	−4.50	8.95	−3.45	27.0	0.29	$R_2 = 0.97$
Frog	−6.79	14.69	−6.88	31.0	0.67	$R_2 = 0.96$
Cat	−5.71	11.52	−4.81	31.9	0.18	$R_2 = 0.99$
Human	−13.43	28.23	−13.96	215.9	193.1	$R_2 = 0.75$

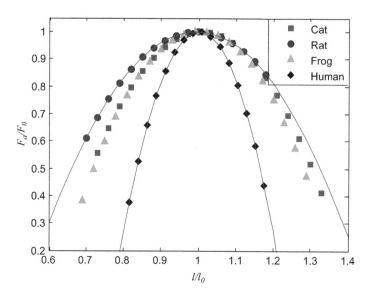

FIGURE 6.24 The dimensionless relationship between active force and length under isometric contraction state of vertebrates.

TABLE 6.4

Passive Force–Length Data of Skeletal Muscles under Isometric Contraction

Vertebrate	k_1	k_2	l_0 (mm)	F_0 (N)	
Frog	0.0006	20.63	31.0	0.67	$R_2 = 0.95$
Cat	0.0301	9.16	31.9	0.18	$R_2 = 0.95$
Human	0.0037	10.43	215.9	193.1	$R_2 = 0.89$

Based on Eq. (6.6), the passive force–length relationships under isometric contraction can be acquired, as illustrated in Figure 6.25. Referring to the figure, passive force of PE is near zero at the resting length and increases quickly when the length exceeds this length. Moreover, passive forces and contraction lengths of the skeletal muscle of different animals are different, but the passive force–length relations all satisfy Eq. (6.6).

Muscle force is the sum of active force and passive force, satisfying Eq. (6.1). The total contraction force–length relationship is illustrated in Figure 6.26. Thus, when the length is shorter than the resting length, contraction force depends mainly on active force. When the length increases, passive force becomes the main component. However, most skeletal muscles in a single joint would not be pulled to the length when passive force is dominant [4]. Moreover, the active force–length curves of different skeletal muscles are almost the same, while there are obvious differences among the passive force–length curves. It is mainly caused by the amount of connective tissue (elastic component)

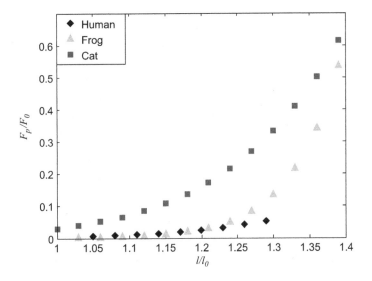

FIGURE 6.25 Dimensionless relationships of passive force and length under isometric contraction of vertebrate skeletal muscles.

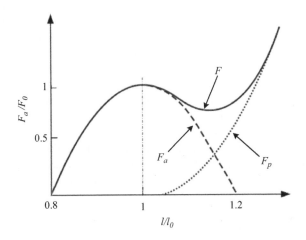

FIGURE 6.26 Dimensionless active force–length, passive force–length, and total force–length relationships of skeletal muscles.

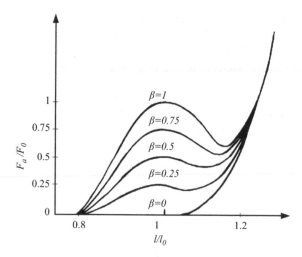

FIGURE 6.27 Dimensionless total force–length relationship under different activation degrees.

in the skeletal muscle. Based on the 4M model (Eq. 6.2), the output force of different skeletal muscles is proportional to the amount of paralleled muscle fibers, and active and passive structures of skeletal muscle match with each other. Thus, in practical bionics, the maximum passive force can be determined by the maximum contraction force and its contraction range, and then the total force–length curve can be acquired.

Active contraction is ignited by the action potential generated from its dominating motoneuron. Action potential frequency determines the skeletal muscle activation degree β indirectly. The higher the firing rate, the larger the contraction force is. When the firing rate exceeds a certain level, contraction force reaches its peak value where skeletal muscle is in the tetanic state (maximum activation degree state). The force–length relation under tetanus is illustrated in Figure 6.26, where $\beta = 1$. Based on the above analysis, force–length relations under different activation degrees can be acquired, as illustrated in Figure 6.27.

6.2.2.2 Isotonic Contraction Modeling

Isotonic contraction involves the force–velocity characteristics of skeletal muscle under constant tension. It can be further divided into concentric contraction and eccentric contraction. In concentric contraction, skeletal muscle does positive work, while in eccentric contraction it generates negative work. The discussion here limits to the concentric contraction process. Under isotonic contraction, contraction force increases when the contraction velocity decreases in the inversely proportional manner. Contraction force is not only related to contraction velocity, but also influenced by length and activation degree. Hill proved the hyperbolic force–velocity relation by experiments [5]. However, the experiment was carried out under the tetanus contraction state, without considering the influence of activation degree. 4M model describes the relationships among load capacity of molecular motor, [ATP], and contraction velocity of sarcomere from microscopic scale, as illustrated in Figure 6.28. Here we limit skeletal muscle length within the resting length and consider the influence of activation degree. In this book, the following relationship is proposed in terms of contraction force, velocity, and activation function combining 4M model and the experimental results of Hill:

$$\left(\frac{F}{F_0} + a \right)\left(\frac{v}{v_0} + b \right) = (1+a)b, \tag{6.7}$$

where $\overline{F}_0 = \beta F_0$.

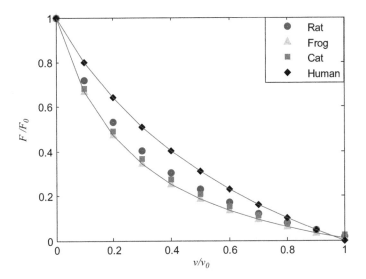

FIGURE 6.28   Dimensionless relationships between passive force and length under isotonic contraction of vertebrate skeletal muscles.

TABLE 6.5
Force–Velocity Data of Vertebrate Skeletal Muscles

Vertebrate	a	F_0 (N)	b	v_0 (mm/s)
Mouse	0.356	4.3	0.38	144
Frog	0.27	0.67	0.28	42
Cat	0.27	0.18	0.30	191
Human	0.81	200	0.81	1,115

F_0 here is the maximum contraction force, and v_0 is the maximum contraction velocity; F is the real-time contraction force, and v is the real-time contraction velocity; β is the activation degree, and $\beta \in [0, 1]$. Parameters a and b are constants, the value of which is not only determined by species, but also by muscle types. Based on the known skeletal muscle data [69,71–73], the model parameters can be acquired, as listed in Table 6.5.

Based on Eq. (6.7), the force–velocity relation under isotonic contraction state can be acquired when $\beta = 1$, as illustrated in Figure 6.28. It can be inferred that human muscle contraction force is larger than that of other three vertebrates under certain velocities. Considering the influence of activation degree and Eq. (6.7), the force–velocity relationship under different activation degrees can be acquired, as illustrated in Figure 6.29.

Considering the relationships among force, velocity, and length, the equation can be obtained as follows:

$$F = \beta \cdot F_0 \cdot f(l) \cdot g(v). \tag{6.8}$$

Based on the above equation, the influence of these quantities can be illustrated in Figure 6.30. It describes the mechanical property of skeletal muscle intuitively. Note that the activation degree here is 1.

In this section, we systematically explain the BID bionic design method with the aim of skeletal muscle bionics. There are four stages, i.e., concept selection, sub-conceptual design, detail design, and iteration and learning. The design method provides detailed principles for multi-objective bionic

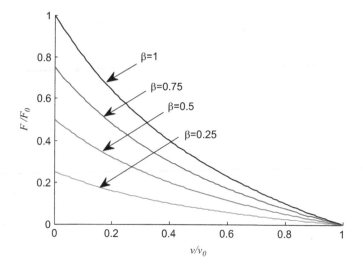

FIGURE 6.29   Dimensionless force–velocity relation under different activation degrees.

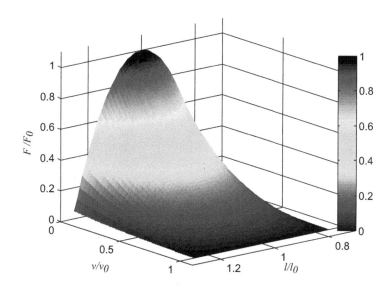

FIGURE 6.30   3D diagram of dimensionless force–velocity–length relationships.

design based on complex creatures. Based on the design method, we presented detailed analysis and identification of musculoskeletal system, simplified the structure and function, developed the biomechanical model for skeletal muscle, and thus laid a foundation for the guiding principles.

6.3   SMA ARTIFICIAL SKELETAL MUSCLE INTEGRATING ACTUATION, SENSING, AND STRUCTURE

Skeletal muscle is a highly integrated actuator integrating actuation, self-sensing, and structure. For decades, conventional motors, such as hydraulic actuator [16–20] and pneumatic AM [3], and smart material actuators [21–26], including PZT, EAP, carbon nanotube, and SMA, have all been applied in AM researches. However, the structure bionics of skeletal muscle under microscopic scale (artificial molecular actuation) is limited by nanotechnology and bionic materials; thus, it is hard to realize. As for macroscopic scale, because of the shortcomings of conventional actuation devices (electric motor, hydraulic, and pneumatic), such as large volume or low power-to-weight ratio, there are problems such as low control accuracy, mismatching with biological muscle's dynamics, and bulkiness in structure for AM. Smart actuation materials, such as PZT and EAPs, are unable to achieve the goal because of the limiting factors such as actuation voltage and environment. Compared with other actuation devices and materials, SMA has many properties similar to skeletal muscle, such as flexibility, large power density, large output force, etc. [27]. Besides the actuation function, SMA also has the self-sensing function, i.e., detecting the length change through the resistance variation. Compared with the rigorous actuation voltage (larger than 1,000 V) of EAP, SMA can run at low actuation voltage (5 V). Thus, SMA has the potential to achieve skeletal muscle bionics.

Guided by BID, the design and realization process of SMA-AM will be presented in detail in this section. Based on the comparison of mechanical property of skeletal muscle and actuation property of SMA, the appropriate simulation of the properties of active force, velocity, activation degree, length of skeletal muscle can be achieved when we overcome the small strain of SMA. As for the passive structure of skeletal muscle, the mechanical property is achieved by bringing in the PET silicon tube. By using forced tube cooling system, the response speed of SMA-AM is increased while maintaining the compactness, large power density, and flexibility of SMA. At last, the bionic mechanical features of SMA-AM are evaluated by experiments.

Besides, although SMA has self-sensing function, it has not been fully recognized. There are few self-sensing models for SMA. Lan in Taiwan, China, established the resistance–strain model using a sixth-order polynomial based on the resistance heating experiments [83,84]. From the perspective of free energy of phase transformation, the resistance varying characters of SMA will be analyzed in this section. The phase transformation dynamics of SMA resistance model will be developed on the basis of determining the phase transformation temperature region and the varying character of latent heat using Differential Scanning Calorimetry (DSC). Through the thermomechanical and electrical experiment, we acquired the resistance varying curves under different thermomechanical loads and proved the correctness of this resistance dynamic model. Then, the "resistance–length" self-sensing model of SMA is developed based on the deduction. At last, the self-sensing model is applied to the single-DOF robot ankle–foot system with SMA-bias spring. Accurate angular tracking has proven the self-sensing function of SMA and laid a theoretical foundation for the realization of the active ankle–foot rehabilitation system based on the SMA-AM integrated with actuation and sensing.

6.3.1 Key Technologies of SMA

No matter what kinds of actuators or smart materials are involved in the research of AM, it should not be purely structural design of actuation materials but ought to be the simulation of the multifunctional character of skeletal muscle through overcoming self-deficiencies. Among them, the most important is the simulation of the integration of flexible structure, actuation and sensing, large power density, and biomechanical properties of skeletal muscle. Only in this way can we simulate the unique motion performance of creatures. Referring to current research status of artificial skeletal muscle, most of the studies of AM are not able to reach this goal. The main reasons are the disunity of bionic design principles and the limitation of bionic materials. Compared with other actuation materials, SMA has many properties that are similar to skeletal muscle. However, to date, there has not been any research on SMA-based bionic design of skeletal muscle based on the structural function and mechanical features of skeletal muscle. This is due to a series of key technical limitations as follows.

6.3.1.1 Low Strain and Low Response Time of SMA

The low strain and low response time are the primary factors limiting the structural design of SMA-AM. Low strain is the inherent character of SMA. Thus, the indirect increase of strain can only be achieved through proper structural design. For example, SMA spring has been used as the actuator [74]. Although the effective deformation can be increased by the spring actuator, the output force of SMA is largely decreased. Most of the existing structural designs increase the strain by sacrificing output force [50–54]. This is not good for the AM design when large output force is required. The response time of SMA is mainly determined by the phase transformation speed of SMA and further determined by the heating and cooling speeds of SMA. Compared with the convenience of heating, such as current heating, increasing the cooling speed of SMA is the key to increase the response speed. The simplistic way is to increase the surface area of SMA, i.e., to select SMA wires with small diameters [54,75]. The smaller the diameter, the shorter the cooling time and faster the response speed we will get. Yee Harn Teh and Roy Featherstone in Australian National University designed a two-DOF SMA actuation device using an SMA wire with the diameter of 0.05 mm [54]. They increased the actuation frequency of SMA to 2 Hz by natural cooling and fast current heating. However, the output force was also small when the diameter of SMA was small. Multiple paralleled SMA wires can be used to increase the output force, but it also increases the design complexity. Besides, the cooling speed of SMA can also be achieved by forced cooling. There are many cooling methods for SMA, such as the bionic hand developed by MIT. Asada [53] used three cooling fans, as illustrated in Figure 6.31. University of Utah used the pipe cooling cycle to achieve the control of SMA actuators [76]. Besides, scholars in MIT used Parr semiconductor to implement forced cooling of SMA segments [77]. Different cooling methods bring different complexities to the design of SMA actuator structure and affect the power density of SMA actuator. Thus, how to increase strain and response speed of SMA and maintain the biomechanical character of skeletal muscle while ensuring the large output force, large power density, and flexibility of SMA is the key to the structural design of SMA-AM.

6.3.1.2   SMA Self-Sensing Character Analysis

The integration of actuation and sensing of AM is the key to integrate bionic design of skeletal muscle. Compared with conventional actuators (electric motor and pneumatic AM for example), SMA has the self-sensing property similar to muscular spindle of skeletal muscle. When the phase of SMA changes, resistance, lattice structure, and length all change at the same time. Thus, there are specific mapping relations between resistance and length. By developing the resistance–length relationship, the length of SMA can be fed back by resistance. Based on this character, the design of SMA-integrated self-sensing actuator can be achieved. Early in the 1980s, Ikuta in Japan used SMA to design the endoscope with the integration of actuation and sensing, as illustrated in Figure 6.31. In China, Professor Tianmiao Wang in Beijing University of Aeronautics and Astronautics developed active operating forceps with SMA by utilizing its self-sensing character. Professor Yuehong Yin in Shanghai Jiao Tong University designed the flexible active stone grabber used in the gall stone operation. Four paralleled SMAs are used as the actuators and sensors to achieve the active grabbing of stone [78].

Although there have been many applications of self-sensing of SMA, they all have the disadvantages of low accuracy, poor robustness, and lack of generality. This is because that SMA resistance is affected by not only phase transformation of SMA, but also multiple factors such as material composition, Martensitic lattice reconstruction, and R-phase [26,79]. Thus, developing an effective

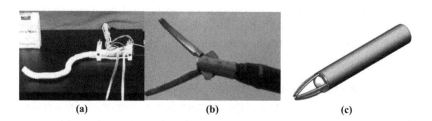

(a)   (b)   (c)

FIGURE 6.31   (a) Active endoscope; (b) active operating forceps; (c) active stone micrograbber.

self-sensing model is the key to solving the above problems. Czech scholars developed the resistance micromechanical model from the perspective of microcrystal by using neuron scattering experiment to analyze NiTi SMA phase change characters [79,80]. It explains the relationships among SMA resistance, stress, and temperature. However, this model cannot be applied directly on self-sensing control. Lan in Taiwan, China, developed the resistance–strain model by sixth-order polynomial based on the resistance heating experiment [81–83]. Through the experiments, they found that the resistance–strain hysteresis is smaller with better degree of linearity when the external load of SMA is larger. Based on the developed self-sensing model, Lan achieved the integrated actuation and feedback of SMA micrograbber. Based on the same experiment method, Song in University of Houston had similar results and applied it in position tracking control [84,85]. However, the self-sensing model based on electric heating experiment will change with SMA wire. Thus, it does not have the generality. How to develop unified self-sensing model and describe resistance changing character of different SMA wire is what has to be solved right now.

6.3.1.3 Hysteresis Nonlinearity Analysis and Control of SMA

In the heating and cooling process of SMA, strong hysteresis nonlinearity is demonstrated by SMA because of lattice phase transition. Different from normal nonlinearity, hysteresis is the common nonlinearity among smart actuation materials (such as PZT and SMA). In practical system, hysteresis is not simple hysteresis relation between input and output, but multi-valued mapping. The strong nonlinearity of SMA largely limits its control accuracy and even leads to instability of SMA actuation systems. Thus, eliminating hysteresis is of great significance to system control. Describing the hysteresis of SMA and developing mathematical model about this property are the keys to solving the above problems. To date, various mathematical models have been developed to describe the hysteresis of SMA and can be divided into two classes. One is the physics-based models, and the representative ones are Tanaka model [86] and Brinson model [87]. This type of model accurately describes the constitutive features and phase transformation characters of SMA, but there are too many unknown material parameters in the model. Thus, it is hard to be applied in control systems.

Phenomenological model is the other type of mathematical model, and the representative ones are Preisach model and Prandtl–Ishlinskii model. However, most of these models are used to describe the hysteresis character of PZT, and only a few have been used to describe that of SMA. This is due to the fact that the hysteresis behavior of SMA is more complex than that of PZT. The hysteresis property of SMA is not only related to actuation frequency, but also depends on external load, and the nonlinearity is saturable and unsmooth, as illustrated in Figure 6.32 [89]. Preisach model is one

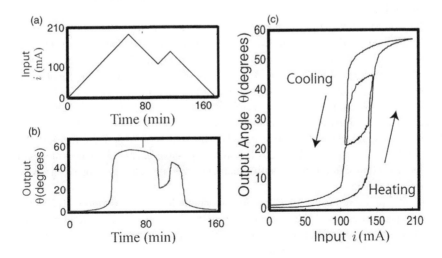

FIGURE 6.32   (a) SMA input signal; (b) output response; (c) hysteresis curve between input and output.

of the most widely used models to describe the hysteresis curve of SMA [88]. American scholar Hughes proved by experiments that SMA hysteresis curve satisfies two features of Preisach model: the congruence property and erase property [90]. Thus, it proved that Preisach model can be used to describe SMA hysteresis. After that, scholars are able to describe and compensate SMA hysteresis by using Preisach model [91–97]. However, it is hard to acquire the analytical solution of Preisach model; thus, it is hard to be applied in real-time control system. Prandtl–Ishlinskii model has analytical solutions; thus, it can be applied in the hysteresis compensation of SMA easily [98–100], but there are many nonlinear weight factors in the model, increasing the computing complexity. Thus, it is not proper to be applied in real-time control system [101] either. Besides, the influence of stress and actuation frequency on SMA hysteresis property is not considered in these models. Model control methods, such as neural network control [102], genetic algorithm [103], variable structure control [104], sliding mode control [105], have all been used to describe the hysteresis phenomenon of SMA, while all these control strategies are aimed at the description and compensation of SMA under specific stress or frequency state without considering the influence of dynamically varying stress and frequency.

For real animals, skeletal muscle is not only able to perform flexion/extension (F/E) activities under different frequency ranges, but also bears different loads and achieves accurate position control. Thus, SMA-AM must have similar abilities. Describing SMA hysteresis property under varying stresses and load to control the hysteresis is the key to realizing SMA-AM.

6.3.2 SMA-BASED AM DESIGN REALIZATION

Although many actuators and smart materials have been applied in AM research and they all have some properties similar to those of skeletal muscle, none of them is able to achieve the comprehensive bionics of biomechanical property of skeletal muscle, i.e., the relationships among force, length, velocity, and activation degree. So far, few scholars have designed AM from this perspective.

In the last section, we proposed the modified 4M model based on the proper analysis and simplification of 4M model. A parabolic model is used to describe the active force–length–activation degree relation of skeletal muscle. An exponential model is proposed to describe the passive force–length relation, and a hyperbolic model is used to describe the tension–velocity–activation relation. Based on the description of the characteristic curves, the force–velocity–activation degree relations of different vertebrates are different from one another. Compared with the bionics of mechanical property of a specific species, determining the bionic region based on the existing data is more proper and feasible.

As for the isotonic contraction property (force–velocity relation), the following parameters can be determined based on the modified 4M model and the known experimental data: $a,b \in [0.27, 0.81]$. The force–velocity envelope curve is illustrated in Figure 6.33, represented by the shadow region. Similarly, for the isometric contraction bionics of active elements (the force–length relation of active element), the following parameter regions can be determined: $a \in [-13.43, -4.5]$; $b \in [8.95, 28.23]$; $c \in [-13.96, -3.45]$. Based on these regions, we can acquire the muscle "envelope" for active force–length curve, as illustrated by the shadow area in Figure 6.34. Besides, the bionics of the isometric properties of passive elements is based on the matching of active force–length properties, i.e., to ensure that the elongation and tensile force of passive elastic element matches the amount of contraction and contraction force of active elements. The muscle envelope of passive elements is illustrated in Figure 6.35.

Note that although the muscle envelope does not include—and it is impossible to include—the biomechanical properties of all the animals, the biomechanical variation trend of animal skeletal muscle has been characterized clearly. It also provides distinct design principles and bionic standards for the design of AM; i.e., the AM contraction mechanical property acquired in muscle contraction experiments should be in the region of muscle envelope.

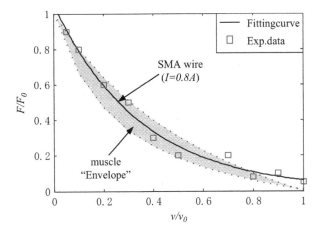

FIGURE 6.33   Force–velocity property of SMA wire under isometric contraction.

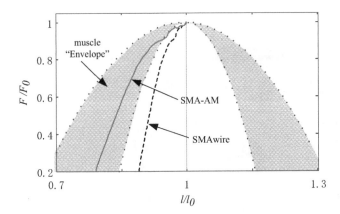

FIGURE 6.34   Force–length property of SMA wire and SMA-AM under isometric contraction.

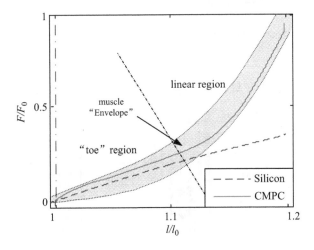

FIGURE 6.35   Force–length curves of silastic tube and CMPC.

6.3.2.1 Bionic Design of Active Elements

SMA has many properties similar to skeletal muscle, such as high power density, large output force, flexibility, and one-way contraction, as well as the self-sensing function similar to muscular spindle. Thus, we select SMA as the active element for skeletal muscle bionics and further study the self-sensing property of SMA to achieve the integrated actuation and sensing functions of AM.

Based on BID, the basic design principle we follow is to achieve the bionics of biomechanical and multi-functional properties and ensure the simplicity and compactness in structure during the design. FlexinolTM equiatomic NiTi SMA wire produced by DYNALLOY Company is selected, as illustrated in Figure 6.36. It has the good property of shape memory, and the detailed parameters are listed in Appendix 6.A.

SMA's active contraction property is similar to that of skeletal muscle fiber. Scholars name SMA wire as bionic muscle based on this property. However, they are not quite clear whether SMA has the bionic mechanical properties, i.e., whether SMA is able to achieve the simulation of isotonic and isometric contractile behaviors of skeletal muscle. To solve the above problems, a series of semi-skeletal muscle contraction experiments have been done using SMA wires. The experiments are divided into two parts, the fast releasing experiment and isometric contraction experiment. The idea is similar to that used in the classic Hill experiment. Detailed experimental devices are illustrated in Figure 6.37.

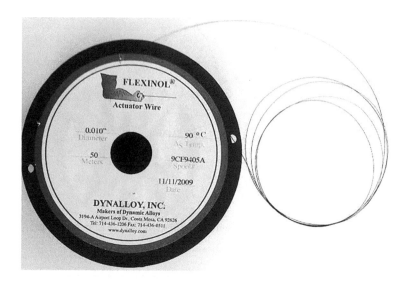

FIGURE 6.36 Flexinol™ equiatomic NiTi SMA.

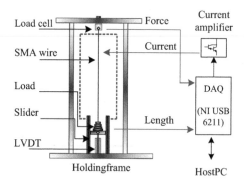

FIGURE 6.37 Schematic diagram of experimental setup.

An SMA wire sample with diameter of 0.25 mm and length of 220 mm is placed vertically with one end fixed to a load cell and the other end connected to external stress. The external stresses are provided by different constant loads varying from 56 to 280 MPa and a helical bias spring with the stiffness of 143 N/m. The contraction force is measured by the load cell, and the displacement is measured by a linear variable differential transformer (LVDT) with the resolution of 0.01 mm. A computer equipped with a data acquisition card (NI USB-6211) generates voltage signal and acquires the measured data. The voltage is used to drive the SMA wire and is amplified by a custom-made current amplifier (CMCA) with a fixed gain of 0.4 A/V, and forced vessel airflow is used to cool the SMA wire using a mini pump. Besides, host PC with an acquisition card with the number NI USB 6211 is applied to achieve the signal control of current amplifier, the contraction force of SMA wire, and the acquisition and control of contraction length data. All the operations are realized in LabVIEW software.

SMA has two phases: the martensite and austenite. When activating SMA through electric heating, SMA wires contract, and martensite phase transformation occurs. While cooling, SMA wire will recover to its original length under external force, and the inverse martensite phase transformation occurs. (Note that SMA length in martensite phase is its maximum. To provide easy comparison, we call the length at this state as the resting length of SMA.)

Release instantly the skeletal muscle in the status of tetanic stimulation and resting length, and skeletal muscle will contract quickly. By measuring skeletal muscle contraction speed under different loads, the contraction force–velocity property under isotonic contraction can be acquired effectively, showing a hyperbolic relation. To analyze the isotonic contraction property of SMA, we perform the SMA fast release experiment under tetanic stimulation with the above device and a single SMA wire. The detailed steps are as follows. Fix the slider at the end of SMA wire and ensure that SMA is at resting length. Then, increase the temperature of SMA to that above the martensite end temperature A_f using current heating. Release instantly the SMA wire, and record the velocity of SMA wire contraction under different loads. Referring to the force–velocity property of SMA under isotonic contraction, it turns out that the force–velocity curve lies within the envelope region of skeletal muscle force–velocity property. It demonstrates that SMA wire has the isometric contraction property similar to skeletal muscle.

Based on the semi-skeletal muscle isometric experiment, we further study the isometric contraction property of SMA. The experiment steps are as follows. Unload the external load. Fix the SMA wire in the region of $[0.9l_0, l_0]$, while l_0 is the resting length of SMA. Then, heat SMA with current to the temperature above A_f, generate tetanic contraction, and record the contraction force. Acquire the force–length property curve under isometric contraction. It can be noted that the contraction force increases with the increase of length and reaches its maximum F_0 at resting length l_0. The force–length curve of SMA wire is hyperbolic, similar to skeletal muscle. However, SMA cannot be used to simulate skeletal muscle force–length property above the resting length. This is because when the length is larger than the resting length, SMA will be broken due to plastic deformation. Besides, the force–length curve of SMA wire is not within the envelope region of skeletal muscle. This is because the maximum strain of SMA is only 10%, lower than the 20%–40% range of skeletal muscle.

Low strain is the inherent property of SMA. Thus, the indirect increase of strain can only be achieved through proper structural design. Although the effective deformation can be increased by the spring actuator, the output force of SMA is largely decreased. Most of the existing structural designs increase the strain by sacrificing output force. This is not expected for the AM design when large output force is required. To increase SMA strain and ensure large output force, inspired by the sliding structure of thick and thin filaments, we achieve the rotation and sliding of multi-paralleled SMA wires through the structure which we name as "muscle frame". It increases the equivalent strain of SMA by nearly 100% (almost 20% for the AM). It is the active element for SMA-AM. The detailed design structure and actuation mechanism are illustrated in Figure 6.38.

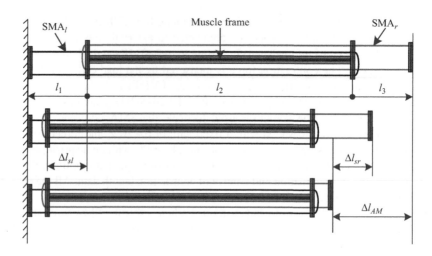

FIGURE 6.38 Structure and contraction mechanism of the parallel rotary SMA-AM.

The parallel SMA wires are arranged into overlapped pattern by the "muscle frame". Besides, the AM length l_{AM} consists of three parts, and the AM strain $\varepsilon_{\mathrm{AM}}$ can be expressed as follows:

$$\begin{cases} l_{\mathrm{AM}} = l_1 + l_2 + l_3 \\ \varepsilon_{\mathrm{AM}} = \dfrac{\Delta l_{\mathrm{AM}}}{l_{\mathrm{AM}}} \end{cases} . \tag{6.9}$$

Besides, length changes of the left and right SMA wires in AM can be described as

$$\begin{cases} \Delta l_{\mathrm{sl}} = (l_1 + l_2)\varepsilon \\ \Delta l_{\mathrm{sr}} = (l_2 + l_3)\varepsilon \end{cases} . \tag{6.10}$$

Combining Eqs. (6.9) and (6.10), the AM strain satisfies the following relationship:

$$\varepsilon_{\mathrm{AM}} = \frac{\Delta l_{\mathrm{sl}} + \Delta l_{\mathrm{sr}}}{l_{\mathrm{AM}}} = \left(1 + \frac{l_2}{l_{\mathrm{AM}}}\right)\varepsilon \leq 2\varepsilon, \tag{6.11}$$

where ε is SMA strain with the maximum about 10%. Thus, the AM strain can be increased to nearly 20% by changing the length of muscle frame l_2 according to Eq. (6.11). Experimental results show that the maximum strain of the designed SMA-AM is 18%. Besides, overstretching protection device is needed to prevent the plastic deformation of SMA, which can be achieved by the AM passive element.

6.3.2.2 Design of AM Passive Element

Skeletal muscle connective tissue is the main component of the passive element. Passive element not only has the function of protecting muscle fibers, but also exhibits nonlinear force–length property. For the sake of easier analysis, elastic force is normalized to the maximum value F_0, and elongation is normalized to $1.2l_0$. It can be inferred that when skeletal muscle length is less than the resting length, passive element is in relaxed state. When it is larger than the resting length, the elastic force–length curve can be divided into two parts. One is the "toe" region. In this region, connective tissues are stretched gradually with small coefficient of elasticity. The other is the linear region. In this region, the stiffness of connective tissue increases quickly and starts to deform with large coefficient of elasticity. In order to mimic the muscle's passive property, we used a silicon tube encapsulated by a polyethylene terephthalate (PET) mesh, which we call as CMPC (custom made passive composite). Note that, the silicon rubber generally has larger strain (about 100%), while the muscle's passive strain is only 10%–20% when the muscle is longer than the resting length. Thus, the PET mesh is used to prevent the overextension of the silicon tube. During the initial tensile test, the PET wire is in relaxed state; thus, the CMPC stiffness is provided by the silicon tube with a muscle-like "toe" region. When the PET mesh is stretched gradually to tensile state, the stiffness increases rapidly with large passive force. By changing the silicon tube length, diameter, and wall thickness and the PET mesh length, we can obtain the desired muscle-like force–length curve. After a series of tests on different tube–PET mesh combinations, the CMPC is selected with the silicon tube length (L) of 250 mm, diameter (D) of 10 mm, wall thickness (W) of 1.5 mm, and PET mesh length (ML) of 263 mm.

6.3.2.3 Bionic Structure Verification

Based on the analysis in the former sections, active contraction element and passive elastic element can be simulated by parallel SMA and CMPC, respectively. The designed AMs are shown in Figure 6.39 with the SMA wires surrounded by the CMPC. Both ends of the CMPC are fixed to hose barbs, glued with cyanoacrylate, and bound with wire ties. In addition, eight parallel overlapped SMA wires with diameter of 0.25 mm are selected as the AM active elements. The AM with total length of 250 mm can provide a maximum contractile force of 230 N. Note that the AM can output the desired contractile force by changing the number of parallel SMA wires. The larger the number, the larger the contractile force.

The total length of SMA-AM is 250 mm with the diameter of 10 mm. As SMA-AM contraction can be achieved by current heating, SMA-AM has a higher force-to-weight ratio and higher compactness structure compared with pneumatic AM. However, the response speed of the AM is severely restricted due to the limited cooling space of the CMPC. Forced vessel airflow cooling method is adopted to improve the response speed while maintaining the AM compactness. We found that the AM cooling time is more than 10 s with free convection cooling, and the cooling time is reduced to 1 s with forced airflow cooling and 0.2 s with forced water-flow cooling method. Compared with water-flow cooling, the airflow cooling method is selected for its simplicity without considering recycle system.

To verify the mechanical property of SMA-AM, we apply the SMA-AM to isometric contraction experiment with the device illustrated in Figure 6.37. The value of heating current represents the phase change degree of SMA and further represents the activation degree of SMA-AM. Thus,

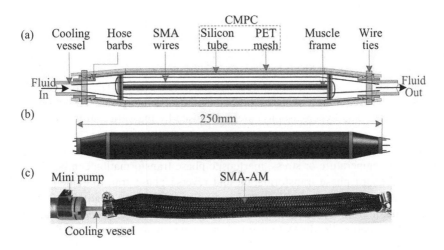

FIGURE 6.39 AM structure and the cooling circuit: (a) schematic; (b) CAD model; (c) picture.

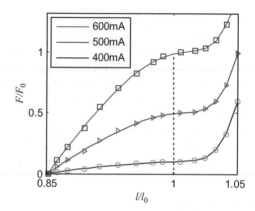

FIGURE 6.40 Experimental results of isometric dimensionless force–length curves of the AM.

the force–length curve of SMA under different activation degree can be acquired by changing current value. Detailed results are illustrated in Figure 6.40. When the current is 600 mA, the AM is fully activated with the highest contraction force. As the current decreases, the contraction force decreases gradually, but the passive force does not change, because the passive force of the CMPC is independent of the active force of SMA wires. Comparing Figure 6.40 with Figure 6.26, we see that the AMs have similar force–length properties with skeletal muscle.

Note that CMPC will store elastic potential energy when stretched. When the tension disappears, it will recover to its original length and release the stored elastic potential energy. Thus, CMPC can not only protect SMA from overstretching and overloading, but it can also mimic the energy storage function of skeletal muscle's connective tissue.

6.3.3 Self-Sensing Properties of SMA

6.3.3.1 SMA Resistivity Phase Transformation Dynamics

Resistivity is a physical parameter representing the conductive property of the material. It is related to material structure, temperature of the conductor, and the external load instead of geometric factors (such as shape, length, and cross-sectional area). From the perspective of microscopic crystal, resistivity mainly depends on the lattice structure of the material. SMA has three lattice structures, i.e., the body-centered cubic structure under austenite state, face-centered cubic structure under martensite state, and rhombohedral structure under R-phase state. Martensite phase transformation is a kind of diffusionless phase transformation of metallic material. During the phase transformation process, lattice atoms move cooperatively following the shearing mechanism, and the lattice structure is changed. Thus, diffusionless phase transformation is sometimes called legion-form phase transformation. The relative displacement accumulation of massive atoms gives rise to the structure change at macroscopic scale. The lattice structure change generated by martensite phase transformation will surely lead to the change of resistivity. The unique material properties of SMA (shape memory effect and hyperelasticity) are just caused by the lattice structure change between different phases.

The main factors influencing SMA phase transformation are temperature and stress. Based on the differences in temperature or stress, martensite phase transformation can be divided into two kinds, i.e., the forward phase transformation and reverse phase transformation. Detailed phase transformation process of SMA is illustrated in Figure 6.41. When heating (unloading), reverse phase transformation from B19′ lattice structure martensite (M) to B2 lattice structure austenite (A) takes place. When cooling (loading), forward phase transformation from B2 to B19′α lattice structure occurs. During the forward phase transformation, sometimes there will be R-phase (R) with rhombohedral lattice structure [106,107].

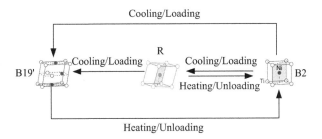

FIGURE 6.41   Phase transformation process of SMA.

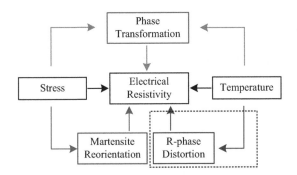

FIGURE 6.42   Relationships between factors influencing SMA resistivity.

For normal alloy, material resistivity depends on material structure, temperature, and external stress. However, for specific SMA material (here we select Flexinol™ equiatomic NiTi SMA wire with the diameter of 0.15 mm, produced by DYNALLOY Company). The resistivity of SMA is related to not only the influencing factors such as normal alloys, but also the phase transformation degree of SMA, reorientation of martensite, and distortion degree of R-phase. Detailed influencing factors relationships of SMA resistivity are illustrated in Figure 6.42. From the figure we kown that SMA resistivity changes linearly with the change of temperature and stress. It is similar to normal alloy materials. SMA resistivity properties are different from ordinary alloy materials. SMA resistivity is closely related to martensite phase transformation caused by stress or temperature. SMA resistivity changes linearly with reorientation of martensite and distortion degree of R-phase. Among them, reorientation of martensite depends on external stress, and distortion degree of R-phase depends on temperature. Thus, for specific SMA, resistivity is directly or indirectly influenced by temperature and stress.

The analysis of SMA resistivity includes parts, i.e., the phase transformation region and non-phase transformation region. In the non-phase transformation region, resistivity is mainly influenced by stress and temperature. Temperature coefficient of resistivity (TCR) and stress coefficient of resistivity (SCR) can be used to denote the direct effects of temperature and stress on the resistivity when no transformation occurs, similar to normal metal. Besides, martensite reorientation degree is proportional to stress, and distortion degree of R-phase is inversely proportional to temperature [79]. Thus, we use positive SCR and negative TCR to indirectly describe the two influencing factors. Detailed parameter values can be acquired through experiments, as illustrated in Tables 6.6 and 6.7. Therefore, the following linear equation can be obtained to express resistivity variations of individual phases outside transformation region:

$$\rho_{iT}^{\sigma} = \rho_{0i}^{0} + \alpha(T - T_{0i}) + \beta_i \sigma, \tag{6.12}$$

where subscript i represents M, A, or R; T is the real-time temperature; and ρ is the external load on SMA wire. ρ_{0i}^{0} is the resistivity of M or A measured at temperature T_{0i} and zero stress; ρ_{iT}^{σ} is the resistivity of M or A at temperature T and zero stress; α_i is the TCR; and β_i is the SCR.

TABLE 6.6

Experimental Material Parameters of SMA Wire

	Martensite	R-phase	Austenite
TCR: αi ($\mu\Omega$cm/°C)	0.08	−0.05	0.05
SCR: βi ($\mu\Omega$cm/MPa)	0.05	0.04	0.04
C_i (MPa/°C)	3.68	—	6.06
T_{0i}: ρ_{0i}^0 ($\mu\Omega$cm)	100.5	104.2	95.2
T_{0i} (°C)	34	58	79

TABLE 6.7

Phase Transformation Parameters of SMA Wires

	$M \rightarrow A$	$A \rightarrow R$	$R \rightarrow M$
Starting temperature of phase transformation (°C)	73	—	44
Maximum temperature of phase transformation (°C)	76	58	39
End temperature of phase transformation (°C)	79	—	34
Latent heat of phase transformation: Q_i (J/g)	24.5	0	11.2
Maximum recoverable strain (%)	4.8	0.8	4

Different from non-phase transformation region, resistivity change in phase transformation region depends mainly on SMA phase transformation degree. However, SMA phase transformation process is complex, as illustrated in Figure 6.41. The existence of R-phase makes the phase transformation structure and resistivity property even more complex. Thus, DSC is applied on TiNi SMA to do thermal cycling test and study the phase transformation process. Then the phase transformation dynamic model can be developed by describing the free energy in SMA phase transformation so as to describe the resistivity variation property in detail. Although R-phase makes the resistivity property more complex, resistivity changes in a similar way between $A \rightarrow$ M and $A \rightarrow R$ in the later thermal, mechanical, and electrical experiments. Thus, to describe it in an easier way, we neglect the existence of R-phase and only consider the resistivity phase transformation property between A and M. The property can be generalized to the situation when R-phase exists.

During the martensite forward and reverse phase transformations, there would be releasing and absorbing of latent heat. DSC is an effective tool for studying latent heat in SMA phase transformation. It can not only determine SMA phase transformation temperature, but also calculate the value and variation trend of latent heat in SMA phase transformation. We describe the varying characteristics of resistivity and develop the model from the perspective of phase transformation free energy via the analysis and simulation of DSC curves. In the DSC experiments, we use the DSC 200 F3 Maia® analyzer produced by Netzsch Company and do the phase transformation testing of Flexinol™ equiatomic NiTi SMA wire produced by DYNALLOY Company. To ensure the accuracy of DSC curve, three identical thermal cyclic loadings on SMA samples have been done. The temperature region of each thermal cycling is −10°C to 120°C. Among them, the heating and cooling velocities are both 10°C/min.

DSC curves tend to be stable and converge after three heat cycles, as illustrated in Figure 6.43. The abscissa is the temperature, and the ordinate is the heat flow. It can be inferred from the figure that there is an endothermic peak curve (red line). The curve represents the martensite reverse phase transformation process ($M \rightarrow A$). In the cooling process, there are two exothermic peaks on the curve (blue line). Among them, one is obvious while the other is not. The curve represents the martensite forward phase transformation process ($A \rightarrow R$ and $R \rightarrow M$). The generation of peak is

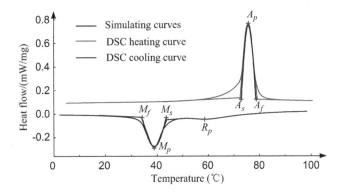

FIGURE 6.43   DSC curves of SMA wire.

caused by the change of latent heat. Here we define M_s, M_p, and M_f as the starting, peak, and end temperatures of the $R \rightarrow M$ phase transformation and define A_s, A_p, and A_f as the starting, peak, and end temperatures of $M \rightarrow A$ phase transformation. R_p is defined as the peak temperature of $A \rightarrow R$ phase transformation. As the released latent heat in $A \rightarrow R$ phase transformation is too small, the starting temperature R_s and end temperature R_f are not detected by DSC. Thus, we neglect the influence of R-phase here. Relevant temperature parameters and data are illustrated in Figure 6.43 and Table 6.7. Besides, the temperature parameters satisfy the following equations:

$$\begin{cases} A_p = \dfrac{A_f + A_s}{2} \\ M_p = \dfrac{M_f + M_s}{2} \end{cases}. \tag{6.13}$$

Whether martensite forward or reverse phase transformation of SMA under a specific temperature will take place largely depends on the value of Gibbs free energy. The driving source of martensite phase transformation is the Gibbs free energy difference ΔG of two phases. Without external load, free energy change ΔG generated by SMA martensite phase transformation satisfies the following equation:

$$\Delta G = \Delta H - T\Delta S, \tag{6.14}$$

where ΔH is the enthalpy change during phase transformation process and ΔS is the entropy change. As elastic potential energy E_s is involved in the SMA phase transformation, ΔH satisfies the following equation:

$$\Delta H = \Delta Q + E_s, \tag{6.15}$$

where ΔQ is the latent heat in phase transformation and can be measured by DSC. Elastic potential energy E_s can be calculated using the following equation [108]:

$$E_s = \frac{|T_f - T_s|}{2} \Delta S, \tag{6.16}$$

where T_i ($i = s, f$) is the phase transformation temperature. ΔS is a constant in a high temperature and load stress region. Combining Eqs. (6.15) and (6.16), we find the derivative of temperature:

$$\frac{d\Delta G}{dT} = \frac{d\Delta Q}{dT} - \Delta S. \tag{6.17}$$

To describe SMA phase transformation latent heat ΔQ, we use cosine function to mimic the heat flow and temperature curve during SMA martensite phase transformation, as denoted by the black line in Figure 6.43. Note that the prerequisite for this method is that DSC has symmetrical characteristic; i.e., the peak temperature satisfies Eq. (6.13). Taking the martensite reverse phase transformation as an example (martensite forward phase transformation has similar properties), the relationship between heat flow and temperature is expressed as

$$f(T) = h\cos\left[a_A(T - A_p)\right] + C_1, \tag{6.18}$$

where T is SMA temperature and h and C_1 are both constants. $a_A = \pi / A_f - A_s$. The latent heat Q of martensite reverse phase transformation is the area surrounded by the temperature region $[As, Af]$ in the DSC curve. It satisfies the following equation:

$$\frac{dQ}{dT} = f(T)\frac{dt}{dT}, \quad A_s < T < A_f. \tag{6.19}$$

Based on the analysis in the last section, in SMA phase transformation region, lattice structure change is caused by martensite phase transformation induced by stress or temperature. In this region, the leading factor that influences SMA resistivity is the lattice structure. Thus, the resistivity during phase transformation mainly depends on the martensite phase transformation induced by stress or temperature. Thus, the direct influence of stress and temperature on resistivity can be neglected. Besides, in Ref. [109], it is proposed that there is a linear relation between the differential of free energy difference on temperature during phase transformation and the differential of martensite phase transformation degree on temperature. Taking the martensite reverse phase transformation as an example, we can get the following equation combining Eqs. (6.18) and (6.19):

$$\frac{d\rho_{M \to A}}{dT} = k\frac{dQ}{dT} + C_2, \tag{6.20}$$

where k is the proportionality coefficient and C_2 is a constant. Substituting Eqs. (6.18) and (6.19) into (6.20), we get

$$\frac{d\rho_{M \to A}}{dT} = H\cos\left[a_A\left(T - A_p\right)\right] + C, \tag{6.21}$$

where H is the proportionality coefficient and $C = kC_1 + C_2$. When $T = A_s$ or A_f, SMA is in the start or end region of phase transformation. There is not any lattice structure change at this time.

Differential resistivity on temperature approximately satisfies $d\rho_{M \to A}/dT = 0$. Integrate Eq. (6.21) to acquire the relationship between resistivity and temperature:

$$\rho_{M \to A} = \frac{\rho_{A_f}^0 - \rho_{A_s}^0}{2}\sin\left[a_A\left(T - A_p\right)\right] + \frac{\rho_{A_f}^0 + \rho_{A_s}^0}{2}, \tag{6.22}$$

where $A_s \le T \le A_f$ and $\rho_{A_s}^0$ and $\rho_{A_f}^0$ are the start and end resistivities of martensite reverse phase transformation process without load. The values of them can be acquired through Eq. (6.12). Based on the above analysis, the resistivity–temperature relation during martensite forward phase transformation process can be acquired in the same way:

$$\rho_{A \to M} = \frac{\rho_{M_s}^0 - \rho_{M_f}^0}{2}\sin\left[a_M\left(T - M\right)_p\right] + \frac{\rho_{M_s}^0 + \rho_{M_f}^0}{2}, \tag{6.23}$$

where $M_f \le T \le M_s$ and $\rho_{M_s}^0$ and $\rho_{M_f}^0$ are the start and end resistivities of martensite forward phase transformation process without load. The values of them can also be acquired through Eq. (6.12), $a_M = \pi / (M_s - M_f)$.

The influence of stress is not considered in the above resistivity analysis. Based on the Clausius–Clapeyron function, when SMA is under external stress, the influence of stress on martensite can be expressed with the following equation:

$$\frac{d\sigma}{dT} = -\frac{\Delta S}{\varepsilon},\qquad(6.24)$$

where σ is the stress and ε is the corresponding strain. ΔS is the entropy change, which can be treated as a constant. Based on the above equation, during the SMA thermal cycle, the phase transformation temperature of SMA will increase linearly when the load is present. Thus, the resistivity of SMA will also change. Besides, we also find that resistivity will change with stress. In Ref. [110], similar results are presented. To accurately describe the relationship between resistivity, temperature, and stress, the following equation is proposed based on the above analysis and Eq. (6.22):

$$\rho_{M\to A} = \frac{\rho_{A_f}^0 - \rho_{A_s}^0}{2}\sin\left[a_A\left(T - A_p\right) + b_A\sigma\right] + \frac{\rho_{A_f}^0 + \rho_{A_s}^0}{2} + \beta_A\sigma,\qquad(6.25)$$

where $A_s \leq T \leq A_p$, $b_A = -a_A/C_A$, C_A is the material constant, representing the stress–temperature coefficient during martensite reverse phase transformation. β_A is the austenite resistivity stress coefficient SCR. In the same way, we can get the relationship of resistivity, temperature, and stress during martensite forward phase transformation:

$$\rho_{A\to M} = \frac{\rho_{M_s}^0 - \rho_{M_f}^0}{2}\sin\left[a_M\left(T - M_p\right) + b_M\sigma\right] + \frac{\rho_{M_s}^0 + \rho_{M_f}^0}{2} + \beta_M\sigma,\qquad(6.26)$$

where $M_f \leq T \leq M_s$, $b_M = -a_M/C_M$, C_M is the material constant, representing the stress–temperature coefficient during martensite forward phase transformation. β_M is the martensite resistivity stress coefficient SCR.

Referring to Figure 6.43, where R-phase exists, martensite forward phase transformation can be divided into two parts, i.e., the phase transformation $A \to R$ and $R \to M$. Thus, based on the analysis above, we have the following equations:

$$\begin{aligned}\rho_{A\to R} &= \frac{\rho_{R_s}^0 - \rho_{R_f}^0}{2}\sin\left[a_R(T - R_p) + b_R\sigma\right] + \frac{\rho_{R_s}^0 + \rho_{R_f}^0}{2} + \beta_R\sigma\\[6pt]\rho_{R\to M} &= \frac{\rho_{M_s}^0 - \rho_{M_f}^0}{2}\sin\left[a_M\left(T - M_p\right) + b_M\sigma\right] + \frac{\rho_{M_s}^0 + \rho_{M_f}^0}{2} + \beta_M\sigma\end{aligned}\qquad(6.27)$$

where $\rho_{R_s}^0$ and $\rho_{R_f}^0$ are the start and end resistivities in $A \to R$ phase transformation region without load, the values of which can still be solved by Eq. (6.12). $aR = \pi/(Rs - Rf)$ and $bR = -aR/CR$ are material parameters. C_M is the force–temperature coefficient in $A \to R$ phase transformation. Equations (6.25–6.27) form the resistivity phase transformation dynamic model under the influence of temperature and stress. The correctness and effectiveness will be verified by the electro-thermo-mechanical experiment introduced in next section.

6.3.3.2 Electro-Thermomechanical Coupling Properties

In order to study resistivity variations during phase transformation, a series of electro-thermomechanical experiments were carried out as shown in Figure 6.44. An SMA wire with a diameter of 0.15 mm and length of 117 mm is connected to different constant loads varying from 28 to 224 MPa and a helical bias spring with the stiffness of 390 N/m. A load cell is connected to the SMA wire to measure the contraction force. A computer equipped with a data acquisition card (NI USB-6211) is used to store and process all the measured data. An LVDT with the resolution of 0.01 mm measures the SMA wire length change. We applied inner heating method by using resistive heating with free

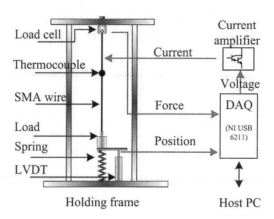

FIGURE 6.44   Schematic diagram of experimental setup.

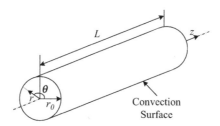

FIGURE 6.45   Size and coordinate of SMA wire.

convection. Heating current generated from current amplifier is used to drive the SMA wire, and the resistivity is computed according to the following equation:

$$\rho = R\frac{S}{l} = \frac{VU}{l^2 I},$$ (6.28)

where R is the resistance of SMA wire, U is the voltage, I is the heating current across the SMA wire, l is the wire length, and V is the wire volume which can be considered as a constant. Besides, for the sake of convenience, we remove the bias spring first and consider only the SMA resistivity properties under constant load.

During the current heating process of SMA, it presents complex electro-thermomechanical coupling properties. Although temperature is the main factor inducing SMA phase transformation, thermocouple can only achieve temperature measurement in stable and slow response temperature variation, but the SMA wire is too thin, so temperature measurement under fast current heating cannot be realized. Moreover, temperature rise and drop caused by SMA latent heat cannot be detected by thermocouple either. From the perspective of real-time feedback control, controlling the heating time and cooling time is more operable and feasible than controlling heating and cooling temperatures. Thus, based on lumped parameter method and energy conservation principle, considering the stable temperature measurement feature of thermocouple, we can analyze SMA heat transfer and develop the thermal transmission model of SMA heat current, thus deriving the relationship between temperature and time.

As illustrated in Figure 6.45, SMA can be described as a long cylinder with the radius of r_0 and length of L. Under the cylindrical coordinate, the heat conduction differential equation can be acquired based on energy conservation principle and Fourier law [111]:

$$V\left[\frac{1}{r}\frac{\partial}{\partial r}\left(kr\frac{\partial T}{\partial r}\right) + \frac{1}{r^2}\frac{\partial}{\partial \theta}\left(k\frac{\partial T}{\partial \theta}\right) + \frac{\partial}{\partial z}\left(k\frac{\partial T}{\partial z}\right)\right] + \frac{dq}{dt} = \frac{dE}{dt},$$ (6.29)

where dq/dt is the input and output heat transmission rate and dE/dt is the energy storage rate of SMA wire. For lathy SMA wire (the SMA wire in the experiment), based on its geometric features and heat transmission properties, without losing correctness, we have the following hypothesis. First, the SMA wire has large length-to-diameter ratio; thus, the temperature change in Z direction can be neglected. Second, SMA wire has unified boundary condition along the circumferential direction; thus, temperature change in θ direction can be neglected. Third, SMA has the same temperature on the whole cross section; thus, temperature change in r direction can be neglected. Hypothesis 3 is based on the following analysis. Based on heat transfer theory, the smaller the B_{iot} (B_i), the smaller the solid thermal resistance will be. When B_i is much less than 1, solid thermal resistance is far less than the convective thermal resistance along the solid boundary. At this point, the temperature in the solid can be viewed as evenly distributed. For the SMA with the diameter of 0.15 mm ($r_0 = 7.5 \times 10^{-5}$ m), Bi ($Bi = h_c r_0 2k$) is approximately 1.8×10^{-4} (far less than 1, and $h_c = 80$ W/m^2 K is the convection coefficient, $k = 17$ W/m K is the thermal conductivity). Based on the above hypothesis, Eq. (6.29) can be simplified as

$$\frac{dq}{dt} = \frac{dE}{dT}. \tag{6.30}$$

That is, SMA energy storage rate is equal to its heat conductive rate. SMA energy storage is achieved by the increase of temperature and absorption of latent heat. When SMA is in the non-phase transformation region, energy storage rate can be expressed as

$$\frac{dE}{dt} = m_f C_p \frac{dT}{dt}, \tag{6.31}$$

where m_f is the mass of SMA wire [kg] and C_p is the constant-pressure specific heat [J/kg °C]. When SMA is in the phase transformation region, because of the release and absorption of latent heat, energy storage rate is described as

$$\frac{dE}{dt} = m_f \left(C_p - Q_i \frac{d\xi}{dT} \right) \frac{dT}{dt}, \tag{6.32}$$

where ξ is the martensite content and Q_i is the latent heat. Subscript i represents $M \rightarrow A$ or $A \rightarrow M$. Based on the DSC experimental results, $A \rightarrow R$ latent heat is small enough to be neglected (as illustrated in Figure 6.43). In the $A \rightarrow M$ region, latent heat belongs to endothermic state. Thus, $d\xi/dT$ is a negative value. SMA heat transfer rate is closely related to SMA heating and cooling methods. Here we take current heating and air cooling as the example. In the process of current heating, heat transfer rate can be described as

$$\frac{dq}{dt} = I^2 R - h_c A_{\mathrm{surf}} (T - T_{\mathrm{amb}}), \tag{6.33}$$

where A_{surf} is the surface area of SMA wire, T_{amb} is the ambient temperature, T is the SMA wire temperature, R is the average resistance of SMA, I is the heating current, and h_c is the coefficient of heat convection. In the air cooling process, heat transfer rate is described as

$$\frac{dq}{dt} = -h_c A_{\mathrm{surf}} (T - T_{\mathrm{amb}}). \tag{6.34}$$

Martensite content ξ reflects martensite phase transformation degree. For temperature-induced martensite phase transformation, the value of ξ completely depends on temperature [112]. Thus, the expression of ξ can be simulated by the above DSC curves. Combining Eq. (6.18) and the boundary

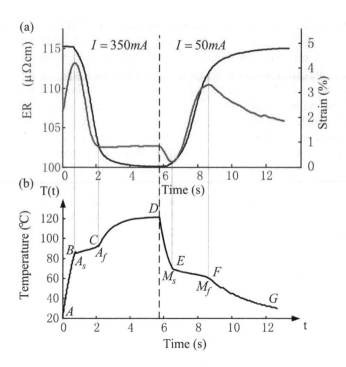

FIGURE 6.46   (a) Resistivity and strain response; (b) temperature response analysis figure in the heating and cooling processes of SMA wire.

condition of ξ (when $T = A_s$, $\xi = 1$ and $d\xi/dT = 0$ and when $T = M_s$, $\xi = 0$ and $d\xi/dT = 0$), the following equations can be obtained:

$$\frac{d\xi}{dT} = -\frac{a_A}{2} \cos\left[a_A \left(T - A_p \right) \right] \quad \text{for} \quad M \to A, \tag{6.35}$$

$$\frac{d\xi}{dT} = -\frac{a_M}{2} \cos\left[a_M \left(T - M_p \right) \right] \quad \text{for} \quad A \to M. \tag{6.36}$$

Based on the above Eqs. (6.30)–(6.36), the SMA temperature response properties under constant heating current can be acquired by numerical analysis. The SMA temperature–time curves in the heating ($I = 350\,\text{mA}$) and cooling ($I = 50\,\text{mA}$) processes are illustrated in Figure 6.46b. Note that the 50 mA current in the cooling process is used to ensure the resistance measurement, and the heat generated can be neglected. In the non-phase transformation region (lines AB, CD and DE, FG), the temperature increases and decreases exponentially. However, in the phase transformation region (line BC, EF), the temperature slope changes quickly, which is caused by the absorption and release of latent heat. BC indicates $M \to A$ when latent heat is in the absorption stage. EF represents $A \to M$ when latent heat is in the release stage. The analytical results in Figure 6.46b are almost the same as the experimental results in Ref. [112]. To provide convenience for further analysis, based on the analytical results, we consider the temperature–time relationship in the phase transformation region as a linear relation expressed by Eq. (6.37) and treat the temperature–time relationship in the non-phase transformation region as exponential relation expressed by Eq. (6.38):

$$T = K_t t + T_s, \tag{6.37}$$

$$T = K_c e^{t/\tau} + T_c, \tag{6.38}$$

where $K_c = T_0 - T_{amb} - I^2 R/hA_{surf}$, $T_c = T_{amb} + I^2 R/hA_{surf}$, and $\tau = -mC_V/hA_{surf}$. Among them, T_0 is the starting temperature of cooling or heating and can be detected by temperature sensor. T_s is the starting temperature of phase transformation, and K_t is the slope of line BC and line EF.

6.3.3.2.1 Thermal Driving Properties

In the heat cycle without load, SMA resistivity and strain response are illustrated by the red line and blue line in Figure 6.46a, respectively. In the heating process, resistivity presents non-monotonic characteristics as it first increases, then decreases, and increases again. In BC segment, SMA undergoes the martensite forward phase transformation ($M \rightarrow A$). In the process, the decrease of resistivity is because resistivity in austenite is smaller than that in martensite. In the segments of AB and CD, there are no phase transformations of SMA. The resistivity increase is due to the increase in temperature. Besides, in the segments of AB and CD, SMA strain changes are small, which can be neglected. In the BC segment, martensite reverse phase transformation makes SMA strain decrease quickly. In the cooling process, the varying trends of SMA resistivity and strain are contrary to the heating process. In the EF segment, resistivity increase is due to martensite forward phase transformation ($A \rightarrow M$). In EF and FG segments, resistivity decrease is caused by the temperature decrease. American scholar Churchill also presented similar experimental results through external heating [113].

SMA phase transformation velocity is influenced by both the heating current value and the cooling methods [111,114,115]. Once the heating current is big enough to ensure that the heating temperature is larger than the end temperature A_f of martensite reverse phase transformation, there will be two extremums in the resistivity curve, as illustrated in Figure 6.47 (points A and B). The two extremum points are the start and end points of martensite reverse phase transformation. Besides, the bigger the current, the faster the resistivity change will be. The resistivity value after reverse phase transformation is also bigger (as the point C).

6.3.3.2.2 Stress Properties

Under different constant stresses (28–224 MPa), the experimental results of strain and resistivity in martensite reverse phase transformation are illustrated in Figure 6.48a and c. It can be inferred that start temperature (denoted by A_1A_2) and end temperature (denoted by B_1B_2) of reverse phase transformation increase with the increase of load stress. Besides, the non-monotonic characteristics of resistivity also increase holistically with the increase of stress. Combining Eqs. (6.12), (6.26), (6.37), and (6.38), we are able to acquire the varying property of SMA resistivity during martensite reverse phase transformation, as illustrated in Figure 6.49a. Compared with Figure 6.49c, it can be noted that the simulation results are almost the same as the experimental results. It proves the correctness of the resistivity phase transformation dynamic model.

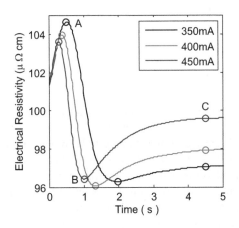

FIGURE 6.47 Resistivity response under different heating currents (constant load of 28 MPa).

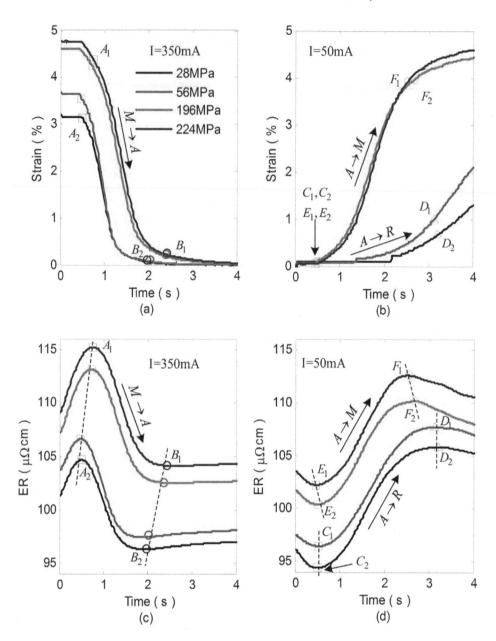

FIGURE 6.48 Experimental results of resistivity and strain of SMA martensite reverse phase transformations ($I = 350\,\text{mA}$ and $I = 50\,\text{mA}$) under different constant loads.

The strain and resistivity experimental results in martensite reverse phase transformation are illustrated in Figure 6.48b and d. Compared with Figure 6.48a, SMA strain curve represents different varying trends. This is caused by the R-phase [27]. When stress is low, there are two phase transformations, $A \rightarrow R$ and $R \rightarrow M$. When stress is high, there is only $A \rightarrow M$ phase transformation. This is because all the phase transformation temperatures will increase with the increase of stress, but the influence of stress on temperature R_s is smaller than that on B_s and A_f. Thus, R-phase content decreases with the increase of stress. When stress reaches a certain value, temperature M_s surpasses R_s, and there would only be $A \rightarrow M$ phase transformation. The strain caused by $A \rightarrow M$ phase transformation is 5%, while that during the $A \rightarrow R$ phase transformation is less than 1%. SMA

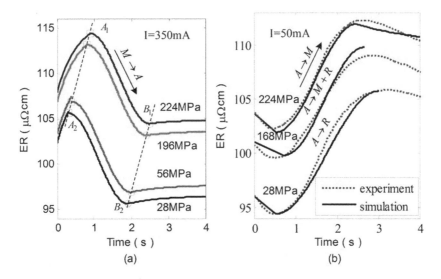

FIGURE 6.49 Results of resistivity simulation of SMA martensite reverse phase transformations ($I = 350$ mA and $I = 50$ mA) under different constant loads.

TABLE 6.8

SMA Martensite Phase Transformation Classification under Stress Influence

Stress (MPa)	Martensite Phase Transformation Process
$\sigma < \sigma_s$	$A \to R \to M$
$\sigma_s < \sigma < \sigma_f$	$A \to R + M$
$\sigma > \sigma_f$	$A \to M$

---

resistivity presents non-monotonic characteristics as it first decreases, then increases, and decreases again, as illustrated in Figure 6.48d. The varying character does not change with the existence of R-phase. Where stress is less than 56 MPa, resistivity increase is caused by $A \to R$ phase transformation (denoted by $C_1C_2 - D_1D_2$). When stress is higher than 196 MPa, resistivity increase is caused by $A \to M$ phase transformation (denoted by $E_1E_2 - F_1F_2$). Moreover, resistivity will still increase holistically with the increase of stress.

To describe SMA phase transformation temperature–stress property when R-phase exists, we make some improvement to Brinson critical stress–temperature analysis [87], as illustrated in Figure 6.49. There are three situations in the cooling process of martensite reverse phase transformation, as illustrated in Table 6.8. When external stress is greater than σ_f, there will not be R-phase (arrow a). When external stress is less than σ_s, two phase transformations occur in a row ($A \to R \to M$) (arrow c). When stress is in between, two phase transformations will occur in mixture ($A \to R + M$) (arrow b) (Figure 6.50).

To prove the correctness of dynamic model of resistivity, 28, 168, and 224 MPa are selected as cases in the analysis. Combining Eqs. (6.12), (6.26), (6.37), and (6.38), we are able to acquire the SMA resistivity varying property during martensite forward phase transformation. Figure 6.49b illustrates the experimental and simulation results of resistivity. It can be inferred that when $A \to R$ and $A \to M$ occur separately, resistivity simulation results agree well with experimental results, thus proving the correctness of dynamic model of resistivity. When $A \to R + M$, the error is relatively high. This is because resistivity is influenced by R-phase and M-phase at the same time.

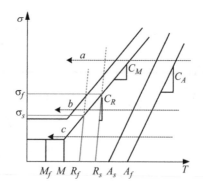

FIGURE 6.50 SMA-improved critical stress–temperature relation.

6.3.3.3 SMA Self-Sensing Model

6.3.3.3.1 Self-Sensing Model

To achieve the self-sensing function of SMA, SMA resistance–length (*R–L*) relation has to be developed. First is the SMA resistivity–strain (ρ–ε) relationship. Based on the former analysis, SMA resistivity and martensite content both depend on phase transformation degree. However, we found that resistivity is also affected by external load, but martensite content is not. Thus, we propose the following equation for the resistivity–martensite content relationship. When there is no *R*-phase, we have

$$\rho_{A\leftrightarrow M} = \rho_A^0 + \left(\rho_M^0 - \rho_A^0\right)\xi + \beta_{A,M}\sigma. \tag{6.39}$$

When *R*-phase is present, we have

$$\begin{cases} \rho A \leftrightarrow R = \rho_A^0 + \left(\rho_R^0 - \rho_A^0\right)\xi_R + \beta_{A,R}\sigma \\ \rho_{R\leftrightarrow M} = \rho_R^0 + \left(\rho_M^0 - \rho_R^0\right)\xi + \beta_{R,M}\sigma \end{cases}. \tag{6.40}$$

The superscript 0 here represents the resistivity with zero load stress. β_i is SCR, which can be regarded as a constant, as listed in Table 6.8. Besides, based on Brinson analysis [87], SMA satisfies the following constitutive model:

$$\sigma - \sigma_0 = E(\varepsilon - \varepsilon_0) + \Theta(T - T_0) + \Omega(\xi - \xi_0), \tag{6.41}$$

where *E* is the Young's modulus, Θ is the thermal coefficient of expansion, and Ω is the transformation tensor of SMA.

$$\Omega = -E\varepsilon_L. \tag{6.42}$$

Here $\varepsilon_L = 4.8\%$ is the maximum residual strain; i.e., the maximum strain caused by phase transformation after stress is removed. The value is a constant when the temperature is less than A_f. Combining Eqs. (6.39)–(6.42), the resistivity–strain (ρ–ε) relationship can be expressed as

$$\rho = \begin{cases} K_{M\rightarrow A}\varepsilon + \rho_A^0 + \beta_A\sigma & \text{for} \quad M \rightarrow A \\ K_{A\rightarrow R}\varepsilon + \rho_A^0 + \beta_A\sigma & \text{for} \quad A \rightarrow R \\ K_{R\rightarrow M}\varepsilon + \rho_R^0 + \beta_R\sigma & \text{for} \quad R \rightarrow M \end{cases}, \tag{6.43}$$

where parameter *K* satisfies

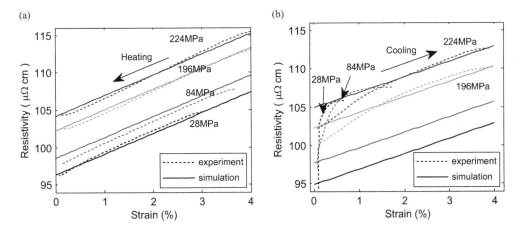

FIGURE 6.51   SMA resistivity–strain experiment and simulation results under different constant loads.

$$\begin{cases} K_{M \to A} = \left(\rho_M^0 - \rho_A^0 \right) \big/ \varepsilon_L \\[2mm] K_{A \to R} = \left(\rho_R^0 - \rho_A^0 \right) \big/ \varepsilon_L^R \\[2mm] K_{R \to M} = \left(\rho_M^0 - \rho_R^0 \right) \big/ \left(\varepsilon_L - \varepsilon_L^R \right) \end{cases} , \qquad (6.44)$$

where $\varepsilon_L^R = 0.8\%$ is the maximum residual strain caused by $A \to R$ phase transformation, which is also a constant that is less than ε_L.

The simulation and experimental results of ρ–ε curves during $M \to A$ and $A \to M$ are shown in Figure 6.51a and b. During $M \to A$, the ρ–ε curves have good linearity. The resistivity value changes linearly with the stress, and the simulation results agree well with the experimental results. However, during $A \to M$, a large error occurs between simulation and experimental results at lower stresses. This is due to the appearance of R-phase during the cooling process. With the increase of the stress, R-phase fraction decreases and the linearity becomes better. Note that the value of resistivity is a constant for a certain given SMA wire with definite composition (such as equiatomic NiTi SMA), treatment process, and thermomechanical conditions, independent of the initial length of SMA wire. Thus, the ρ–ε expression of Eq. (6.43) is suitable for SMA wires with different initial lengths.

The experimental resistance–length (R–L) curves are shown in Figure 6.52a. When the applied stress is large, R-phase is inhibited, the linearity of R–L curve is quite good, and the hysteresis gap of heating and cooling path is also small. However, when the applied stress is small, the R–L curve has two different steps with very different slopes during cooling caused by R-phase, which is not proper for self-sensing application. The simplest way is to exert certain pre-stress. Besides, heat treatment can also achieve the restraining of R-phase [27]. Here we are only concerned with the case without R-phase. Assuming the initial length of SMA wire is l_0, then

$$\varepsilon = \frac{l - l_0}{l_0}. \qquad (6.45)$$

Combining Eqs. (6.28), (6.43), and (6.45), the following resistance–length equations can be acquired:

$$\begin{cases} R_h = \frac{1}{V} \left(\frac{K_A}{l_0} l^3 + H_A l^2 \right) \quad \text{for} \quad M \to A \\[3mm] R_c = \frac{1}{V} \left(\frac{K_M}{l_0} l^3 + H_M l^2 \right) \quad \text{for} \quad A \to M \end{cases} , \qquad (6.46)$$

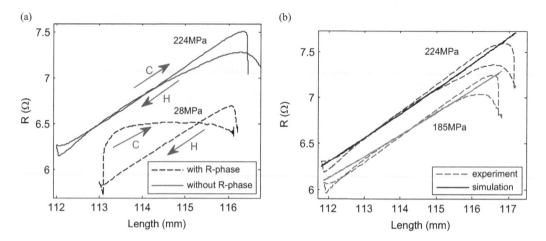

FIGURE 6.52 SMA resistance–length experiment and simulation results.

in which parameter H satisfies

$$\begin{cases} H_A = \beta_A \sigma + \rho_{A_f}^0 - K_A \\ H_M = \beta_M \sigma + \rho_{M_s}^0 - K_M \end{cases}. \tag{6.47}$$

Besides, R_h and R_c are the SMA resistance values in the heating and cooling processes, respectively. As the hysteresis in cooling and heating curves is small, we can compute the average of the curves with the following equation:

$$R = \frac{R_h + R_c}{2}. \tag{6.48}$$

Combining Eqs. (6.46)–(6.48), we acquire the resistance–length simulation results under different constant loads, as illustrated in Figure 6.52b. It can be inferred that simulation results and experimental results are quite consistent with each other. Note that the above self-sensing model is based on SMA resistivity–strain relationships; thus, it has good generality and versatility and can be applied on SMA wires with different sizes.

6.3.3.3.2 Stress Factor in Self-Sensing Model

The above self-sensing model was deduced under constant stress. In practice, the artificial skeletal muscle generally contracts against variable stresses. In order to demonstrate the correctness of the self-sensing model under variable stress conditions, the same experiment is performed by adding a bias spring under the constant load, as shown in Figure 6.53. The R–L curves with and without bias spring are shown in Figure 6.53. The differences between the two curves are minimal, and they have the same slope. Thus, the self-sensing model can predict the R–L relationships under both constant and variable stresses, and self-sensing can be achieved for the AM.

6.3.4 Application of SMA Self-Sensing Model

To further demonstrate the self-sensing capability of the AM, we build a one-DOF robotic ankle–foot actuated by the AM and bias spring, as shown in Figure 6.54. Note that we focus on the verification of SMA self-sensing function; thus, current heating and conventional air cooling methods are applied. Different cooling methods mainly influence the coefficient of heat convection in the model in Figure 6.33, but they do not affect SMA self-sensing function [111].

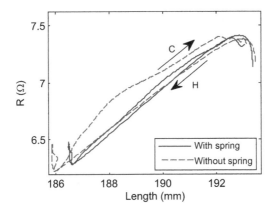

FIGURE 6.53 Experimental results of R–L relationships under constant (without spring) and variable (with spring) loads.

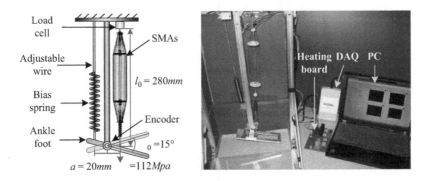

FIGURE 6.54 One-DOF robotic ankle-foot actuated by artificial skeletal muscle.

The bias spring serves two purposes: (1) to provide enough restoring force for the AM and (2) to simulate variable load conditions. The current heating and data processing methods are similar to the previous experiments. Before experiments, an initial restoring force of 32 N, corresponding to the pre-transformation stress of 112 MPa, is applied on the AM to inhibit the appearance of R-phase. In addition, it is reasonable to assume that all the 16 SMA wires in the AM maintain the same tension force because of their uniform distribution around the artificial parallel element (APE) and the same initial length. Therefore, only one of the 16 SMA wires rather than the whole AM was selected as the self-sensor in our experiments.

Fuzzy-tuned proportional-integral-derivative (PID) controller is implemented in the LabVIEW environment to control the robotic ankle–foot. The PID parameters are tuned between $K_P = 0.1$–0.5, $K_I = 0.01$–0.06, and $K_D = 0.001$–0.002 by using MAX-MIN fuzzy reasoning method. The control diagram is shown in Figure 6.55.

When the angle of robotic ankle changes, the AM length change can be determined according to the following equation:

$$l - l_0 = \frac{a}{2}\sin(\theta - \theta_0), \tag{6.49}$$

where l is the AM length, θ is the angular position, and $a/2$ is the moment arm of the robotic ankle–foot. The subscript 0 denotes the initial length and angle value, as shown in Figure 6.54.

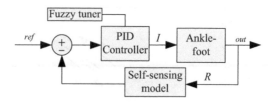

FIGURE 6.55   Fuzzy PID control diagram.

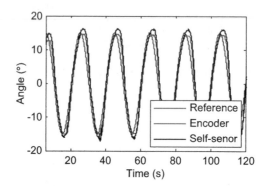

FIGURE 6.56   Sinusoidal tracking response of 0.05 Hz.

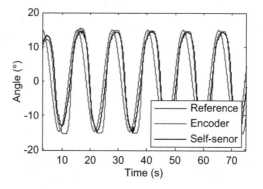

FIGURE 6.57   Sinusoidal tracking response of 0.08 Hz.

The resistance of the selected SMA wire is measured as the feedback signal and then converted to the ankle angle combining the self-sensing model (Eqs. 6.47 and 6.48) and Eq. (6.49). An encoder is used to measure the actual ankle angle. Furthermore, the actual angle is also used for the feedback control as a comparison. Figure 6.56 shows the results of sinusoidal tracking response experiments using the self-sensor and encoder respectively at 0.05 Hz. The actual angle with the two feedback methods can accurately follow the reference angle, which demonstrates the validity of the self-sensing method. When the sinusoidal frequency increases to 0.08 Hz as shown in Figure 6.57, a small phase lag appears between the actual angle and the reference angle, while the two actual angle curves coincide well with each other, because both resistance and length change of SMA wires are closely related to SMA transformation, which further demonstrates the validity of the self-sensing model.

Figure 6.58 shows the experimental frequency response of the AM ranging from 0.01 to 1 Hz. The limited bandwidth of SMA (approx. 0.17 Hz) resulting from SMA slow heat-transfer rate is

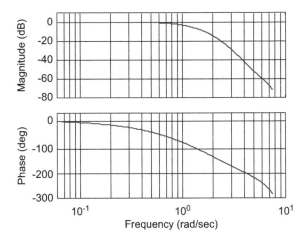

FIGURE 6.58 Experimental frequency response of the artificial skeletal muscle.

the major challenge for its application to robotic ankle–foot. Here we only focus on its self-sensing capability. In general, the self-sensing model can predict the length change of SMA wires within SMA bandwidth, which is robust to the external load. Thus, the self-sensing capability of the AM can be achieved.

6.4 HYSTERESIS PROPERTIES OF SMA-AM

Based on the above sections, SMA multi-functional property makes SMA-AM achieve the function of integrated actuation and self-sensing. However, in the heating process of SMA, lattice phase transformation has strong hysteresis nonlinearity. The phenomenon largely limits the control accuracy of SMA-AM and even leads to instability of the actuation system. Thus, in practical applications, eliminating SMA hysteresis is of great significance to system control, and accurately describing SMA hysteresis properties and developing a mathematical model that is able to characterize these properties are the keys to solving the above problems.

Hysteresis is the common nonlinearity among smart actuation materials (such as PZT and SMA). In practical system, hysteresis is not simple hysteretic relation between input and output but multi-valued mapping. The larger the input signal range, the larger the hysteresis interval of SMA output signal is. To date, various mathematical models have been developed to describe the hysteresis of SMA, and they can be divided into two classes. One is the physics-based model, the representatives being Tanaka model [86] and Brinson model [87]. This model accurately describes the constitutive feather and phase transformation characters of SMA. But there are too many unknown material parameters in the model. Thus, it can be hard to apply this in control systems. The other is the phenomenological model [88], the representatives being Duhem model [116], Preisach model [90], and Prandtl–Ishlinskii model. However, most of these models are used to describe the hysteresis character of PZT, and only a few have been used to describe that of the SMA. This is due to the fact that the hysteresis of SMA is more complex than that of PZT. The hysteresis character of SMA is related to not only actuation frequency, but also external load. And the nonlinearity is saturable and unsmooth [89]. Although there have been scholars achieving the simulation of SMA's saturable hysteresis property by the improvement of Prandtl–Ishlinskii model, a comprehensive description of SMA hysteresis properties under different stresses and frequencies is still hard to achieve. Besides, it is hard to acquire analytical solution of most phenomenological models; thus, it is hard to apply them in the real-time control system.

Besides the above mathematical models, scholars have achieved the description and compensation of SMA hysteresis by applying many modern control methods. Song in University of Houston applied neural network to achieve the hysteresis model of SMA under specific spring load [102]. Hysteresis compensation is achieved by Korean scholar K. K. Ah by integrating genetic algorithm and Preisach model [88]. Similar control methods include variable structure control [104], sliding mode control [105], etc. But all these control strategies are aimed at the description and compensation of SMA under a specific stress or frequency state without considering the influence of varying stresses and frequencies.

To achieve an accurate description of SMA hysteresis properties, based on the analysis of the varying properties of SMA hysteresis under different loads and actuation frequencies, we propose the Sigmoid-based hysteresis (SBH) model. Compared with the existing models, the outstanding advantage of SBH model is that the double influences of external load and actuation frequency are both considered. Parameter identification of this model is simple, and physical concepts are also clear. Experimental results show that it is able to describe SMA hysteresis curves effectively. Besides, the reverse SBH model can also be acquired easily. Based on this model, we develop the feedforward control system to achieve hysteresis compensation. Experimental results show that SBH model is able to compensate for SMA hysteresis curves effectively and lays the foundation for the accurate and quick control of SMA-AM.

6.4.1 SMA Hysteresis Properties and Research Survey

6.4.1.1 Description of Hysteresis Property

Hysteresis property is a common nonlinear phenomenon in smart actuation materials. It reflects the inherent material property related to input signal and output signal. Hysteresis properties of different smart materials have similarities as well as differences. Take the PZT and SMA for example; their typical hysteresis curves are illustrated in Figure 6.59a and b. What they have in common is the multi-value property between the input and output of hysteresis curve, i.e., for the same input signal $u(t)$, the output signal $y(t)$ is multi-valued. Besides, hysteresis output curve not only depends on the current input, but also depends on historical inputs. Thus, hysteresis presents a certain nonlocal memory effect. When exposed to different amplitudes of input signal $u(t)$, smart materials have different sizes of hysteresis loops. The hysteresis loop under the maximum input signal is called the major hysteresis loop, as illustrated by the large cyclic curve in Figure 6.59. The hysteresis loop under the small input signal is called the minor hysteresis loop, as illustrated by the small cycling curve in Figure 6.59.

Hysteresis curves of both PZT and SMA have the congruence property and erase property, which are two main hysteresis properties. Congruence property refers to the consistency of the hysteresis loops; i.e., when the input signal's maximum and minimum values are the same, the hysteresis

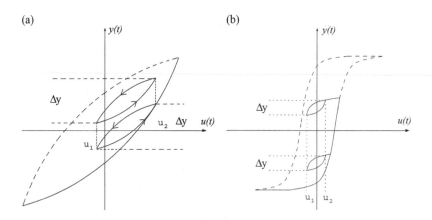

FIGURE 6.59 Hysteresis curves of (a) PZT; (b) SMA.

loops' shapes are also identical. Erase property refers to the fact that local maximum (minimum) value will erase the historical maximum (minimum) value that is smaller or larger than the current values [117].

To better describe the complex nonlinear property in hysteresis curves, scholar I. D. Mayerogyz proposes a general definition based on the common hysteresis properties; i.e., the hysteresis system can be described as the hysteresis transducer between input and output signals, as illustrated in Figure 6.60. Here $u(t)$ is the system input, and $y(t)$ is the system output. Input and output signals present nonlinear and nonsmooth properties of nonlocal memory and multi-valued mapping. $H(.)$ is the hysteresis transducer instead of a function. For 1D hysteresis system, $H(.)$ satisfies the following relation:

$$H(.): C_m[0,T] \times \varsigma_0 \to C_m[0,T],$$ (6.50)

where ς_0 is the initial system state and $C_m[0,T]$ is the piecewise continuous monotonic function space.

The general definition describes the common properties of hysteresis curves. For SMA, it has more complex nonlinear varying properties, as illustrated in Figure 6.59a and b. Compared with PZT, SMA presents saturated nonlinearity near the input signal extremum. Besides, SMA hysteresis curve is influenced by not only input signal frequency, but also external loads [89]. This is what other materials do not have.

To establish proper SMA hysteresis model, SMA's detailed and special hysteresis varying properties have to be clarified first. Due to the complex nonlinear properties and slow response speed of SMA, most SMA hysteresis studies are limited by specific load. The frequency-dependent property of SMA hysteresis, i.e., the influence of actuation frequency on SMA hysteresis, is rarely considered. The actuation condition of SMA-AM is current heating and forced tube airflow cooling. Current heating and forced airflow cooling are able to increase SMA response speed largely.

One purpose of our research is the rehabilitation application of SMA-AM under large loads. Thus, the influences of load and actuation frequency on SMA hysteresis have to be considered. With a single SMA wire, an experimental device similar to SMA-AM heating and cooling equipment is used to further study the SMA hysteresis properties.

The detailed experimental device is illustrated in Figure 6.61. An SMA wire sample with the diameter of 0.15 mm and length of 220 mm is placed vertically with one end fixed to a load cell and the other end connected to external stress. The external stresses are provided by different constant

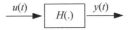

FIGURE 6.60 Hysteresis system.

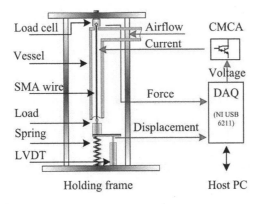

FIGURE 6.61 Schematic diagram of the experimental setup.

loads varying from 56 to 280 MPa and a helical bias spring with stiffness of 143 N/m. The contractile force is measured by the load cell, and the displacement is measured by a linear variable differential transformer (LVDT) with a resolution of 0.01 mm. A computer equipped with a data acquisition card (NI USB-6211) generates voltage signal and acquires the measured data. Voltage is used to drive the SMA wire, and forced vessel airflow is used to cool the SMA wire to acquire SMA hysteresis curve; the input signal of heating current control of SMA wire under the LabVIEW environment is as follows:

$$\begin{cases} U(t) = A\big[1 + \sin(2\pi ft)\big] \\ I(t) = C_I U(t) \end{cases}, \tag{6.51}$$

where $U(t)$ is the control voltage, A is voltage amplitude, f is actuation frequency, $C_I = 0.4$ A/V is the gain coefficient, and $I(t)$ is the heating current.

The actuation frequency, amplitude, and external stress are selected as 0.1 Hz, 0.6 V, and 56 MPa, respectively. Voltage/current–time curve and displacement–time curve of SMA wire acquired by the experiment are illustrated in Figures 6.62 and 6.63. On comparing the two figures,

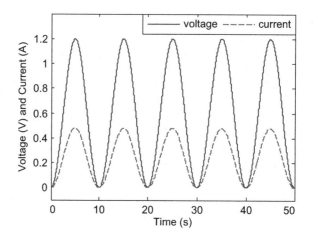

FIGURE 6.62 Actuation voltage and measured current–time curve.

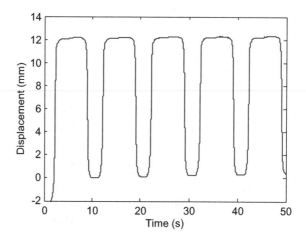

FIGURE 6.63 SMA wire displacement–time curve under sinusoidal heating current.

although actuation voltages are both sinusoidal, SMA displacement curve has non-sinusoidal properties with different widths due to SMA hysteresis. SMA wire voltage–displacement diagram is illustrated in Figure 6.64. It can be inferred from the figure that there is a hysteresis gap with the value of about 0.35 V between the heating curve (arrow H) and cooling curve (arrow C). Besides, both the heating and cooling curves have the shape similar to sigmoidal curve and its saturable hysteresis property.

6.4.1.1.1   Stress Effect on SMA Hysteresis

To study the stress effect on SMA hysteresis, the external load on SMA wire is changed to repeat the above experiment. Loads are classified into constant load and continuous load. Temporarily, only hysteresis property under different constant stresses is considered; thus, the bias spring is removed. SMA voltage–displacement (V–D) curves are shown in Figure 6.65 under different stresses ranging from 56 to 280 MPa. Referring to the figure, SMA hysteresis gap decreases, and the maximum displacement increases gradually with the increase of stress. Besides, all the hysteresis curves have properties similar to those of sigmoidal curve.

The same experiments were performed by adding the bias spring under a constant stress of 112 MPa. The V–D hysteresis curves are shown in Figure 6.66 with and without bias spring. As can

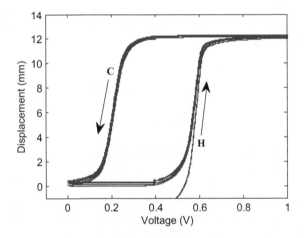

FIGURE 6.64   SMA voltage–displacement hysteresis curve.

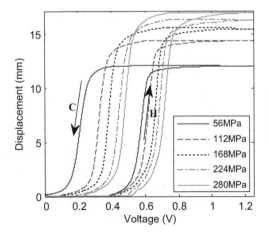

FIGURE 6.65   SMA hysteresis curve under different constant loads.

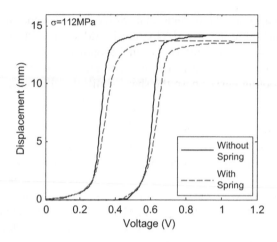

FIGURE 6.66 Comparisons of SMA hysteresis loops with and without bias spring.

be seen, the hysteresis gap is not affected by the stress state as long as prestress is determined, but the curve slope at phase transformation regions and the maximum displacement decreases when a bias spring is added. Besides, the larger the spring stiffness, the greater the reduction of curve slope and the greater the displacement will be.

6.4.1.1.2 Frequency Effect on SMA Hysteresis

To further explore the effect of driving frequency on SMA hysteresis, a sinusoidal driving voltage is applied to the SMA sample with the frequency ranging from 0.1 to 1 Hz and the amplitude of 1 V based on Eq. (6.17). Note that the SMA wire is cooled constantly by the forced vessel airflow under a prestress of 84 MPa during the experiment.

The experimental V–D curves are shown in Figure 6.67. As can be seen, the hysteresis gap increases and the curve slope decreases with the increase of driving frequency. Besides, the hysteresis curves also present a similar sigmoidal shape at frequencies below 0.6 Hz, while they become smooth at the end of phase transformation regions (denoted by two circles) at higher frequencies. This phenomenon is caused by SMA's slow heat transfer rate. More effective cooling and heating methods can be used to enhance heat transfer rate [111]. Here we mainly focus on the hysteresis properties under forced air cooling condition.

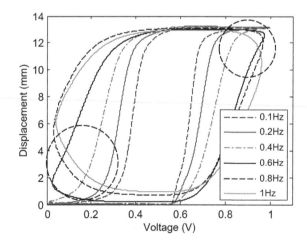

FIGURE 6.67 SMA hysteresis curves under different driving frequencies.

6.4.1.1.3 Minor Hysteresis Loop Properties

When heating current is not able to bring about complete phase transformation, there would be minor hysteresis loop. Thus, two sets of partially martensitic transformation experiments are performed under 56 and 168 MPa to explore the minor hysteresis properties, and the detailed V–D curves are shown in Figure 6.68 with different transformation degrees. As can be seen, all the first-order descending (FOD) reversal curves present similar sigmoidal shape with different maximum displacements. The minor hysteresis properties can be effectively represented by introducing two suitable scaling constants, which will be explained below.

It can be noted that FOD reversal curves are selected as the case studies for the symmetry of first-order ascending (FOA) and FOD [116]. FOD/FOA reversal curves are parts of minor loops attached to the ascending/descending branch of the major hysteresis curves, as illustrated in Figure 6.69.

6.4.1.2 Hysteresis Model

Developing a mathematical model that is able to reflect hysteresis properties accurately is the key to study the hysteresis system. To date, existing mathematical models developed to describe the

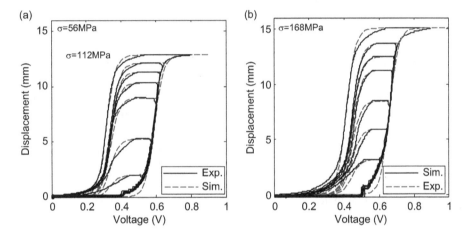

FIGURE 6.68 Comparisons of SMA minor hysteresis loops based on the experimental results and the simulation results.

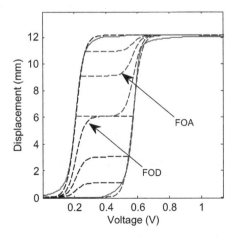

FIGURE 6.69 Descriptions of minor hysteresis loops of SMA FOD and FOA.

hysteresis of SMA can be divided into two classes, the physics-based hysteresis model and phenomenological hysteresis model

6.4.1.2.1 Physics-Based Model

The physics-based hysteresis model of SMA is a mathematical model based on material properties and is developed from thermodynamics, conservation of energy, and stress–temperature relation [86,87,118–120]. The most representative one is the exponential model proposed by Japanese scholar Tanaka. Based on the qualitative research on SMA's stress–strain properties, he pointed out that SMA's martensite content, stress, and temperature should satisfy the following relationship:

$$
\xi = \begin{cases} \exp\left[A_a \left(T - A_s \right) + B_a \sigma \right] & M \to A \\ 1 - \exp\left[A_m \left(T - M_s \right) + B_m \sigma \right] & A \to M \end{cases}.
\tag{6.52}
$$

The input of the model is temperature, and the martensite content is the output, considering the influence of stress on output. A_a, A_m, B_a, and B_m are all material parameters. M_s and A_s are the phase transformation temperatures. After that, Liang proposed the cosine form based theoretical model on the basis of Tanaka model, proposing that during SMA phase transformation, martensite content is the cosine function of temperature and stress, as illustrated by Eq. (6.53):

$$
\xi = \begin{cases} \dfrac{\xi_M}{2} \cos\left[\alpha_A \left(T - A_s \right) + b_A \sigma \right] + \dfrac{\xi_M}{2} & M \to A \\ \dfrac{1 - \xi_A}{2} \cos\left[a_M \left(T - M_f \right) + b_M \sigma \right] + \dfrac{1 + \xi_A}{2} & A \to M \end{cases}.
\tag{6.53}
$$

Liang's model assumes that material parameters are constant and the temperature variation region satisfies

$$
A_s \le T \le A_f \quad \text{or} \quad M_f \le T \le M_s.
\tag{6.54}
$$

Stress variation region satisfies

$$
\begin{cases} C_A \left(T - A_s \right) - \dfrac{\pi}{|b_A|} \le \sigma \le C_A \left(T - A_s \right) & M \to A \\ C_M \left(T - M_f \right) - \dfrac{\pi}{|b_M|} \le \sigma \le C_M \left(T - M_f \right) & A \to M \end{cases}.
\tag{6.55}
$$

All the involved parameters are material parameters. After that, based on Liang's model, American scholar Brinson divided martensite content into two parts, stress-induced martensite ξ_S and temperature-induced martensite ξ_T, so we have the following relationship:

$$
\xi = \xi_S + \xi_T.
\tag{6.56}
$$

Based on the different induced forms of martensite, input temperature, and external stress variation region, Brinson proposed a more detailed mathematical model.

When $T > A_s$ and $C_A (T - A_f) < \sigma < C_A (T - A_s)$,

$$
\begin{cases}
\xi = \dfrac{\xi_0}{2} \cos\left[\alpha_A (T - A_s) - \dfrac{\sigma}{C_A} \right] + \dfrac{\xi_0}{2} \\[3mm]
\xi_S = \xi_{S0} - \dfrac{\xi_{S0}}{\xi_0} (\xi_0 - \xi) \\[3mm]
\xi_T = \xi_{T0} - \dfrac{\xi_{T0}}{\xi_0} (\xi_0 - \xi)
\end{cases}
\tag{6.57}
$$

When $T > Ms$ and $\sigma_s^{cr} + C_M (T - M) < \sigma < \sigma_f^{cr} + C_M (T - M_s)$,

$$
\xi_S = \frac{1 - \xi_{S0}}{2} \cos\left\{ \frac{\pi}{\sigma_s^{cr} - \sigma_f^{cr}} \left[\sigma - \sigma_f^{cr} - C_M (T - M_s) \right] \right\} + \frac{1 + \xi_{S0}}{2},
$$

$$
\xi_T = \xi_{T0} - \frac{\xi_{T0}}{1 - \xi_{S0}} (\xi_S - \xi_{S0}).
\tag{6.58}
$$

When $T < M_s$ and $\sigma_s^{cr} < \sigma < \sigma_f^{cr}$,

$$
\xi_S = \frac{1 - \xi_{S0}}{2} \cos\left[\frac{\pi}{\sigma_s^{cr} - \sigma_f^{cr}} (\sigma - \sigma_f^{cr}) \right] + \frac{1 + \xi_{S0}}{2},
$$

$$
\xi_T = \xi_{T0} - \frac{\xi_{T0}}{1 - \xi_{S0}} (\xi_S - \xi_{S0}) + \Delta.
\tag{6.59}
$$

The subscript 0 here represents the initial value and the superscript cr represents the critical stress. Besides, when $M_f < T < M_s$ and $T < T_0$,

$$
\Delta = \frac{1 - \xi_{T0}}{2} \left\{ \cos\left[a_M (T - M_f) \right] + 1 \right\}. \text{ In other situations, } \Delta = 0.
$$

Based on the above analysis, SMA physics-based model describes clearly the hysteresis properties when output is martensite content and input is temperature. Load stress is also considered. However, these models describe only the SMA major hysteresis loop properties but are not able to describe SMA hysteresis properties under limited input. Moreover, the model is too complex with too many material parameters. Martensite content cannot be measured directly either. Thus, physics-based model of SMA is not proper to be applied in real-time feedback control.

6.4.1.2.2 *Phenomenological Model*
Phenomenological hysteresis model is not limited by the practical physical meaning. It is based on the variation law and phenomenological property of hysteresis curves and applies only mathematical methods to develop mathematical models, which are able to characterize the hysteresis curve. Based on the different forms, it can be further divided into differential hysteresis model and operator hysteresis model.

6.4.1.2.2.1 Differential Hysteresis Model
Differential hysteresis model describes the relationships between input and output of hysteresis curves by developing differential functions. Duhem model is one of the most representative ones in differential hysteresis models [121]. Based on Duhem model, the input–output relationship of hysteresis curve is

$$\begin{cases} \dot{v} = g_+\big(u(t), v(t)\big)\dot{u}_+(t) - g_-\big(u(t), v(t)\big)\dot{u}_-(t) \\ v(0) = v_0 \end{cases}, \tag{6.60}$$

in which

$$\dot{u}_{\pm}(t) = \frac{|\dot{u}(t)| \pm \dot{u}(t)}{2}, \tag{6.61}$$

where $u(t)$ is input and $v(t)$ is output. $g_+, g_- \in C^0 (R^2)$. $u(t)$ and $v(t)$ are both continuously differentiable functions in $[0,T]$. Duhem model also follows the following principles. When input $u(t)$ is an increasing function, output $v(t)$ will increase along a certain path. When input $u(t)$ is a decreasing function, output $v(t)$ will decrease along another path. The slopes are denoted by functions g_+ and g_-.

Scholar S. M. Dutta describes SMA hysteresis properties using Duhem model [116]. SMA hysteresis curve can be divided into major and minor hysteresis loops based on different input amplitudes. Gaussian probability density distribution function is applied to construct the path slope function as follows:

$$g_{+/-}(u) = \frac{1}{\sigma_{+/-}\sqrt{2\pi}} \exp\left(-\frac{\left(u - \mu_{+/-}\right)^2}{2\sigma_{+/-}^2}\right), \tag{6.62}$$

where μ is the average value and σ^2 is the variance. Subscripts $+$ and $-$ represent the increase and decrease curves. Major hysteresis loop output v is described as

$$v_{+/-}(u) = h_{+/-}(u) = \int_{-\infty}^{u} g_{+/-}(u')du' = \frac{1}{2}\left[1 + erf\left(\frac{u - \mu_{+/-}}{\sigma_{+/-}\sqrt{2}}\right)\right]. \tag{6.63}$$

Thus, SMA major hysteresis loop can be described by the following differential function:

$$\frac{dv}{du} = \begin{cases} \dfrac{1}{\sigma_+\sqrt{2\pi}} \exp\left(-\dfrac{\left(u - \mu_+\right)^2}{2\sigma_+^2}\right), & \dot{u} \geq 0 \\[4mm] \dfrac{1}{\sigma_-\sqrt{2\pi}} \exp\left(-\dfrac{\left(u - \mu_-\right)^2}{2\sigma_-^2}\right), & \dot{u} < 0 \end{cases}. \tag{6.64}$$

SMA minor hysteresis loop can be described by a proper metric function based on the slope function, and the following relationship can be obtained:

$$g_{i+/-}(u) = \frac{n_{i+/-}}{\sigma_{+/-}\sqrt{2\pi}} \exp\left(-\frac{\left(u - \mu_{+/-}\right)}{2\sigma_{+/-}^2}\right), \tag{6.65}$$

where $n_{i+/-} \in [0,1]$, $i = 1, \dots, N$. Based on the above differential model, typical SMA hysteresis curve can be drawn, as illustrated in Figure 6.70. Note that $n_{i+/-} = 1$ represents the SMA main hysteresis curve.

Based on the above analysis, as there are input signal derivatives in differential hysteresis model, hysteresis can be described no matter whether the frequency is related or not. However, it is often hard to compute the reverse differential model of this kind; thus, it is not proper to be applied in the control based on reverse hysteresis model compensation.

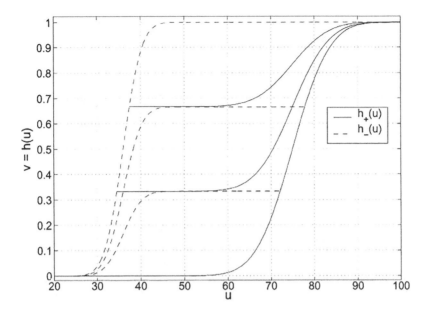

FIGURE 6.70 Duhem-model–based SMA hysteresis curve.

6.4.1.2.2.2 Operator Hysteresis Model   Operator hysteresis model achieves qualitative description of hysteresis curve through the weighted stack of operators. Compared with differential model, operator model is able to describe major and minor hysteresis loops more accurately. Preisach model is the most representative one among the existing operator hysteresis models.

Preisach model was first proposed by German scholar F. Preisach in 1930s. It is a pure mathematical model and one of the most widely used models. The core idea of Preisach model is the Relay operator, as illustrated in Figure 6.71. The Relay operator is represented by a couple of switching thresholds (α, β), where $\alpha > \beta$. $u(t)$ is the input of Relay operator, and $\hat{\gamma}_{\alpha\beta}[u(t)]$ is the output. On the Relay operator plane, input is irreversible on vertical axis and is reversible on lateral axis. Based on the different values of $u(t)$, operator output is +1 or −1. Basic hypothesis of Preisach model is that system output is the weighted stack of numerous paralleled Relay operators. The mathematical description of Preisach model is given in Eq. (6.66) and is shown in Figure 6.72.

$$f(t) = P[u](u) = \int\int_{\alpha \geq \beta} \mu(\alpha, \beta)\hat{\gamma}_{\alpha\beta}[u(t)]\,d\alpha\,d\beta, \tag{6.66}$$

where $\mu(\alpha, \beta)$ is the weighted function and $f(t)$ is model output.

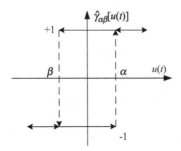

FIGURE 6.71 Relay hysteresis operator.

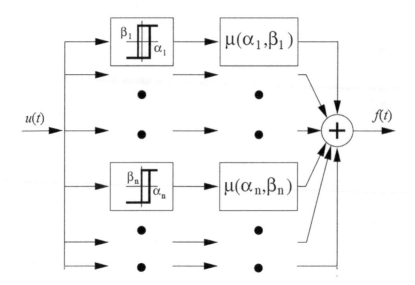

FIGURE 6.72   Preisach model.

Based on Eq. (6.66), the output of Preisach model can be uniquely determined by the weighted function $\mu(\alpha, \beta)$. Thus, when applying Preisach model to describe SMA hysteresis properties, the key is to acquire the weighted function. However, in practical applications, the double integral of Preisach model makes the computation complex. Besides, the difficulty in acquiring analytic reverse model limits its application. After that, a series of operator hysteresis models have been proposed, such as the Prandtl–Ishlinskii and Krasnosel'skii–Pokrovkiim models. Although the model's function is relatively simple, a series of models have rarely been applied in the description of SMA hysteresis properties. The root cause is that the hysteresis properties of SMA are more complex and volatile than those of PZT, such as the saturated nonlinear property, the effects of stress and frequency, etc.

6.4.1.3   SBH Model of SMA

6.4.1.3.1   Hysteresis Description of SBH Model

As can be seen in Figures 6.64–6.69, all the SMA hysteresis curves are sigmoidal. The main distinctions are hysteresis gap, curve slope, and maximum displacement. As the two branches of curves are both sigmoidal, sigmoidal function is used to construct SMA hysteresis model. By introducing a few set of parameters, sigmoid-based hysteresis (SBH) model is proposed. The two branches are expressed as

$$y = \frac{k(\sigma, f)}{1 + e^{-\alpha(\sigma, f)[u - r_+(\sigma, f)]}} \quad \text{for } \dot{u} \geq 0, \tag{6.67a}$$

$$y = \frac{k(\sigma, f)}{1 + e^{-\alpha(\sigma, f)[u - r_-(\sigma, f)]}} \quad \text{for } \dot{u} < 0, \tag{6.67b}$$

where u is the input voltage and y is the output displacement. k, $a_{+/-}$, and $r_{+/-}$ are model parameters. k represents the maximum displacement. $a_{+/-}$ and $r_{+/-}$ represent curve slopes and voltage values at peak transformations of $M \to A$ and $A \to M$. Besides, the hysteresis gap is defined as follows:

$$\Delta r(\sigma, f) = r_+(\sigma, f) - r_-(\sigma, f). \tag{6.68}$$

The hysteresis curves expressed by Eq. (6.67) refer to the major hysteresis properties. We found that the minor hysteresis properties can be represented by multiplying the major hysteresis curves' expressions in Eq. (6.67) by two suitable scaling constants $\beta_{+/-}$, where $\beta_{+/-} \in [0,1]$. Hence, we get

$$y = \beta_+ \frac{k(\sigma, f)}{1 + e^{-a(\sigma, f)[u - r_+(\sigma, f)]}} \quad \text{for } \dot{u} \geq 0, \tag{6.69a}$$

$$y = \beta_- \frac{k(\sigma, f)}{1 + e^{-a(\sigma, f)[u - r_-(\sigma, f)]}} + (1 - \beta_-)k(\sigma, f) \quad \text{for } \dot{u} < 0. \tag{6.69b}$$

The coupled influence of external load and driving frequency on SMA hysteresis has been considered by the proposed SBH. Besides, sigmoid function is simple in form and has completely reversible analytic solution; thus, it is easier to apply this model in real-time control systems compared with other hysteresis models.

6.4.1.3.2 Parameter Identification, Fitting, and Verification of SBH Model

To demonstrate the effectiveness of the above SBH model, the primary problem is parameter identification. Parameters involved in the hysteresis model are all functions of stress and driving frequency. Based on the above experimental data, we identify the model parameters though linear regression. The identification algorithm is completed offline through MATLAB optimization toolbox. The curves of model parameters k, a, r, external stress, and driving frequency are illustrated in Figures 6.73–6.75.

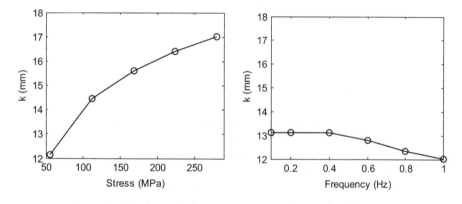

FIGURE 6.73   Relation curves of SMA hysteresis displacement and stress/frequency.

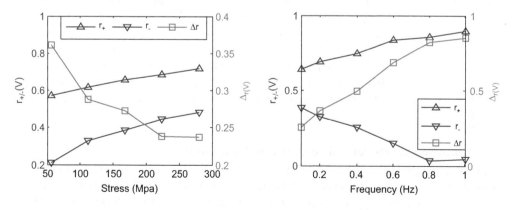

FIGURE 6.74   Relation curves of SMA hysteresis gap and stress/frequency.

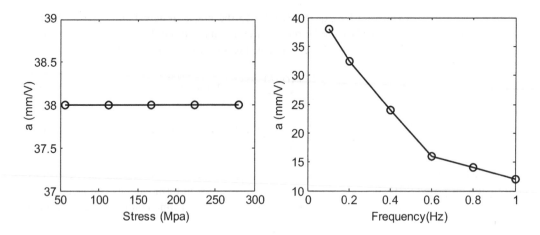

FIGURE 6.75   Curve slope relation with stress and frequency curves.

Based on the data fitting methods, we can fit the hysteresis model parameters and develop the function of frequencies with maximum displacement, curve slope, hysteresis gap, and stress. Detailed relationships are given in Eqs (6.70)–(6.72):

$$k(\sigma, f) = \left(13.16 - 1.196 f^{2.23}\right)\left(28.62 - 39.4\sigma^{-0.22}\right), \tag{6.70}$$

$$\Delta r(\sigma, f) = \left(0.139 + 1.151 f - 0.422 f^2 - 0.422 f^2\right) \cdot \left(2.109\sigma^{-0.57} + 0.151\right), \tag{6.71}$$

$$a(\sigma, f) = 43.38 e^{-1.453 f}. \tag{6.72}$$

To prove the effectiveness and generality of SBH model, based on the hysteresis experimental data, comparisons have been made between the simulation and experimental results under different stresses and driving frequencies, as illustrated in Figure 6.76. In a relatively large variation range (56–280 MPa), simulation and experimental results agree well, indicating that SBH is able to describe stress-related hysteresis properties well. Note that near the inflection point, there is certain error, and the larger the stress, the bigger the error is. However, the error can be eliminated by feedback control.

Figure 6.77 illustrates the comparison of experimental results at driving frequencies of 0.1–1 Hz. Referring to the figure, when the frequency is less than 0.6 Hz, SBH is able to describe the effect of frequency well. When the frequency is higher than 0.6 HZ, because of incomplete phase transformation, there are big errors in the branch ends of hysteresis curves. In fact, the errors can be reduced or eliminated by increasing heat-transfer velocity. Besides, by changing the scaling constant in SBH model, the effectiveness of SBH in describing SMA minor hysteresis loop can also be proved. The simulation and experimental results coincide well, as illustrated in Figure 6.68.

6.4.1.4   Inverse SBH Model and Feedforward Compensation

To demonstrate the effectiveness of the SBH model for hysteresis compensation, we design a feedforward controller based on the inverse SBH model. The control scheme is shown in Figure 6.78. y_d is the desired displacement, y_a is the actual displacement, u is the control voltage acquired from the reverse model, and I is the heating current after current amplification.

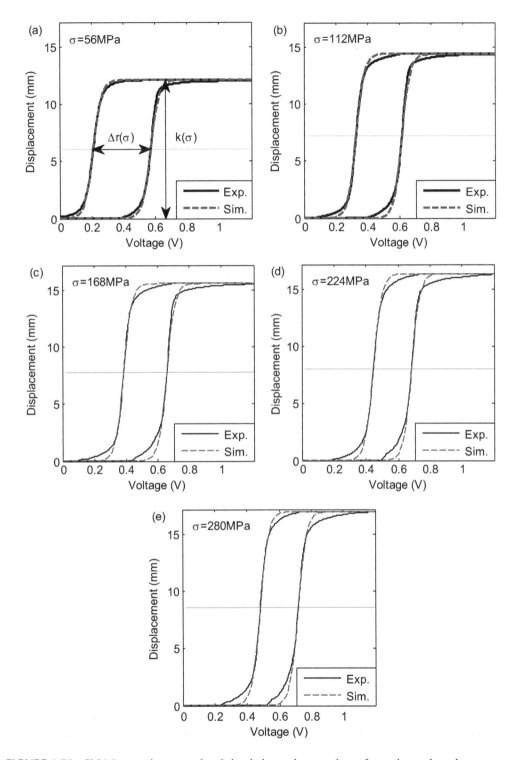

FIGURE 6.76 SMA hysteresis stress-related simulation and comparison of experimental results.

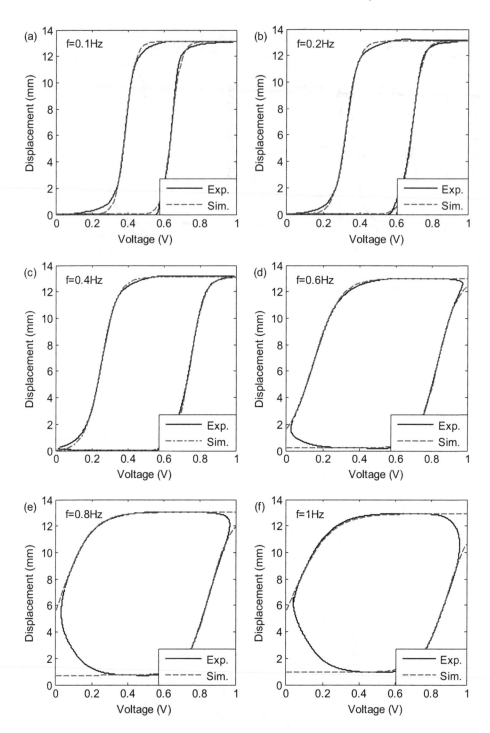

FIGURE 6.77   SMA hysteresis frequency-related simulation and comparison of experimental results.

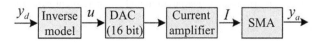

FIGURE 6.78   Feedforward controller diagram based on inverse hysteresis model.

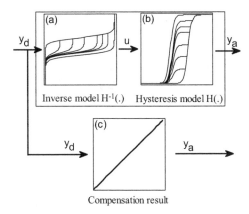

FIGURE 6.79   Inverse hysteresis compensation flow chart of SMA.

Figure 6.79 shows the flow chart of the inverse hysteresis compensation. For the hysteresis model $H(.)$ and the inverse model $H^{-1}(.)$, the following equation can be obtained if the exact inverse model exists:

$$\begin{cases} y_a = H(u) \\ u = H^{-1}(y_d) \end{cases} \Rightarrow y_a = y_d . \tag{6.73}$$

Ideally, the actual displacement y_a should follow the desired displacement y_d precisely, and the hysteresis can be eliminated by inverse hysteresis compensation, as shown in Figure 6.79c.

Due to the continuous and monotonic properties of the SBH model, the exact inverse model can be formulated analytically. The detailed expression of the inverse hysteresis model is obtained as

$$u = H^{-1}\left(y^d\right) =$$

$$\begin{cases} \dfrac{1}{a_+(\sigma,f)}\left[\ln y_d - \ln\left(\beta_+ k(\sigma,f) - y_d\right)\right] + r_+(\sigma,f) & \text{for } \dot{y}_d \geq 0 \\ \dfrac{1}{a_-(\sigma,f)}\left[\ln\left(y_d - (1-\beta_-)k(\sigma,f)\right) - \ln\left(\beta_- k(\sigma,f) - y_d\right)\right] + r_-(\sigma,f) & \text{for } \dot{y}_d < 0 \end{cases} \tag{6.74}$$

To verify the effectiveness of the proposed inverse model, several experimental tests are conducted to track a 10 mm peak-to-peak triangular trajectory. Three conditions are selected (56 MPa/0.1 Hz, 112 MPa/0.1 Hz, and 84 MPa/0.4 Hz) as the cases. The feedforward controller based on $H^{-1}(\cdot)$ is applied in the test setup with LabVIEW software as previously described.

Figure 6.80a illustrates the comparison of desired trajectory y_d (red dotted line) and the actual trajectory y_a (blue solid line) and the tracking error after the inverse hysteresis compensation (green dash-dotted line). It can be inferred from the figure that the feedforward controller based on the inverse SBH model largely decreases the hysteresis nonlinear error. Detailed maximum tracking error (MTE) and root mean square (RMS) are listed in Table 6.9. Figure 6.80b illustrates the control signal u. Because of the forward controller, voltage u is sigmoidal instead of triangular wave. To better illustrate the hysteresis compensation effect, Figure 6.80c illustrates the relation between the input and output of forward controller. It can be seen from the figure that because of the compensation effect of the forward controller, the desired trajectory and the actual trajectory are nearly linear. Thus, it proves that the proposed SBH model greatly reduces the influence of hysteresis nonlinearity. We can change the external stress and the driving frequency and then repeat the above experiments.

The results demonstrate that the inverse-SBH–based feedforward controller well compensates the hysteresis. Three different external conditions are included in the experiments (56 MPa/0.1 Hz,

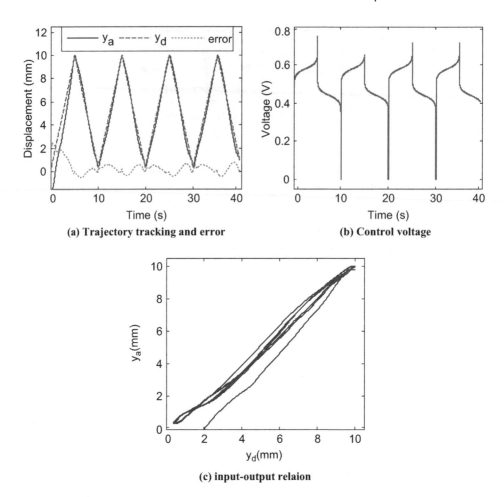

FIGURE 6.80 SMA trajectory tracking experimental results (56 MPa and 0.1 Hz). (a) comparison of desired trajectory and the actual trajectory and the tracking error after the inverse hysteresis compensation; (b) the control signal; (c) the relation between the input and output of forward controller.

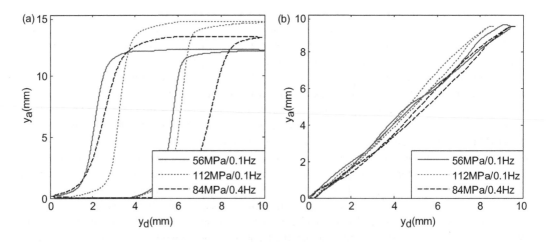

FIGURE 6.81 Comparison before and after SMA hysteresis compensation under different conditions. (a) before compensation; (b) after compensation.

TABLE 6.9
Trajectory Tracking Errors under Different External Conditions

Applied Condition	MTE (mm)	RMSTE (mm)
56 MPa/0.1 Hz	0.55	0.28
112 MPa/0.1 Hz	0.62	0.37
84 MPa/0.4 Hz	0.68	0.36

112 MPa/0.1 Hz, and 84 MPa/0.4 Hz). Experimental results before and after compensation are illustrated in Figure 6.81a and b. Comparing the two figures, the hysteresis decreases obviously, and then a good linear relation is achieved between the input and output. To quantitatively describe the compensation effect of forward controller, the detailed MTE and root mean square tracking error (RMSTE) are illustrated in Table 6.9. It can be inferred that compared with the maximum hysteresis error of 14.2 mm before compensation, the error after the compensation decreases to 0.68 (95%).

6.5 SMA-AM APPLICATION IN ANKLE–FOOT REHABILITATION SYSTEM

SMA artificial muscle (SMA-AM) not only has integrated actuation and self-sensing properties similar to skeletal muscle, but also has the properties of large output force and large power density. To verify the above properties of SMA-AM and explore its clinical application, SMA-AM is selected as the main actuator to design the active ankle–foot rehabilitation system. It is expected to be applied in the orthopedic rehabilitation of foot drop. Foot drop is the normal complication of strike and cerebral palsy. Its typical clinical manifestation is that the patient's toe touches the ground first in the later stage of gait swing phase, while heel should touch the ground first in normal gait. Foot drop can easily lead to gait instability and fall. The main reason for foot drop is that the front muscle group of tibia becomes invalid; i.e., front muscle group of tibia is unable to achieve normal contraction [121].

The most direct and effective method to treat foot drop is to wear ankle–foot orthosis (AFO) [125]. Passive AFO is common in clinical application [122–124]. This kind of AFO has the features of low cost and portability. It is usually composed of light leather or resin without any actuation control elements, as illustrated in Figure 6.82. Most passive AFOs limit ankle–foot range of motion by binding so as to prevent foot drop. However, the long-time use of the passive AFO will lead to dependence. Besides, the fact that front muscle group of tibia does not move will aggravate the myophagism, which is even worse for the treatment of foot drop. Thus, passive AFO is unable to train the front muscle group of tibia.

The other type is active AFO, as illustrated in Figure 6.83. Active AFO achieves the control of ankle joint flexion–dorsiflexion through active actuation. Electric and pneumatic muscles are the main actuation sources of existing AFOs. Compared with passive AFO, active AFO not only provides assistive force for ankle joint, but also achieves the training of front muscle group of

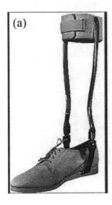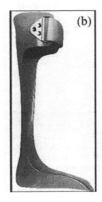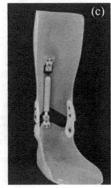

FIGURE 6.82 Passive AFO: (a) metal leather; (b) leaf spring; (c) resin.

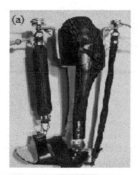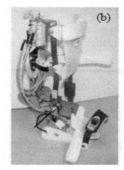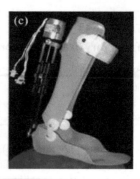

FIGURE 6.83 Active AFO: (a) Michigan pneumatic AM; (b) Arizona electric spring AM; (c) MIT electric spring AM.

tibia. Thus, it will compensate the shortcomings of passive AFOs. However, limited by the application conditions of actuators, active AFO has the disadvantages of being complex and cumbersome. These will largely increase the discomfort of patients. Thus, active AFO is still at the stage of experimental research, and there is still a gap in its practical application.

It has been well recognized that an ideal AFO system should not only have the function of active actuation as the active AFOs, but also should be light, flexible, and comfortable as passive AFOs. Thus, SMA-AM is promising to realize the ideal AFO system. To further study the system properties of SMA-AFO, a comprehensive dynamic model, which is able to systematically reflect the multi-field coupling properties of SMA-AM actuation system, needs to be established, considering the properties of SMA thermal actuation, circuit, heat transfer, hysteresis, self-sensing, and mechanical vibration. Based on the above-mentioned comprehensive modeling, a sliding-mode controller is designed, and Lyapunov function is applied to prove the stability of SMA closed-loop control system. Finally, experiments prove the correctness of the comprehensive dynamic model and the effectiveness of the controller. Accurate and fast tracking of the joint angle of SMA-AFO is achieved under the conditions of self-sensing and large output force when the response frequency reaches 1 Hz. The experimental results indicate that the system has satisfied the application requirements of ankle–foot rehabilitation.

6.5.1 SMA-AFO

SMA-AFO is mainly composed of three parts: the actuation-sensing system, ankle–foot orthopedic system, and control system, as illustrated in Figure 6.84.

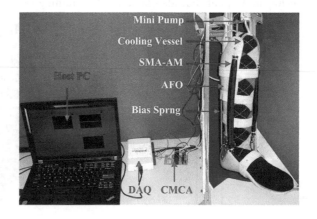

FIGURE 6.84 SMA-AM active ankle–foot rehabilitation system (SMA-AFO).

6.5.1.1   Actuating–Sensing System

Based on the analysis in former sections, SMA-AM has the properties of integrated actuation and self-sensing. Thus, the actuators and sensors of SMA-AFO are all provided by SMA-AM. Eight SMA wires with a diameter of 0.25 mm act as the actuator of SMA-AM. Its maximum contraction force is 230 N. Two parallel SMA-AMs are selected as the actuators with the maximum contraction force of 460 N. Total length of SMA-AM is 250 mm, and the designed maximum contraction length is 45 mm.

Based on human gait data [126], ankle-joint flexion–dorsiflexion range of motion is −15° to 15° in normal gait. The maximum torque of ankle in swing phase is 7.5 Nm, provided mainly by tibialis anterior, extensor digitorum longus, and extensor pollicis longus. To satisfy these requirements, the SMA-AFO joint torque can be computed though the following equations:

$$
\begin{cases}
l - l_0 = a \sin(\theta - \theta_0) \\
T = Fa
\end{cases}, \tag{6.75}
$$

where θ is the joint angle of SMA-AFO, T is the torque, l is the length of SMA-AM, F is the contraction force of the two SMA-AMs, a is joint torque arm, and subscript 0 represents the initial value. Here, the torque arm is selected as 40 mm, and the maximum output torque of SMA-AFO is 18.4 Nm, satisfying the torque requirement of ankle joint in swing phase.

Note that the focus of this chapter is to verify the actuation property of SMA-AM and explore primarily the clinical application. Joint torques are different for different disease conditions; thus, the assistive torques required for different patients are also different. They can be achieved by adding and reducing number of parallel SMA wires, which will not be discussed here.

The unique self-sensing property of SMA-AM is able to achieve the integrated actuation and sensing of SMA-AFO; thus, the structure of SMA-AFO can be simplified further. Based on the analysis in Section 6.3, the contraction length of SMA-AM can be obtained by the following self-sensing model:

$$
\begin{cases}
R_h = \dfrac{1}{V}\left(\dfrac{K_A}{l_0} l_3 + H_A l^2\right) & \text{for } M \to A \\[3mm]
R_c = \dfrac{1}{V}\left(\dfrac{K_M}{l_0} l_3 + H_M l^2\right) & \text{for } A \to M
\end{cases}. \tag{6.76}
$$

Further, combining Eqs. (6.75) and (6.76), the real-time joint angle of SMA-AFO can be acquired.

6.5.1.2   AFO

To ensure the portability and comfort features of SMA-AFO, standard polypropylene material is selected to develop the orthoses for calf and foot. Frames of the two parts are connected by a metal hinge joint. It realizes AFO free rotation in the sagittal plane and limits the movement in the coronal plane. On the two sides of the head of AFO, one end of SMA-AM is connected to the hinge joint and is symmetrically distributed. The other end is connected with a mini pump through a cooling vessel to realize the real-time forced air cooling of SMA-AM. A bias spring is fixed at the back of AFO. The bias spring serves two purposes, i.e., to provide enough restoring force for the AM and to simulate variable load conditions.

6.5.1.3   Control System

The control system of SMA-AFO is composed of three parts: the constant current source operational circuit, data acquisition card, and host PC. The operational circuit can amplify the signal from data acquisition card and drive SMA-AM, as illustrated in Figure 6.85. The data acquisition

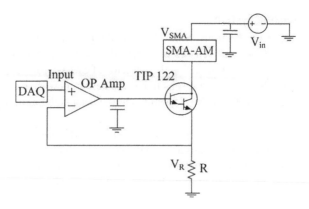

FIGURE 6.85 SMA-AFO operational circuit.

card (NI-USB-6211) is able to realize two channels of analog output and eight channels of differential analog input. All the data is stored in the host PC after digital filtering; the details are illustrated in Figure 6.84.

6.5.2 COMPREHENSIVE DYNAMIC MODEL OF SMA-AFO SYSTEM

To further analyze the system property of SMA-AFO, a comprehensive thermomechanical and electrodynamic model that describes SMA-AFO system property is proposed from the perspective of thermoelectric properties, SMA physical structure, hysteresis property, and mechanical vibration. It also lays a foundation for further model-based sliding-mode controller design. Detailed model diagram of SMA-AFO system is illustrated in Figure 6.86.

6.5.2.1 Thermoelectric Property

SMA-AM satisfies the following heat-transfer model under current heating and forced tube air cooling:

$$\rho c \frac{n_s \pi d_0^2 l_0}{4} \frac{dT}{dt} = \frac{u^2}{R} - \pi d_0 l_0 h_c (T - T_{amb}), \qquad (6.77)$$

where R is the resistance of single SMA wire, d_0 and l_0 are the initial diameter and length of SMA wire, T_{amb} is environment temperature, ρ is SMA wire density, n_s is the number of parallel SMA

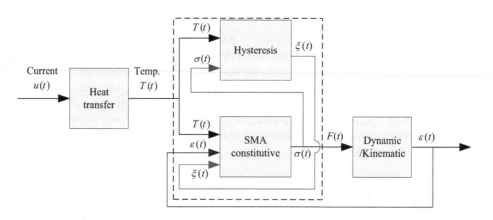

FIGURE 6.86 SMA-AFO model diagram.

TABLE 6.10
SMA-AM Parameter Values

Par.	Value	Par.	Value	Par.	Value	Par.	Value
ρ	6,500 kg/m³	a_1	165 W/m² °C	b_1	1,400 J/kg °C	n_1	10°C
l_0	250 mm	a_2	0.5 W/m² °C²	b_2	1,000 J/kg °C	n_2	0.5°C
d_0	0.25 mm	a_3	300 W/m² °C	m_1	62°C	n_s	16
T_{amb}	20°C	a_4	150 W/m² °C²	m_2	88°C	R	20 Ω/m
E	51.5 GPa	Ω	−1.12 GPa	Θ	0.55 MPa/°C	k	10

wires in SMA-AM, $c(\cdot)$ is specific heat, and hc $(\cdot)$ is convection coefficient. In Eq. (6.77), $c(\cdot)$ and hc $(\cdot)$ satisfy the following equations [127,128]:

$$h_c = \begin{cases} a_1 - a_2 T & \dot{T} \geq 0 \\ a_3 + a_4 \operatorname{erf}\left(\dfrac{T - m_1}{n_1}\right) & \dot{T} < 0 \end{cases}, \tag{6.78}$$

$$c = b_1 + b_2 \operatorname{erf}\left(\frac{T - m_2}{n_2}\right), \tag{6.79}$$

where $a_1, a_2, a_3, a_4, b_1, b_2, m_1, n_1, m_2$, and n_2 are all constants, the values of which are listed in Table 6.10.

6.5.2.2   SMA Physics-Based Property

SMA physics-based property refers to its material properties. The physics-based model describes the relationship between martensite content, strain, temperature, and stress [86,87,118] as follows:

$$\sigma - \sigma_0 = E(\varepsilon - \varepsilon_0) + \Theta(T - T_0) + \Omega(\xi - \xi_0), \tag{6.80}$$

where E is the Young's modulus, Θ is the thermal coefficient of expansion, and Ω is the transformation tensor of SMA. When there is no martensite, SMA strain ε and martensite content ξ are distributed reciprocally, as per the following equation:

$$\xi = k\varepsilon, \tag{6.81}$$

where k is constant; thus, the physics-based model illustrated in Eq. (6.80) can be simplified as

$$\sigma = Q\varepsilon + \Theta T + f_0, \tag{6.82}$$

where $Q = E + k\Omega$ and $f_0 = \sigma_0 + Q\varepsilon_0 + \Theta T_0$. Subscript 0 means that it is the initial value. Detailed parameters can be found in Table 6.10.

6.5.2.3   Hysteresis Properties

Under the influence of input signal, SMA output presents complex nonlinear saturated hysteresis properties. The hysteresis relationship between SMA-AM displacement $x(t)$ and input voltage $u(t)$ has been discussed in detail before, and the SBH model is also developed. The general expression is as follows:

$$x(t) = H[u(t)]. \tag{6.83}$$

SMA strain ε and SMA-AM displacement $x(t)$ are distributed reciprocally and satisfy the following equation:

$$\varepsilon = \frac{x_0 - x}{x_0}, \tag{6.84}$$

where x_0 is the initial displacement of SMA-AM. Thus, SMA strain and input voltage satisfy the following hysteresis relationship:

$$\varepsilon(t) = H\big[u(t)\big]. \tag{6.85}$$

6.5.2.4 Mechanical Properties

Based on the structural property of SMA-AFO system, SMA-AFO system can be expressed as mass-spring–damping system. Based on Newton's laws of motion, we have

$$J\ddot{\theta} + c_b\dot{\theta} + k_b\theta = F_A a, \tag{6.86}$$

where F_A is output force of SMA-AM. J, c_b, and k_b are the equivalent moment of inertia, damping, and stiffness, respectively. Note that SMA-AM active contraction force is provided by parallel SMA wires; thus, the F_A in the above equation satisfies the following equation:

$$F_A = \frac{n_s \pi d_0^2}{4}\sigma. \tag{6.87}$$

Combining Eqs. (6.77), (6.82), and (6.87), we get

$$\bar{J}\ddot{\theta} + \bar{c}_b\dot{\theta} + \bar{k}_b\theta = H\big[u(t)\big] + g\big[u(t)\big], \tag{6.88}$$

where $\bar{J} = \dfrac{4J}{Q n_s a \pi d_0^2}$, $\bar{c}_b = \dfrac{4c_b}{Q n_s a \pi d_0^2}$, $\bar{k}_b = \dfrac{4k_b}{Q n_s a \pi d_0^2}$, and $g\big[u(t)\big] = \dfrac{\Theta f(u) + f_0}{Q}$. $f(u)$ here is exactly Eq. (6.77). Based on Eq. (6.88), the comprehensive dynamic model of SMA-AFO system can be described as a second-order linear dynamic model with hysteresis nonlinear factors.

6.5.3 Sliding-Mode Control of SMA-AFO System

Accurate and fast tracking control is the prerequisite of SMA-AFO rehabilitation application. The inherent hysteresis nonlinearity and parameter uncertainty of SMA-AM are the difficulties for the control of SMA-AFO. Based on the comprehensive dynamic model in the last section, the model-based sliding-mode algorithm is developed to realize the angular tracking control of SMA-AFO. SMA self-sensing model is applied to achieve the integrated actuation of SMA-AFO. Lyapunov function is also used to conduct the analysis and verification of the global stability of SMA-AFO closed-loop control system.

6.5.3.1 Mechanism of Sliding-Mode Control

For a nonlinear system or system with unknown and uncertain parameters, controlling first-order system is much easier than controlling nth-order system [129]. The basic mechanism of sliding control is to transfer the nth-order system to first-order system equivalently by bringing in a sliding-mode plane.

Consider the following signal input dynamical system:

$$x^{(n)} = f(\mathbf{x}) + b(\mathbf{x})u, \tag{6.89}$$

where scalar x is the output which we are interested in. u is the control input. $\mathbf{x} = [x, \dot{x}, \dots x^{(n-1)}]^T$ is the state vector. Besides, it is known that function $f(x)$ is not accurate, but its inaccurate region is known. Similarly, control gain $b(x)$ is known as inaccurate, while its value range is limited by a function of x. The aim of sliding-mode control is to ensure that practical x follows the track of the ideal state $\mathbf{x}_d = [x_d, \dot{x}_d, \dots x_d^{(n-1)}]^T$ when $f(x)$ and $b(x)$ are both inaccurately modeled in system described by Eq. (6.89).

Define the following sliding-mode plane:

$$s(t) = \left(\frac{d}{dt} + \lambda \right)^{n-1} \tilde{\mathbf{x}}, \tag{6.90}$$

where γ is a positive constant and $\tilde{\mathbf{x}} = \mathbf{x} - \mathbf{x}_d = [\tilde{x}, \dot{\tilde{x}}, \dots \tilde{x}^{(n-1)}]^T$ is the tracking error vector.

Equation (6.90) can be simplified as

$$s(t) = \Lambda^T \tilde{\mathbf{x}}, \tag{6.91}$$

where $\Lambda^T = \left[c_{n-1} \lambda^{n-1}, \dots c_1 \lambda^1, c_0 \right]$, and it satisfies

$$c_i = \left(\begin{array}{c} n-1 \\ i \end{array} \right) = \frac{(n-1)!}{(n-i-1)! i!}, \quad i = 0, 1, \dots, n-1. \tag{6.92}$$

Thus, given the initial state $\mathbf{x}_d(0) = \mathbf{x}(0)$, the problem of tracking n-dimensional vector $\mathbf{x}_d$ is transformed into the problem of turning scalar s into 0. In fact, as there is $\tilde{x}^{(n-1)}$ in Eq. (6.90), one-time derivation of s is enough to bring out the controlled variable u. One step further, the boundary of s can be transferred directly into that of the tracking error $\mathbf{x}$; i.e., scalar s is the practical measurement of tracking quality. Thus, the control of nth-order system (Eq. 6.90) can be effectively transformed into the control of the first-order system (Eq. 6.91) particularly when

$$\tilde{\mathbf{x}}(0) = 0,$$

$$\forall t \geq 0, |s(t)| \leq \Phi \Rightarrow \forall t \geq 0, |\tilde{x}^{(i)}(t)| \leq (2\lambda)^i \varsigma, i = 0, 1, \dots, n-1, \tag{6.93}$$

where $\varsigma = \Phi / \lambda^{n-1}$. When $\tilde{\mathbf{x}}(0) \neq 0$, the boundary Eq. (6.93) can be progressively acquired with the time constant $(n-1)/\lambda$.

By selecting control signal u in Eq. (6.89), we can ensure that the following equation can be satisfied outside the surface $S(t)$:

$$\frac{1}{2} \frac{d}{dt} s^2 \leq -\eta |s|. \tag{6.94}$$

In this way, the problem can be simplified as the first-order problem of turning s into constant 0, where $\eta > 0$. Essentially, what Eq. (6.94) expresses is that the square of the distance to the surface with the measurement of s^2 decreases along all the system trajectories [129], as illustrated in Figure 6.87. Once the trajectory enters the surface, it will stay in that surface. The trajectories outside the surface will still move toward the surface, as indicated by the arrows in Figure 6.87. It is the sliding condition of sliding-mode control.

6.5.3.2 Controller Design

For SMA-AFO system, the difficulty of sliding-mode control is the inherent hysteresis nonlinearity of SMA. The sliding-mode control and SMA-AFO system based on self-sensing and actuation is illustrated in Figure 6.88.

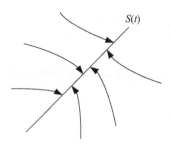

FIGURE 6.87 Sliding prerequisite.

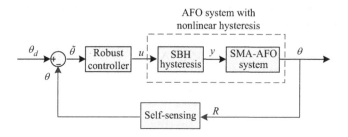

FIGURE 6.88 Control diagram of SMA-AFO system.

We define $\theta_1 = \theta$ and $\theta_2 = \dot{\theta}$, and the comprehensive dynamic model of SMA-AFO system can be described as

$$\begin{cases} \theta_2 = \dot{\theta}_1 \\ \dot{\theta}_2 = -\dfrac{\overline{c}_b}{J}\theta_2 - \dfrac{\overline{k}_b}{J}\theta_1 + \dfrac{1}{J}H[u(t)] + \dfrac{1}{J}g[u(t)] \end{cases}, \tag{6.95}$$

where $H[u(t)]$ is the hysteresis nonlinear term. Note that SMA presents different hysteresis curves under different loads and driving frequencies. To design a sliding-mode controller with good robustness and the ability to deal with disturbance, the hysteresis nonlinear term is divided into linear term q_1, hysteresis term q_2, and disturbance term $d(t)$ (stress, measurement errors) based on Refs. [130–132], as illustrated in the following equation:

$$H[u(t)] = q_1 u(t) + q_2[u(t)] + d(t). \tag{6.96}$$

Thus, Eq. (6.95) turns into

$$\begin{cases} \theta_2 = \dot{\theta}_1 \\ \dot{\theta}_2 = \dfrac{\overline{c}_b}{J}\theta_2 - \dfrac{\overline{k}_b}{J}\theta_1 + \dfrac{1}{J}\left(q_1 u(t) + q_2[u(t)]\right) + \psi(t) \end{cases}, \tag{6.97}$$

where $\psi(t) = \dfrac{1}{J}\left(d(t) + g[u(t)]\right)$. Based on the former analysis, $\psi(t)$ is bounded. We define its bound value as Ψ. Besides, in order to deduce further sliding-control algorithm, the following hypotheses are made. First, the desired trajectory vector $\theta_d = [\theta_d, \dot{\theta}_d]$ is continuous. Second, SMA hysteresis term satisfies the following property:

$$\zeta(u - u_0) \le q_2[u(t)] \le \zeta(u + u_0), \tag{6.98}$$

where $\zeta > 0$ and $u_0 > 0$. Based on the former analysis, for SMA with nonlinear saturated hysteresis properties, it is easy to get its nonlinear boundary using the known linear functions. Third, there is a maximum known constant term q_{min}, satisfying $q_1 \geq q_{min}$. The value can be acquired through data identification.

In the design of sliding-mode controller, the system's dynamic property is completely determined by the sliding-mode plane. Here, we define the sliding-mode plane of SMA-AFO system as

$$s(t) = \begin{bmatrix} \lambda & 1 \end{bmatrix} \begin{bmatrix} \tilde{\theta}_1 \\ \tilde{\theta}_2 \end{bmatrix}, \quad \lambda > 0, \tag{6.99}$$

where $\tilde{\theta} = \theta - \theta_d = \begin{bmatrix} \tilde{\theta}_1, \tilde{\theta}_2 \end{bmatrix}^T$ is the system tracking error vector. To eliminate the flutter caused by model inaccuracy and disturbance, we define the following modified sliding mode plane:

$$s_\tau = s - \tau sat\left(\frac{s}{\tau}\right), \tag{6.100}$$

where $\tau > 0$ and $sat(x)$ has the following form:

$$sat(x) = \begin{cases} 1 & for \ x \geq 1 \\ x & for \ -1 < x < 1 \\ -1 & for \ x \leq -1 \end{cases}. \tag{6.101}$$

Based on Eqs. (6.97) and (6.99), set $\dot{s}(t) = 0$:

$$\begin{aligned} \dot{s}(t) &= \left(\dot{\theta}_2 - \ddot{\theta}_d\right) + \lambda\left(\dot{\theta}_1 - \dot{\theta}_d\right) \\ &= \lambda\left(\dot{\theta}_1 - \dot{\theta}_d\right) - \frac{\overline{c}_b}{\overline{J}}\theta_2 - \frac{\overline{k}_b}{\overline{J}}\theta_1 + \frac{1}{\overline{J}}\left(q_1 u(t) + q_2[u(t)]\right) + \psi(t) - \ddot{\theta}_d. \end{aligned} \tag{6.102}$$

To acquire the control principle satisfying the sliding conditions, we first define $\tilde{\Psi} = \hat{\Psi} - \Psi$, where $\hat{\Psi}$ is the estimation of Ψ. Thus, the control principle is expressed as follows:

$$u = \left(\varphi(\theta, t) - u_0\right)\text{sgn}(s_\tau), \tag{6.103}$$

where $\varphi(\theta, t)$ satisfies

$$\varphi(\theta, t) = \frac{\beta \overline{J}}{\zeta + q_{min}}\left(\left|\lambda\left(\dot{\theta}_1 - \dot{\theta}_d\right)\right| + \left|\frac{\overline{c}_b}{\overline{J}}\theta_2 + \frac{\overline{k}_b}{\overline{J}}\theta_1 + \ddot{\theta}_d\right| + \frac{1}{\beta}\hat{\Psi}\right). \tag{6.104}$$

The parameter Ψ satisfies

$$\dot{\hat{\Psi}} = \kappa|s_\tau|, \tag{6.105}$$

where β and κ are both positive constants.

6.5.3.3 Stability Analysis

Stability analysis is an important component of system controller design. To prove that the above closed-loop system is globally stable, we propose the following function:

$$V(t) = \frac{1}{2}s_\tau^2 + \frac{1}{2\kappa}\tilde{\Psi}^2. \tag{6.106}$$

Differentiating both sides of the equation, we have

$$\dot{V}(t) = s_\tau \dot{s}_\tau + \frac{1}{\kappa}\tilde{\Psi}\dot{\tilde{\Psi}}. \tag{6.107}$$

Based on the definition of s_τ in Eq. (6.100), when $|s| \le \tau$, $s_\tau = 0$. When $|s| > \tau$, $s_\tau \dot{s}_\tau = s_\tau \dot{s}$. Thus, we have

$$
\begin{aligned}
s_\tau \dot{s} = s_\tau & \left[\lambda(\dot{\theta}_1 - \dot{\theta}_d) - \frac{\bar{c}_b}{J}\theta_2 - \frac{\bar{k}_b}{J}\theta_1 + \frac{1}{J}(q_1 u(t) + q_2[u(t)]) + \psi(t) - \ddot{\theta}_d \right] \\
& \le |s_\tau|\mathrm{sgn}(s_\tau)\left(\frac{1}{J}q_1 u(t) + \frac{1}{J}q_2[u(t)] \right) + |s_\tau|\left(\left| \lambda(\dot{\theta}_1 - \dot{\theta}_d) \right| \right. \\
& \left. + \left| \frac{\bar{c}_b}{J}\theta_2 + \frac{\bar{k}_b}{J}\theta_1 + \ddot{\theta}_d \right| \right) + |s_\tau|\Psi.
\end{aligned}
\tag{6.108}
$$

Based on Eq. (6.103), when $s_\tau > 0$, the control principle can be simplified as $u = \varphi(\theta, t) - u_0$. Thus, inequality (6.98) can be expressed as

$$\zeta(\varphi(\theta,t) - 2u_0) \le q_2[u(t)] \le \zeta\varphi(\theta,t). \tag{6.109}$$

When $s_\tau < 0$, the control principle can be simplified as $u = -\varphi(\theta, t) + u_0$. Thus, inequality (6.98) becomes

$$-\zeta\varphi(\theta,t) \le q_2[u(t)] \le \zeta(-\varphi(\theta,t) + 2u_0). \tag{6.110}$$

Based on (6.109) and (6.110), we have

$$\zeta(\varphi(\theta,t) - 2u_0) \le \mathrm{sgn}(s_\tau)q_2[u(t)] \le \zeta\varphi(\theta,t). \tag{6.111}$$

Thus, inequality (6.108) is transformed into

$$
\begin{aligned}
s_\tau \dot{s} \le & \frac{1}{J}|s_\tau|(q_1 + \zeta)\varphi(\theta,t) - \frac{1}{J}|s_\tau|q_1 u_0 + |s_\tau|\left(\left| \lambda(\dot{\theta}_1 - \dot{\theta}_d) \right| \right. \\
& \left. + \left| \frac{\bar{c}_b}{J}\theta_2 + \frac{\bar{k}_b}{J}\theta_1 + \ddot{\theta}_d \right| \right) + |s_\tau|\Psi.
\end{aligned}
\tag{6.112}
$$

Based on Eqs. (6.104) and (6.105), if $\hat{\Psi}(0) \ge 0$, $\varphi(\theta,t)$ would be negative. Thus, we get

$$|s_\tau|(q_1 + \zeta)\varphi(\theta,t) \le |s_\tau|(q_{\min} + \zeta)\varphi(\theta,t). \tag{6.113}$$

Further, we have

$$s_\tau \dot{s} \leq \frac{1}{J}|s_\tau|(q_{\min} + \zeta)\varphi(\theta,t) - \frac{1}{J}|s_\tau|q_1 u_0 + |s_\tau|\left(\left|\lambda(\dot{\theta}_1 - \dot{\theta}_d)\right|\right.$$
$$\left. + \left|\frac{\overline{c}_b}{J}\theta_2 + \frac{\overline{k}_b}{J}\theta_1 + \ddot{\theta}_d\right|\right) + |s_\tau|\Psi. \tag{6.114}$$

Based on the definition of $\varphi(\theta,t)$, the above inequality can be written as

$$s_\tau \dot{s} \leq -\beta|s_\tau|\left(\left|\lambda(\dot{\theta}_1 - \dot{\theta}_d)\right| + \left|\frac{\overline{c}_b}{J}\theta_2 + \frac{\overline{k}_b}{J}\theta_1 + \ddot{\theta}_d\right| + \frac{1}{\beta}\hat{\Psi}\right)$$
$$- \frac{1}{J}|s_\tau|q_1 u_0 + |s_\tau|\left(\left|\lambda(\dot{\theta}_1 - \dot{\theta}_d)\right|\right.$$
$$\left. + \left|\frac{\overline{c}_b}{J}\theta_2 + \frac{\overline{k}_b}{J}\theta_1 + \ddot{\theta}_d\right|\right) + |s_\tau|\Psi \tag{6.115}$$
$$\leq (1,\beta)|s_\tau|\left(\left|\lambda(\dot{\theta}_1 - \theta_d)\right| + \left|\frac{\overline{c}_b}{J}\theta_2 + \frac{\overline{k}_b}{J}\theta_1 + \ddot{\theta}_d\right|\right)$$
$$\frac{1}{J}|s_\tau|q_1 u_0 - |s_\tau|\tilde{\Psi}.$$

Combining Eqs. (6.105), (6.107), and (6.115), the Lyapunov function satisfies

$$\dot{V}(t) \leq (1-\beta)|s_\tau|\left(\left|\lambda(\dot{\theta}_1 - \dot{\theta}_d)\right| + \left|\frac{\overline{c}_b}{J}\theta_2 + \frac{\overline{k}_b}{J}\theta_1 + \ddot{\theta}_d\right|\right)$$
$$- \frac{1}{J}|s_\tau|q_1 u_0. \tag{6.116}$$

When $\beta > 1$, $\dot{V}(t) \leq -\frac{1}{J}|s_\tau|q_1 u_0 \leq 0$. Thus, s_τ is bounded, and for all t, it satisfies $\dot{V}(t) \leq 0$. Based on Barbalat's lemma [129], $\dot{V}(t) \to 0$. Thus, when $t \to \infty$, $s_\tau \to 0$. The global stability is guaranteed.

6.5.4 EXPERIMENTAL STUDY

To verify the correctness of the above comprehensive dynamic model and the effectiveness of the sliding-mode controller, the angle tracking control experiment under different driving frequencies is conducted on the SMA-AFO system that is illustrated in Figure 6.84. The control diagram is shown in Figure 6.86. Note that the bias spring serves two purposes: to provide enough restoring force for the AM and to simulate variable load conditions. Besides, self-sensing function of SMA is applied to realize the closed-loop feedback of SMA-AFO system. To make a comparison, the sliding-mode controller and the conventional PID controller are used to implement the same angle tracking control experiment.

To analyze the performance of the designed sliding-mode controller quantitatively, we define two groups of tracking error criteria:

1. $e_{\text{mte}} = \dfrac{\max\left(|\theta(t) - \theta_d(t)|\right)}{\theta_d(t)}$: the maximum angle tracking error, describing the instantaneous tracking performance in the form of percentage.

2. $e_{\text{rms}} = \dfrac{\sqrt{(1/T) \displaystyle\int_0^T |\theta(t) - \theta_d(t)|^2 \, dt}}{\theta_d(t)}$: the RMS value of angle tracking error, describing the average performance of the tracking function of the controller, where T is the total tracking time.

Note that during the experiment, the SMA-AFO system is always under forced tube cooling. Sinusoidal angle tracking experiment using conventional PID feedback control is done first with the driving frequencies of 0.2, 0.5, and 1 Hz. Then the tracking experiment with sliding-mode controller follows. The experimental results are shown in Figures 6.89–6.91. It can be inferred from the figures that the tracking performance of SBH is much better than that of conventional PID controller. Detailed maximum angle tracking errors e_{mte} and RMS errors e_{rms} are illustrated in Table 6.11. On the one hand, the proposed control strategy reduces the MTE by up to 75% at 0.2 Hz, 77% at 0.5 Hz, and 82% at 1 Hz, compared with the PID controller. On the other hand, the tracking performance decreases with the increase of tracking frequency.

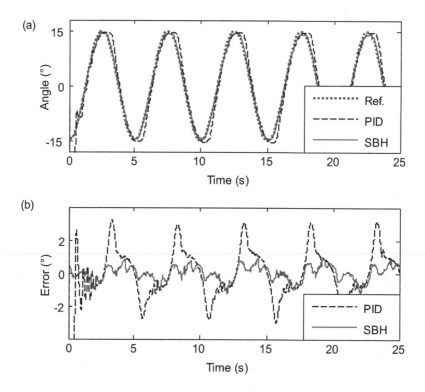

FIGURE 6.89   Tracking response of 0.2 Hz sinusoidal signal. (a) Tracking trajectory; (b) error.

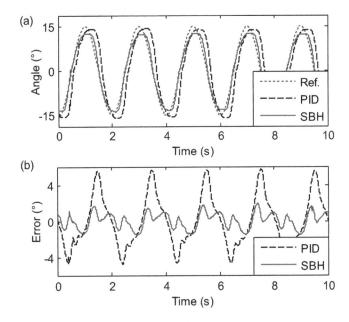

FIGURE 6.90   Tracking response of 0.5 Hz sinusoidal signal. (a) Tracking trajectory; (b) error.

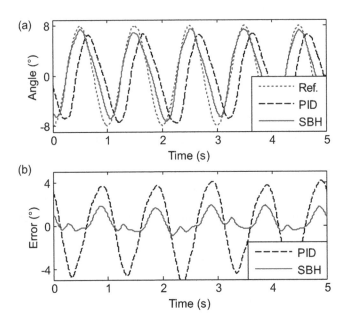

FIGURE 6.91   Tracking response of 1 Hz sinusoidal signal. (a) Tracking trajectory; (b) error.

When the frequency increases to 1 Hz, which is equivalent to the normal step frequency, a large phase lag appears between the actual and the reference angle for the PID controller with MTE more than 5°. However, the phase lag is greatly reduced for the proposed controller with MTE about 1°, which is suitable for ankle–foot rehabilitation. It should be noted that the tracking peak-to-peak

TABLE 6.11

SMA-AM Parameter Values

Frequency (Hz)	Controller	MTE (%)	RMSTE (%)
0.2	PID	15.9	7.2
	SBH	4.0	1.6
0.5	PID	35.8	17.8
	SBH	8.3	4.2
1.0	PID	67.5	37.5
	SBH	12.1	6.8

magnitude is reduced from 30° at 0.2 Hz to 16° at 1 Hz, due to the limitation of power source, which can be improved by using a stronger power source. Here we only focus on the AM actuation capability. In general, the AM presents good actuation capability while maintaining the compactness and large force-to-weight ratio by introducing forced vessel cooling and hysteresis compensation methods. The AFO response frequency is increased from 0.08 to 1 Hz, and the RMS tracking error is reduced by up to 82%, which basically satisfies the initial ankle–foot rehabilitation requirements. To further demonstrate the actual tracking properties of SMA-AFO, human normal ankle–foot gait curve is selected as the tracking reference to conduct the ankle–foot tracing experiment with sliding-mode controller. The results are illustrated in Figure 6.92. It can be noted that SMA-AM is able to track the complex gait curve with varying external loads, laying a foundation for further application of SMA-AFO rehabilitation.

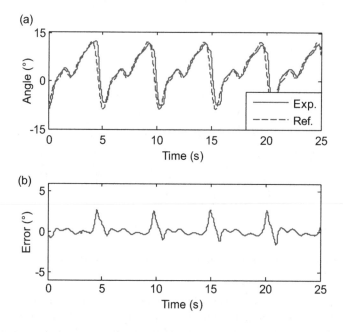

FIGURE 6.92 Tracking response of gait curve. (a) Tracking trajectory; (b) error.

APPENDIX 6.A

Properties	Flexinol Name	025	037	050	075	100	125	150	200	250	300	375
Physical	Wire Diameter (µm)	25	37	50	75	100	125	150	200	250	300	375
	Minimum Ben Radius (mm)	1.3	1.85	2.5	3.75	5.0	6.25	7.5	10.0	12.50	15.0	18.75
	Cross-sectional Area (µm²)	490	1,075	1,960	4,420	7,850	12,270	17,700	31,420	49,100	70,700	110,450
Electrical	Linear Resistance (Ω/m)	1,770	860	510	200	150	70	50	31	20	13	8
	Recommended Current[a] (mA)	20	30	50	100	180	250	400	610	1000	1,750	2,750
	Recommended Power[a] (W/m)	0.71	0.78	1.28	2.0	4.86	4.4	8.00	12.0	20.0	39.8	60.5
Strength[b]	Max. Recovery Weight @ 600 MPa (g)	29	65	117	250	469	736	1,056	1,860	2,933	4,240	6,630
	Rec. Recovery Weight @ 190 MPa (g)	7	20	35	80	150	230	330	590	930	1,250	2,000
	Rec. Deformation Weight @ 35 MPa (g)	2	4	8	815	28	43	62	110	172	245	393
Speed	Typical Contraction Speed[c] (s)	1.0	1.0	1.0	1.0	1.0	1.0	1.0	1.0	1.0	1.0	1.0
	LT Relaxation Speed[c] (s)	0.16	0.25	0.3	0.5	0.8	1.6	2.0	3.5	5.5	8.0	13.0
	LT Alloy Thermal Cycle Rate (cyc/min)	52	48	46	40	33	23	20	13	9	7	4
	HT Relaxation Speed[c] (s)	n.a.	0.09	0.1	0.2	0.4	0.9	1.2	2.2	3.5	6	10
	HT Alloy Thermal Cycle Rate (cyc/min)	n.a.	55	55	50	43	32	27	19	13	9	5

		LT Alloy	HT Alloy
Thermal	Activation Start Temp. (°C)	68	88
	Activation Finish Temp. (°C)	78	98
	Relaxation Start Temp. (°C)	52	72
	Relaxation Finish Temp. (°C)	42	62
	Annealing Temp. (°C)	300	300
	Melting Temp. (°C)	1,300	1,300
	Specific Heat (cal/g°C)	0.077	0.077
	Heat Capacity (Joule/g°C)	0.32	0.32
	Latent Heat (Joule/g)	24.2	24.2

(Continued)

		LT Alloy	HT Alloy
Material	Density (g/cc)	6.45	(~43 ton/in^2)
	Maximum Recovery Force (MPa)	600	(~2.5 ton/in^2)
	Recommended Deformation Force (MPa)	35	(~71 ton/in^2)
	Breaking Strength (MPa)	1,000	
	Poisson's Ratio	0.33	
	Work Output (Joule/g)	1	
	Energy Conversion Efficiency (%)	5	
	Maximum Deformation Ratio (%)	8	
	Recommended Deformation Ratio (%)	3-5	
Phase Related	Phase	*Martensite*	*Austenite*
	Resistivity (μΩcm)	76	82
	Young's Modulus (GPa)	28	75
	Magnetic Susceptibility (μemu/g)	2.5	3.8
	Themal Conductivity (W/cm°C)	0.08	0.18

[a] In still air, at 20°C.

[b] To obtain force in Newtons, multiply mass in grams by 0.0098.

[c] Depends greatly on local beating and cooling conditions. See text.

REFERENCES

1. MacIntosh B R, Gardiner P F, MacComas A J. *Skeletal Muscle: Form and Function*. Champaign, IL: Human Kinetics, 2006.
2. Gels E P. *Electroactive Polymer (EAP) Actuators as Artificial Muscles: Reality, Potential, and Challenges*, Bellingham, WA: SPIE Press, 2004.
3. Klute G K, Czerniecki J M, Hannaford B. Artificial muscles: Actuators for biorobotic systems. *Int. J. Robot. Res.*, April 2002, 21: 295–309.
4. Nordin M, Frankel V H. *Basic Biomechanics of the Musculoskeletal System*. Philadelphia, PA: Lippincott Williams & Wilkins, 2001.
5. Hill A. The heat of shortening and the dynamic constants of muscle. *Proc. R. Soc. Lond. B*, 1938, 126: 136–195.
6. Huxley H, Hanson J. Changes in the cross-striations of muscle during contraction and stretch and their structural interpretation. *Nature*, 1954, 173: 973–976.
7. Huxley A F. Muscle structure and theories of contraction. *Prog. Biophys. Biophys. Chem.*, 1957, 7: 255–318.
8. Huxley, H E. The Mechanism of Muscular Contraction. *Science*, 1969, 164(3886):1356-1366.
9. Yin Y, Guo Z. Collective operation mechanism of molecular motor and dynamic mechanical model of sarcomere. *Sci. China Technol. Sci.*, 2011, 54(8), 1533–1540 (in Chinese).
10. Guo Z, Yin Y. Bioelectrochemical principle of variable frequency control on skeletal muscle contraction-Operation mechanism of molecular motor based biomechanical mechanism of skeletal muscle (I). *Sci. China Technol. Sci.*, 2012, 42(8): 672–679 (in Chinese).
11. Yin Y, Chen X. Bioelectrochemical principle of variable frequency control on skeletal muscle contraction- Operation mechanism of molecular motor based biomechanical mechanism of skeletal muscle (II). *Sci. China Technol. Sci.*, 2012, 42(8): 901–910 (in Chinese).
12. Yin Y, Guo Z, Chen X, Fan Y. Operation mechanism of molecular motor based biomechanical research progresses on skeletal muscle. *Chin. Sci. Bull.*, 2012, 30: 2794–2805 (in Chinese).
13. Chen X, Yin Y. Dynamic system of muscle spindle afferent nerve postsynaptic response-Markov model. *Chin. Sci. Bull.*, 2013, 58(9): 793–802 (in Chinese).
14. Herr H M, Kornbluh R D. New horizons for orthotic and prosthetic technology: artificial muscle for ambulation. *Smart Structures and Materials*, McHenry, IL, 2004, pp. 1–9.

15. Madden J D, Vandesteeg N A, Anquetil P A, et al. Artificial muscle technology: Physical principles and naval prospects. *IEEE J. Oceanic Eng.*, 2004, 29: 706–728.

16. Yin Y H, Hu H, Xia Y C. Active tracking of unknown surface using force sensing and control technique for robot. *Sens. Actuators A Phys.*, May 1 2004, 112: 313–319.

17. Alfayad S, Ouezdou F B, Namoun F, Gheng G. High performance integrated electro-hydraulic actuator for robotics—Part I: Principle, prototype design and first experiments. *Sens. Actuators A Phys.*, September 10 2011, 169: 115–123.

18. Alfayad S, Ouezdou F B, Namoun F, Gheng G. High performance integrated electro-hydraulic actuator for robotics. Part II: Theoretical modelling, simulation, control & comparison with real measurements. *Sens. Actuators A Phys.*, September 10 2011, 169: 124–132.

19. Fan Y, Guo Z, Yin Y. SEMG-based neuro-fuzzy controller for a parallel ankle exoskeleton with proprioception. *Int. J. Robot. Autom.*, 2011, 26: 450.

20. Yin Y H, Fan Y J, Xu L D. EMG and EPP-integrated human-machine interface between the paralyzed and rehabilitation exoskeleton. *IEEE Trans. Inf. Technol. Biomed.*, July 2012, 16: 542–549.

21. Brock D L. Review of artificial muscle based on contractile polymers, No. AI-M-1330. Massachusetts Institute of Tech Cambridge Artificial Intelligence Lab, 1991.

22. Pelrine R, Kornbluh R D, Pei Q, et al. Dielectric elastomer artificial muscle actuators: toward biomimetic motion. *SPIE's 9th Annual International Symposium on Smart Structures and Materials*, San Diego, CA, 2002, pp. 126–137.

23. Pei Q, Pelrine R, Rosenthal M A, Stanford S, Prahlad H, Kornbluh R D. Recent progress on electroelastomer artificial muscles and their application for biomimetic robots. *Smart Structures and Materials*, San Diego, CA, 2004, pp. 41–50.

24. Foroughi J, Spinks G M, Wallace G G, et al. Torsional carbon nanotube artificial muscles. *Science*, October 28 2011, 334: 494–497.

25. Zhang J, Zhu J. 4M-Model based bionic design of artificial skeletal muscle actuated by SMA. In *Intelligent Robotics and Applications*, Su CY., Rakheja S., Liu H. (eds.). Lecture Notes in Computer Science. Berlin, Heidelberg: Springer, 2012, 7508: 123–130.

26. Zhang J J, Yin Y H. SMA-based bionic integration design of self-sensor–actuator-structure for artificial skeletal muscle. *Sens. Actuators A Phys.*, 2012, 181: 94–102.

27. Otsuka K, Wayman C M. *Shape Memory Materials.* Cambridge, UK: Cambridge University Press, 1999.

28. Cen 岑 H, Chen W. Conception and evolvement of bionics. *J. Mach. Des.*, 2007, 1–2: 66 (in Chinese).

29. Robinson D W. *Design and Analysis of Series Elasticity in Closed-Loop Actuator Force Control.* Cambridge, MA: Massachusetts Institute of Technology, 2000.

30. Blaya J A, Herr H. Adaptive control of a variable-impedance ankle-foot orthosis to assist drop-foot gait. *IEEE Trans. Neural Syst. Rehabil. Eng.*, March 2004, 12: 24–31.

31. Au S K, Weber J, Herr H. Biomechanical design of a powered ankle-foot prosthesis. *2007 IEEE 10th International Conference on Rehabilitation Robotics, Vols 1 and 2*, Noordwijk, Netherlands, 2007, pp. 298–303.

32. Au S K, Herr H M. Powered ankle-foot prosthesis—the importance of series and parallel motor elasticity. *IEEE Robot. Autom. Mag.*, September 2008, 15: 52–59.

33. Paluska D, Herr H. The effect of series elasticity on actuator power and work output: Implications for robotic and prosthetic joint design. *Rob. Auton. Syst.*, August 31 2006, 54: 667–673.

34. Hirai K, Hirose M, Haikawa Y, Takenaka T. The development of Honda humanoid robot. *Robotics and Automation, 1998. Proceedings of 1998 IEEE International Conference on*, Vancouver, BC, 1998, pp. 1321–1326.

35. Nelson G, Blankespoor K, Raibert M. Walking BigDog: Insights and challenges from legged robotics. *J. Biomech.*, 2006, 39: S360.

36. Chou C-P, Hannaford B. Static and dynamic characteristics of McKibben pneumatic artificial muscles. *Robotics and Automation, 1994. Proceedings of 1994 IEEE International Conference on*, San Diego, CA, 1994, pp. 281–286.

37. Chou C-P, Hannaford B. Measurement and modeling of McKibben pneumatic artificial muscles. *IEEE Trans. Robot. Autom.*, 1996, 12: 90–102.

38. Klute G K, Hannaford B. Fatigue characteristics of McKibben artificial muscle actuators. *Intelligent Robots and Systems, 1998. Proceedings of 1998 IEEE/RSJ International Conference on*, Victoria, BC, 1998, pp. 1776–1781.

39. Klute G K, Czerniecki J M, Hannaford B. McKibben artificial muscles: Pneumatic actuators with biomechanical intelligence. *Advanced Intelligent Mechatronics, 1999. Proceedings of 1999 IEEE/ASME International Conference on*, Atlanta, GA, 1999, pp. 221–226.

40. Saga N, Nagase J, Saikawa T. Pneumatic artificial muscles based on biomechanical characteristics of human muscles. *Appl. Bionics Biomech.*, 2006, 3: 191–197.
41. Saga N, Saikawa T. Development of a pneumatic artificial muscle based on biomechanical characteristics. *Adv. Robotics*, 2008, 22: 761–770.
42. Pack R T, Christopher J L Jr, Kawamura K. A rubbertuator-based structure-climbing inspection robot. *Robotics and Automation, 1997. Proceedings of 1997 IEEE International Conference on*, Albuquerque, NM, 1997, pp. 1869–1874.
43. Park Y L, Chen B-r, Young D, et al. Bio-inspired active soft orthotic device for ankle foot pathologies. *Intelligent Robots and Systems (IROS), 2011 IEEE/RSJ International Conference on*, San Francisco, CA, 2011, pp. 4488–4495.
44. Ferris D P, Czerniecki J M, Hannaford B. An ankle-foot orthosis powered by artificial pneumatic muscles. *J. Appl. Biomech.*, May 2005, 21: 189–197.
45. Ferris D P, Gordon K E, Sawicki G S, Peethambaran A. An improved powered ankle-foot orthosis using proportional myoelectric control. *Gait Posture*, Jun 2006, 23: 425–428.
46. Shorter K A. *The Design and Control of Active Ankle-Foot Orthoses*. Atlanta, GA: Georgia Institute of Technology, 2011.
47. Shorter K A, Li Y, Morris E A, Kogler G F, Hsiao-Wecksler E T. Experimental evaluation of a portable powered ankle-foot orthosis. *Engineering in Medicine and Biology Society, EMBC, 2011 Annual International Conference of the IEEE*, Boston, MA, 2011, pp. 624–627.
48. Ashley S. Artificial muscles. *Sci. Am.*, 2003, 289: 52–59.
49. Lagoudas D C. *Shape Memory Alloys: Modeling and Engineering Applications*. Berlin, Germany: Springer, 2008.
50. Shaw J A. Material instabilities in a nickel-titanium shape-memory alloy, *PhD dissertation*, The University of Texas at Austin. 1997.
51. Pfeiffer C, DeLaurentis K, Mavroidis C. Shape memory alloy actuated robot prostheses: Initial experiments. *Icra '99: IEEE International Conference on Robotics and Automation, Vols 1–4, Proceedings*, Detroit, MI, 1999, pp. 2385–2391.
52. Ebron V H, Yang Z W, Seyer D J, et al. Fuel-powered artificial muscles. *Science*, March 17 2006, 311: 1580–1583.
53. Price, A, Jnifene, A, Naguib, H E. Biologically inspired anthropomorphic arm and dextrous robot hand actuated by smart material based artificial muscles—art. no. 61730X. *Proc. SPIE—Int. Soc. Opt. Eng.*, 2006, 6173: X1730–X1730.
54. Cho K-J, Rosmarin J, Asada H. SBC Hand: A lightweight robotic hand with an SMA actuator array implementing C-segmentation. *Robotics and Automation, 2007 IEEE International Conference on*, Rome, Italy, 2007, pp. 921–926.
55. Teh Y H, Featherstone R. An architecture for fast and accurate control of shape memory alloy actuators. *Int. J. Robot. Res.*, May 2008, 27: 595–611.
56. Tong J, Moayad B Z, Ma Y H, et al. Effects of biomimetic surface designs on furrow opener performance. *J. Bionic Eng.*, September 2009, 6: 280–289.
57. Oka K, Aoyagi S, Arai Y, Isono Y, Hashiguchi G, Fujita H. Fabrication of a micro needle for a trace blood test. *Sens. Actuators A Phys.*, April 1 2002, 97–98: 478–485.
58. Bobbert M F, van Ingen Schenau G J. Isokinetic plantar flexion: Experimental results and model calculations. *J. Biomech.*, 1990, 23: 105–119.
59. Bahler A S. Series elastic component of mammalian skeletal muscle. *Am. J. Physiol.—Legacy Content*, 1967, 213: 1560–1564.
60. Guo Z, Yin Y. Coupling mechanism of multi-force interactions in the myosin molecular motor. *Chin. Sci. Bull.*, 2010, 55: 3538–3544.
61. Yin Y, Guo Z. Collective mechanism of molecular motors and a dynamic mechanical model for sarcomere. *Sci. China Technol. Sci.*, 2011, 54: 2130–2137.
62. Guo Z, Yin Y. A dynamic model of skeletal muscle based on collective behavior of myosin motors—Biomechanics of skeletal muscle based on working mechanism of myosin motors (I). *Sci. China Technol. Sci.*, 2012, 55: 1589–1595.
63. Yin Y, Chen X. Bioelectrochemical control mechanism with variable-frequency regulation for skeletal muscle contraction—Biomechanics of skeletal muscle based on the working mechanism of myosin motors (II). *Sci. China Technol. Sci.*, 2012, 55: 2115–2125.
64. Guo Z. Myosin II-based biomechanics principle of skeletal muscle and its application in human-machine interaction for exoskeleton. Shanghai, Shanghai Jiao Tong University, Shanghai, China, 2012. (in Chinese).

65. Editors of Wikipedia (2000–2015). Wikipedia Online. Retrieved August 8, 2012, from Wikipedia Online on the World Wide Web: http://en.wikipedia.org/wiki/Muscle_contraction.

66. Linke W A, Ivemeyer M, Mundel P, Stockmeier M R, Kolmerer B. Nature of PEVK-titin elasticity in skeletal muscle. *Proc. Nat. Acad. Sci. USA*, July 7 1998, 95: 8052–8057.

67. Cook G, Stark L. The human eye-movement mechanism: Experiments, modeling, and model testing. *Arch. Ophthalmol.*, 1968, 79: 428.

68. Bahler A S. Modeling of mammalian skeletal muscle. *IEEE Trans. Biomed. Eng.*, 1968, 4: 249–257.

69. Wilkie D. The mechanical properties of muscle. *Br. Med. Bull.*, 1956, 12: 177–182.

70. McCrorey H, Gale H, Alpert N. Mechanical properties of the cat tenuissimus muscle. *Am. J. Physiol.*, 1966, 210: 114–120.

71. Ralston H, Polissar M, Inman V, Close J, Feinstein B. Dynamic features of human isolated voluntary muscle in isometric and free contractions. *J. Appl. Physiol.*, 1949, 1, 526–533.

72. Winter D A. *Biomechanics and Motor Control of Human Movement*. Hoboken, NJ: Wiley.com, 2009.

73. Abbott B, Wilkie D. The relation between velocity of shortening and the tension-length curve of skeletal muscle. *J. Physiol.*, 1953, 120: 214–223.

74. Lan C C, Lin C M, Fan C H. A self-sensing microgripper module with wide handling ranges. *IEEE-ASME Trans. Mech.*, February 2011, 16: 141–150.

75. Costanza G, Tata M E, Calisti C. Nitinol one-way shape memory springs: Thermomechanical characterization and actuator design. *Sens. Actuators A Phys.*, January 2010, 157: 113–117.

76. Grant D. Accurate and rapid control of shape memory alloy actuators, *PhD Thesis*, McGill University, 2001.

77. Pierce M D, Mascaro S A. A biologically inspired wet shape memory alloy actuated robotic pump. IEEE/ASME Trans. Mech., 2012, 18(2): 536–546.

78. Wang T M, Shi Z Y, Liu D, Ma C, Zhang Z H. An accurately controlled antagonistic shape memory alloy actuator with self-sensing. *Sensors*, June 2012, 12: 7682–7700.

79. Yin Y, Zhang J, Zhu J. Active stone micro gripper. CN102973306A (in Chinese).

80. Novak V, Sittner P, Dayananda G N, Braz-Fernandes F M, Mahesh K K. Electric resistance variation of NiTi shape memory alloy wires in thermomechanical tests: Experiments and simulation. *Mater. Sci. Eng.*, May 25 2008, 481: 127–133.

81. Sittner P, Novak V, Lukas P, Landa M. Stress-strain-temperature behavior due to B2-R-B19 ' transformation in NiTi polycrystals. *J. Eng. Mater. Technol.*, Jul 2006, 128: 268–278.

82. Lan C C, Fan C H. An accurate self-sensing method for the control of shape memory alloy actuated flexures. *Sens. Actuators A Phys.*, September 2010, 163: 323–332.

83. Lan C C, Fan C H. Investigation on Pretensioned Shape Memory Alloy Actuators for Force and Displacement Self-Sensing. *IEEE/RSJ 2010 International Conference on Intelligent Robots and Systems (Iros 2010)*, Taipei, China, 2010, pp. 3043–3048.

84. Lan C C, Lin C M, Fan C H. A Self-Sensing Microgripper Module With Wide Handling Ranges. *IEEE-ASME Trans. Mech.*, February 2011, 16: 141–150.

85. Cui D, Song G B, Li H N. Modeling of the electrical resistance of shape memory alloy wires. *Smart Mater. Struct.*, May 2010, 19: 055019.

86. Ma N, Song G, Lee H J. Position control of shape memory alloy actuators with internal electrical resistance feedback using neural networks. *Smart Mater. Struct.*, August 2004, 13: 777–783.

87. Tanaka K. A thermomechanical sketch of shape memory effect: One-dimensional tensile behavior. *Res. Mechan.*, 1986, 18: 251–263.

88. Brinson L. One-dimensional constitutive behavior of shape memory alloys: Thermomechanical derivation with non-constant material functions and redefined martensite internal variable. *J. Intell. Mater. Syst. Struct.*, 1993, 4: 229–242.

89. Mayergoyz I D. *Mathematical Models of Hysteresis and Their Applications*. Pittsburgh, PA: Academic Press, 2003.

90. Leang K K, Ashley S, Tchoupo G. Iterative and feedback control for hysteresis compensation in SMA. *J. Dyn. Syst. Meas. Control-Tran. ASME*, Jan 2009, 131: 014502.

91. Hughes D, Wen J T. Preisach modeling of piezoceramic and shape memory alloy hysteresis. *Smart Mater. Struct.*, June 1997, 6: 287–300.

92. Gorbet R B, Wang D W L, Morris K A. Preisach model identification of a two-wire SMA actuator. *1998 IEEE International Conference on Robotics and Automation, Vols 1–4*, Leuven, Belgium, 1998, pp. 2161–2167.

93. Hasegawa T, Majima S. A control system to compensate the hysteresis by Preisach model on SMA actuator. *Mhs '98, Proceedings of the 1998 International Symposium on Micromechatronics and Human Science*, Nagoya, Japan, 1998, pp. 171–176.

94. Wang Y F, Su C Y, Hong H, Hu Y M. Modeling and compensation for hysteresis of shape memory alloy actuators with the Preisach representation. *2007 IEEE International Conference on Control and Automation, Vols 1–7*, Guangzhou, China, 2007, pp. 2731–2736.

95. Zhang Y, Yan S, N Ma. Preisach based SMA resistance-strain hysteresis model. *J. Vib. Shock*, 2008, 184: 146–148 (in Chinese).

96. Nguyen B K, Ahn K K. Feedforward control of shape memory alloy actuators using fuzzy-based inverse Preisach model. *IEEE Trans. Contr. Syst. Technol.*, Mar 2009, 17: 434–441.

97. Liu W, Chen Z, Hou S, Shen N, Jiao Y. Preisach based SMA temperature-displacement hysteresis simulation research. *J. Vib. Shock*, 2012, 31(16): 83–87(in Chinese).

98. Liu W, Chen Z, Huang S, Jiao Y. SMA hysteresis model. *J. Jilin Univ. (Engineering and Technology Edition)*, 2012, 42(3): 719–725 (in Chinese).

99. Feng Y, Y Hu, C Su. Adaptive control of a class of nonlinear systems with Prandtl-Ishlinskii hysteresis. *Acta Automatica Sinica*, 2006, 32(3): 450–455 (in Chinese)

100. M. Al Janaideh, Rakheja S, Su C Y. A generalized Prandtl-Ishlinskii model for characterizing the hysteresis and saturation nonlinearities of smart actuators. *Smart Mater. Struct.*, April 2009, 18: 045001.

101. Sayyaadi H, Zakerzadeh M R. Position control of shape memory alloy actuator based on the generalized Prandtl-Ishlinskii inverse model. *Mechatronics*, Oct 2012, 22: 945–957.

102. Gu G Y, Zhu L M. High-speed tracking control of piezoelectric actuators using an ellipse-based hysteresis model. *Rev. Sci. Instrum.*, August 2010, 81: 085104.

103. Song G, Chaudhry V, Batur C. A neural network inverse model for a shape memory alloy wire actuator. *J. Intell. Mater. Syst. Struct.*, Jun 2003, 14: 371–377.

104. Ahn K K, Kha N B. Modeling and control of shape memory alloy actuators using Preisach model, genetic algorithm and fuzzy logic. *Mechatronics*, Apr 2008, 18: 141–152.

105. Elahinia M H. *Nonlinear Control of a Shape Memory Alloy Actuated Manipulator*. Philadelphia, PA: Villanova University, 2001.

106. Song G, Chaudhry V, Batur C. Precision tracking control of shape memory alloy actuators using neural networks and a sliding-mode based robust controller. *Smart Mater. Struct.*, Apr 2003, 12: 223–231.

107. He Z, Gall K R, Brinson L C. Use of electrical resistance testing to redefine the transformation kinetics and phase diagram for shape-memory alloys. *Metall. Mater. Trans. A*, Mar 2006, 37A: 579–587.

108. Wayman C, Cornelis I, Shimizu K. Transformation behavior and the shape memory in thermally cycled TiNi. *Scripta Metallurgica*, 1972, 6: 115–122.

109. Wollants P, Roos J, Delaey L. Thermally- and stress-induced thermoelastic martensitic transformations in the reference frame of equilibrium thermodynamics. *Prog. Mater. Sci.*, 1993, 37: 227–288.

110. Z Xu. *Martensitic Transformation and Martensite*. Beijing,China: Science Press, 1999.

111. Pozzi M, Airoldi G. The electrical transport properties of shape memory alloys. *Mater. Sci. Eng. A*, Dec 15 1999, 273: 300–304.

112. Bergman T L, Lavine A S, Incropera F P, Dewitt D P. *Introduction to Heat Transfer*. Hoboken, NJ: John Wiley & Sons, Incorporated, 2011.

113. Bhattacharyya A, Sweeney L, Faulkner M. Experimental characterization of free convection during thermal phase transformations in shape memory alloy wires. *Smart Mater. Struct.*, 2002, 11: 411.

114. Churchill C B, Shaw J A. Shakedown response of conditioned shape memory alloy wire. *The 15th International Symposium on: Smart Structures and Materials & Nondestructive Evaluation and Health Monitoring*, San Diego, CA, 2008, pp. 69291F-69291F–12.

115. Brailovski V, Trochu F, Daigneault G. Temporal characteristics of shape memory linear actuators and their application to circuit breakers. *Mater. Des.*, 1996, 17: 151–158.

116. Potapov P L, dA Silva E P. Time response of shape memory alloy actuators. *J. Intell. Mater. Syst. Struct.*, Feb 2000, 11: 125–134.

117. Dutta S M, Ghorbel F H. Differential hysteresis modeling of a shape memory alloy wire actuator. *IEEE-ASME Trans. Mech.*, Apr 2005, 10: 189–197.

118. Gu G. Control of piezoceramic actuated micro/nanopositioning stages with hysteresis compensation. Shanghai, Shanghai Jiao Tong University, Shanghai,China, 2012 (in Chinese)

119. Liang C, Rogers C. One-dimensional thermomechanical constitutive relations for shape memory materials. *J. Intell. Mater. Syst. Struct.*, 1990, 1: 207–234.

120. Elahinia M H, Ahmadian M. An enhanced SMA phenomenological model: I. The shortcomings of the existing models. *Smart Mater. Struct.*, 2005, 14: 1297.

121. Elahinia M H, Ahmadian M. An enhanced SMA phenomenological model: I. The experimental study. *Smart Mater. Struct.*, 2005, 14: 1309.

122. Shorter K A, Xia J C, Hsiao E T-Wecksler, Durfee W K, Kogler G F. Technologies for powered ankle-foot orthotic systems: Possibilities and challenges. *IEEE-ASME Trans. Mech.*, Feb 2013, 18: 337–347.

123. Yamamoto S, Ebina M, Kubo S, Hayashi T, Akita Y, Hayakawa Y. Development of an ankle-foot orthosis with dorsiflexion assist, part 2: Structure and evaluation. *J. Prosthet. Orthot.*, 1999, 11: 24–28.

124. Lefort H T a G. Dynamic Orthosis: Eur. Patent WO2004008987, 2005.

125. Boehler A W, Hollander K W, Sugar T G, Shin D. Design, implementation and test results of a robust control method for a powered ankle foot orthosis (AFO). *Robotics and Automation, 2008. ICRA 2008. IEEE International Conference on*, Pasadena, CA, 2008, pp. 2025–2030.

126. Zhang J, Yin Y, Zhu J. Sigmoid-based hysteresis modeling and high-speed tracking control of SMA-artificial muscle. *Sens. Actuators A Phys.*, 2013, 201: 264–273.

127. Whittle, M W. Gait *Analysis: An Introduction*. Oxford, UK: Butterworth-Heinemann, 2014.

128. McNichols J, Cory J. Thermodynamics of nitinol. *J. Appl. Phys.*, 1987, 61: 972–984.

129. Lienhard J H. *A Heat Transfer Textbook*. New York: Courier Dover Publications, 2011.

130. Slotine J-J E, Li W, *Applied Nonlinear Control*. vol. 199. Upper Saddle River, NJ: Prentice Hall, 1991.

131. Oh J, Bernstein D S. Semilinear Duhem model for rate-independent and rate-dependent hysteresis. *IEEE Trans. Automat. Contr.*, 2005, 50: 631–645.

132. Bashash S, Jalili N. Robust adaptive control of coupled parallel piezo-flexural nanopositioning stages. *IEEE/ASME Trans. Mech.*, 2009, 14: 11–20.

Conclusion

With the fast development of economy, people have more requirements for better quality of life, and more attention is paid to life and health. On one hand, social problems are caused by the aging of population, and there is greater need for smart rehabilitation devices. As the typical application of robot technology, exoskeleton robotics is an important field of human–machine interaction. It has great research value and promising application prospect in the field of military and medicine and is also the research hotspot over the world. On the other hand, the generation mechanism of human–machine interactive force, which is closely related to exoskeleton robot, is also the aporia in the research of rehabilitation engineering and biomechanics. Thus, it is worth an in-depth study. Besides, biomechanical model of skeletal muscle is also significant in its bionics.

The generation and regulatory mechanism of muscle contraction force is first deeply discussed in this book. Biomechanical model is also summarized in multi-scales, including the force generation model based on collective operation mechanism of molecular motors, the bioelectrochemical variable-frequency control mechanism of muscular contraction, and the semiphenomenological model of sarcomere. To provide easy, in-time, safe, and effective access to rehabilitation treatment, the exoskeleton robot for lower-limb rehabilitation system and its related hardware devices are discussed in this book. The differential electromyogram (EMG) feature extraction algorithm and multi-source signal fusion algorithm based on artificial fuzzy neural network are proposed to realize the real-time and accurate identification of human motor intent. The oscillator model of EMG and the energy kernel feature extraction method are also introduced. The coordinated control of exoskeleton robot is also achieved by the bidirectional human–machine interactive interface with motion control channel and information feedback channel. The progressive compound rehabilitation strategy and IoT-based smart rehabilitation system for different patients' requirements are established. For different patients of lower-limb diseases, corresponding rehabilitation strategy and robot control strategy are generated, and robot experiments were carried out using human–machine interface, and part of the practical clinical application was achieved. At last, this book introduces shape memory alloy (SMA) as the bionic actuator of skeletal muscle. The modified 4M model of skeletal muscle and bionic design principles to guide SMA-AM design are developed after analyzing the structure, function, and biomechanical properties of muscle. Besides, to further realize the integrated actuating and control of SMA-AM, extensive research is conducted on the key problems including SMA self-sensing and hysteresis compensation, and SMA-AM has been preliminarily applied in SMA ankle–foot rehabilitation system.

Theory and application are well combined in this book. The bionic nature, mathematical and mechanical mechanism of force sensing and control are also introduced in an intelligible manner. Because of the limited space, the emphasis is on the key achievements in the field, as well as the related work and achievements of the author's research group. However, of course, there are still a lot of important studies on this topic, but they are not included in this book. This book has a large span in content; thus, there may be inevitably some mistakes in its narrative. We greatly welcome readers' comments and criticisms. At last, we sincerely hope that this book will provide necessary help to researchers in the fields of molecular motor, biomechanics, biomedicine, robotics, and bionics.

PROSPECT

The bionic nature of force sensing, control, the biomechanical mechanism of force generation, and related applications have been systematically introduced in this book. Although a lot of outstanding achievements have been made by the scholars and research groups, and firm foundation has been laid for future research, there are still lots of problems that should be further studied. The summary is as follows.

1. Biomechanics and modeling of skeletal muscle

Nowadays, the microscopic operation mechanism research of skeletal muscle is mainly focused on theoretical analysis. The experimental verification of multi-field coupling mechanism of molecular motor has to be studied further. Continuous progress has been made on the microforce detecting devices with the accuracy of pN, such as optical tweezers, atomic force microscopy, and confocal laser scanning microscopy. They can be applied to the nanomechanics of molecular level and provide technical support for further molecular motor experiments. Devices such as atomic force microscopes and optical tweezers can be used to detect the mutual force between molecular motor and actin filaments and further verify the multi-force coupling mechanism of molecular motors to explain their motion mechanism. Meanwhile, experimental platforms in the microscale and nanoscale with the object of muscle fiber can be used to analyze the control mechanism of firing rate on muscular contraction.

2. Clinical application of exoskeleton rehabilitation system

Around the world, although there are preliminary clinical experiments on the treatment of stroke patients with exoskeleton robots, the portion of patients taking such kind of treatment is still small. Thus, the clinical results still lack universal significance. More clinical contrast tests should be implemented to demonstrate the effectiveness of the system and to find the potential problems to improve the system, so that the lower-extremity exoskeleton robot system can be effectively applied in clinical situation. New rehabilitation methods and strategies should be explored, e.g., integrating functional electric stimulation (FES) system into exoskeleton robot to realize the rehabilitation of patients with joint diseases. The active and intelligent control of exoskeleton robot has always been the key difficulty in exoskeleton technology. New methods should be proposed to overcome current shortcomings. Besides, many problems should be discovered and solved in practical applications of exoskeleton robot.

3. Novel human–machine interface research

As one of the motion control signal sources, although sEMG is able to reflect human motion intention in advance, it is controversial to use only the sEMG signal to perform intent identification because the fuzziness of sEMG signal is strong and is affected by human status and environmental factors. Thus, information such as angle and interactive force should be integrated to complete the multi-source signal fusion to identify motion intention. However, the accuracy could be improved by other methods, such as bringing in another physiological signal, such as electroencephalogram (EEG) signal, EMG signal, and even neural signal. Extensive research on the operation mechanism of human motoneuron system should be carried out to develop more accurate motion control model. These research areas are all of great significance for improving the accuracy of motion intention identification. Meanwhile, information feedback method based on force sensing should be improved. Feedback methods that are able to reflect multi-dimensional information should be developed so that the exoskeleton system could be a virtual part of human body.

4. Research on bionic design methodology

Bionic design is the design methodology to solve engineering problems with inspiration from nature. Bionic design of skeletal muscle is conducted from three aspects in this book: the structure, function, and biomechanical properties. Compared to the existing artificial muscles (AMs), deeper bionics of skeletal muscle is achieved by SMA-AM in the book. However, to achieve the complex actuating property and environmental adaptivity like real skeletal muscle, deeper analysis is necessary on neural control system and contractile mechanism of skeletal muscle. Besides, more work should be focused on the detailed steps and methodology of bionic design, i.e., what bionics is and how bionic design should be done. This is a very interesting research topic in both biological and engineering domains.

5. Clinical application of SMA bionic muscle in rehabilitation system

After solving the self-sensing and hysteresis problems of SMA-AM, SMA-AFO (ankle–foot orthosis) is designed in this book, and the application properties of SMA-AM have been preliminarily explored. Compared with the existing AFOs, the biggest advantage of SMA-AFO is that it integrates the portability of passive AFO and the assistive force feature of active AFO. However, to apply SMA-AFO to clinical rehabilitation, the following problems should be solved further: first, power supply. In practical application, battery should be applied to replace cable power supply gradually to realize the portability, active force assistance, and wearing comfort. Second, generation of clinical rehabilitation strategy, i.e., designing different types of SMA-AFOs and generating proper rehabilitation strategies for different ankle–foot patients. Third, application extension of SMA-AM. SMA-AM properties of large power density, large output force, and flexibility can also be applied to the medical devices such as active prosthesis and exoskeleton robots.

Index

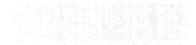

T - #0623 - 101024 - C0 - 254/178/21 - PB - 9781032401195 - Gloss Lamination